Health Science Library
Frimley P

Class Mark:
Book Number:

CW01263173

20360

Essentials in Ophthalmology   **Medical Retina**

F. G. Holz   R. F. Spaide
Editors

Essentials in Ophthalmology

G. K. Krieglstein   R. N. Weinreb
Series Editors

Glaucoma

Cataract and Refractive Surgery

Uveitis and Immunological Disorders

Vitreo-retinal Surgery

Medical Retina

Oculoplastics and Orbit

**Pediatric Ophthalmology,
Neuro-Ophthalmology, Genetics**

Cornea and External Eye Disease

Editors   Frank G. Holz
　　　　　Richard F. Spaide

Medical Retina

With 91 Figures, Mostly in Colour
and 13 Tables

Springer

Series Editors

Günter K. Krieglstein, MD
Professor and Chairman
Department of Ophthalmology
University of Cologne
Kerpener Straße 62
50924 Cologne
Germany

Robert N. Weinreb, MD
Professor and Director
Hamilton Glaucoma Center
Department of Ophthalmology
University of California at San Diego
9500 Gilman Drive
La Jolla, CA 92093-0946
USA

Volume Editors

Frank G. Holz, MD
Professor and Chairman
Department of Ophthalmology
University of Bonn
Ernst-Abbe-Straße 2
53127 Bonn
Germany

Richard F. Spaide, MD
Assistant Clinical Professor
Vitreous, Retina, and Macula Consultants
of New York, and
LuEsther T. Mertz Retinal Research Center
Manhattan Eye, Ear, and Throat Hospital
460 Park Avenue
New York, NY 10022
USA

ISBN 978-3-540-33671-6
Springer Berlin Heidelberg New York

ISSN 1612-3212

Library of Congress Control Number: 2007927503

This work is subject to copyright. All rights are reserved, whether the whole or part of the material is concerned, specifically the rights of translation, reprinting, reuse of illustrations, recitation, broadcasting, reproduction on microfilms or in any other way, and storage in data banks. Duplication of this publication or parts thereof is permitted only under the provisions of the German Copyright Law of September 9, 1965, in its current version, and permission for use must always be obtained from Springer-Verlag. Violations are liable for prosecution under the German Copyright Law.

Springer is a part of Springer Science + Business Media

springer.com

© Springer-Verlag Berlin Heidelberg 2007

The use of general descriptive names, registered names, trademarks, etc. in this publication does not imply, even in the absence of a specific statement, that such names are exempt from the relevant protective laws and regulations and therefore free for general use.

Product liability: The publishers cannot guarantee the accuracy of any information about dosage and application contained in this book. In every individual case the user must check such information by consulting the relevant literature.

Editor: Marion Philipp, Heidelberg, Germany
Desk Editor: Martina Himberger, Heidelberg, Germany
Production: LE-TeX Jelonek, Schmidt & Vöckler GbR, Leipzig, Germany
Cover Design: WMXDesign GmbH, Heidelberg, Germany

Printed on acid-free paper
24/3180Wa   5 4 3 2 1 0

Foreword

The series *Essentials in Ophthalmology* was initiated two years ago to expedite the timely transfer of new information in vision science and evidence-based medicine into clinical practice. We thought that this prospicient idea would be moved and guided by a resolute commitment to excellence. It is reasonable to now update our readers with what has been achieved.

The immediate goal was to transfer information through a high quality quarterly publication in which ophthalmology would be represented by eight subspecialties. In this regard, each issue has had a subspecialty theme and has been overseen by two internationally recognized volume editors, who in turn have invited a bevy of experts to discuss clinically relevant and appropriate topics. Summaries of clinically relevant information have been provided throughout each chapter.

Each subspecialty area now has been covered once, and the response to the first eight volumes in the series has been enthusiastically positive. With the start of the second cycle of subspecialty coverage, the dissemination of practical information will be continued as we learn more about the emerging advances in various ophthalmic subspecialties that can be applied to obtain the best possible care of our patients. Moreover, we will continue to highlight clinically relevant information and maintain our commitment to excellence.

G. K. Krieglstein
R. N. Weinreb
Series Editors

Preface

Clinicians and basic scientists from the fields of ophthalmology and vision research have made tremendous progress in understanding the pathogenesis of retinal diseases, developing novel diagnostic techniques, and instituting new treatments for retinal conditions.

This multi-authored volume provides concise updates on the relevant and most challenging topics in medical retina. It is a practical and useful publication that will help all ophthalmologists, whether in training or in practice, to manage patients with retinal diseases.

The first two chapters on microperimetry and scanning laser fundus imaging highlight the advances in diagnostic technology that have contributed significantly to our understanding of the pathophysiology and treatment of various diseases. The following chapters address the latest developments in the area of age-related macular degeneration including an update on genetic factors, current management strategies using anti-VEGF therapy, the role of combination treatments, and nutritional supplementation. The atrophic form of late AMD, i.e., geographic atrophy, is also addressed. Furthermore, current treatment approaches to diabetic macular edema and retinal vein occlusions are described. Finally, there is a discussion of the novel insights into Stargardt's disease and idiopathic macular teleangiectasia, as well as perspectives on the expanding field of artificial vision.

Time and effort have been generously given by the contributing authors, to whom we, as editors, are extremely grateful. We are indebted to the editorial and production staff at Springer for their commitment to a timely publication in this rapidly moving field.

Frank G. Holz
Richard F. Spaide

Contents

Chapter 1
Microperimetry in Macular Disease
Klaus Rohrschneider

1.1	Introduction	1
1.2	Instruments	2
1.2.1	Scanning Laser Ophthalmoscope	2
1.2.1.1	Fundus Perimetry (Microperimetry)	3
1.2.2	Micro Perimeter 1	4
1.2.2.1	Static Threshold Fundus Perimetry	4
1.2.2.2	Kinetic Fundus Perimetry	6
1.2.3	Comparison Between SLO Perimetry and MP 1	6
1.2.4	Accuracy of Fundus Perimetry	6
1.2.4.1	Static Threshold Perimetry	6
1.2.4.2	Kinetic Perimetry	7
1.2.5	Fundus-related Perimetry Versus Cupola Perimetry	7
1.3	Clinical Implementation	8
1.3.1	Macular Holes	8
1.3.2	Age-related Macular Degeneration	10
1.3.2.1	Geographic Atrophy of the RPE	10
1.3.2.2	Choroidal Neovascularization in AMD	10
1.3.3	Diabetic Retinopathy	10
1.3.4	Central Serous Chorioretinopathy	14
1.3.5	Stargardt's Disease	15
1.3.6	Vitelliform Macular Dystrophy (Best's Disease)	16
1.4	Conclusion	16

Chapter 2
New Developments in cSLO Fundus Imaging
Giovanni Staurenghi, Grazia Levi, Silvia Pedenovi, Chiara Veronese

2.1	Introduction	21
2.2	Near Infrared Imaging	22
2.2.1	Introduction	22
2.2.2	The Effect of Wavelength on Imaging in the Human Fundus	22
2.2.3	Comparison of Light Tissue Interactions for Visible and Near Infrared Wavelengths Using SLO	22
2.2.4	Mode of Imaging	22
2.2.5	Contrast of the Fundus	23
2.2.6	Fundus Features	23
2.2.7	Imaging of Pathological Features in Direct and Indirect Mode	23
2.3	Blue Autofluorescence Imaging	23
2.3.1	Autofluorescence and the Eye	24
2.3.1.1	Fluorescence of the Retinal Pigment Epithelium	24
2.3.1.2	How to Evaluate RPE Autofluorescence	24
2.3.2	Fundus Autofluorescence Changes in Early AMD	25
2.3.3	Fundus Autofluorescence Changes in Choroidal Neovascularization in AMD	26
2.3.4	Fundus Autofluorescence Changes in Geographic Atrophy in AMD	26
2.3.5	Fundus Autofluorescence in Acute and Chronic Recurrent Central Serous Chorioretinopathy	27

2.3.6	Fundus Autofluorescence in Stargardt's Macular Dystrophy-Fundus Flavimaculatus	27	4.1.1	Historical Perspective	53
			4.1.2	VEGF Isoforms	54
			4.1.3	VEGF Expression	54
			4.1.4	VEGF Receptors	54
2.3.7	Fundus Autofluorescence in Patients with Macular Holes	28	4.1.5	VEGF Activity	55
			4.2	Current Anti-VEGF Therapies	55
			4.2.1	Aptamers: Pegaptanib Sodium (Macugen)	55
2.4	Wide-Field Contact Lens System	28	4.2.2	Monoclonal Antibodies: Ranibizumab (Lucentis)	56
2.4.1	Introduction	28			
2.4.2	Materials and Methods	29	4.2.3	Monoclonal Antibodies: Bevacizumab (Avastin)	58
2.4.2.1	Structure of a Wide-Field Contact Lens System	29	4.3	Anti-VEGF Therapy: Practical Considerations	60
2.4.2.2	Limit and Advantage of a Wide-Field Contact Lens System	29	4.3.1	Intravitreal Injection Technique	60
			4.3.2	Safety Considerations	60
2.4.2.3	Technique for Performing the Examination	29	4.3.3	Bevacizumab (Avastin) Preparation: Compounding Pharmacies	61
2.4.3	Other Techniques of Execution of Wide-field Fluorescein Angiograms	30	4.4	Future Anti-VEGF Therapies	61
			4.4.1	VEGF Trap	61
2.4.4	Clinical Application	31	4.4.2	Small Interfering RNAs	62
			4.4.3	Receptor Tyrosine Kinase Inhibitors	63
			4.5	Conclusion	64

Chapter 3
Genetics of Age-Related Macular Degeneration: Update

Hendrik P.N. Scholl, Monika Fleckenstein, Peter Charbel Issa, Claudia Keilhauer, Frank G. Holz, Bernhard H.F. Weber

3.1	Introduction: Genetic Influence on AMD	35
3.2	Analysis of Candidate Genes for AMD	36
3.3	Linkage and Association Studies in AMD	38
3.4	Complement Factor H Gene	38
3.5	**LOC387715**	43
3.6	Factor B	44
3.7	Gene–Gene and Gene–Environment Interaction in AMD	45
3.8	Conclusions	46

Chapter 4
Anti-VEGF Treatment for Age-Related Macular Degeneration

Todd R. Klesert, Jennifer I. Lim

4.1	Basic Science	53

Chapter 5
Intravitreal Injections: Techniques and Sequelae

Heinrich Heimann

5.1	Introduction	67
5.2	Complications of Intravitreal Injections	68
5.2.1	Methodology	69
5.2.2	Perioperative Complications	69
5.2.2.1	Conjunctival Hemorrhage	69
5.2.2.2	Conjunctival Scarring	72
5.2.2.3	Pain	72
5.2.2.4	Punctate Keratitis and Corneal Edema	72
5.2.2.5	Vitreous Reflux	72
5.2.2.6	Traumatic Cataract	72
5.2.2.7	Cataract Progression	73
5.2.2.8	Retinal Perforation	73
5.2.2.9	Vitreous Floaters	74
5.2.2.10	Vitreous Hemorrhage	74
5.2.2.11	Retinal Toxicity	74
5.2.2.12	Intraocular Inflammation	74

5.2.2.13	Uveitis and Pseudo-endophthalmitis	75
5.2.2.14	Endophthalmitis	76
5.2.2.15	Retinal Artery and Vein Occlusion	78
5.2.2.16	Retinal Detachment	78
5.2.2.17	Acute Rise in Intraocular Pressure	79
5.2.2.18	Ocular Hypertension and Glaucoma	79
5.3	Surgical Technique for Intravitreal Injection	80
5.3.1	Guidelines and Preferred Practice Survey	81
5.3.2	Preoperative Assessment and Preparation	81
5.3.2.1	Concomitant Eye Diseases	81
5.3.2.2	Preoperative Assessment	81
5.3.2.3	Preoperative Medication	81
5.3.2.4	Location	81
5.3.2.5	Preparation of the Eye and Ocular Adnexa	81
5.3.2.6	Preparation of the Surgeon	84
5.3.2.7	Preparation of the Drug	84
5.3.3	Injection	84
5.3.3.1	Syringe and Needle	84
5.3.3.2	Position of the Injection	84
5.3.3.3	Entry Path	84
5.3.3.4	Advancement of Needle and Injection	84
5.3.4	Postoperative Assessment	84
5.3.4.1	Assessment Immediately Following the Injection	84
5.3.4.2	Topical Therapy	85
5.3.4.3	Follow-up Examinations	85

Chapter 6
Combination Therapies for Choroidal Neovascularization
Richard F. Spaide

6.1	Introduction	90
6.2	Angiogenesis	90
6.2.1	Development of CNV	91
6.2.2	Cancer and Angiogenesis	91
6.3	Normalization of Tumor Vasculature	92
6.4	Two-Component Model of CNV	94
6.5	Two-Component Model and Therapy	94
6.5.1	Are There Cytokines to Block Other Than VEGF?	95
6.6	Combination Therapies	96
6.6.1	Anti-VEGF Biologics and Photodynamic Therapy	96
6.6.2	Anecortave Acetate and Photodynamic Therapy	97
6.6.3	Intravitreal Triamcinolone and Photodynamic Therapy	97
6.6.4	Triamcinolone and Anti-VEGF Therapy	97
6.6.5	Triamcinolone and Anecortave Acetate	98
6.7	Conclusion	99

Chapter 7
Nutritional Supplementation in Age-related Macular Degeneration
Hanna R. Coleman, Emily Y. Chew

7.1	Introduction	105
7.2	Risk Factors	105
7.3	Age-Related Eye Disease Study	106
7.4	Lutein/Zeaxanthin	106
7.5	Zinc	106
7.6	Vitamin E	107
7.7	Dietary Fat Intake	107
7.8	Age-Related Eye Disease Study 2	107
7.9	Conclusion	108

Chapter 8
New Perspectives in Geographic Atrophy Associated with AMD
Steffen Schmitz-Valckenberg, Monika Fleckenstein, Hendrik P.N. Scholl, Frank G. Holz

8.1	Introduction	114
8.1.1	Basics	114
8.1.2	Development and Spread of Atrophy	115
8.2	Fundus Autofluorescence Imaging in Geographic Atrophy	116
8.3	Quantification of Atrophy Progression	117

8.4	Risk Factors	118
8.4.1	Genetic Factors	118
8.4.2	Systemic Risk Factors	118
8.4.3	Ocular Risk Factors	119
8.5	Development of CNV in Eyes with GA	122
8.6	Visual Function in GA Patients	123
8.6.1	Measurement of Visual Acuity	123
8.6.2	Contrast Sensitivity	124
8.6.3	Reading Speed	124
8.6.4	Fundus Perimetry	124

Chapter 9
Diabetic Macular Edema: Current Treatments

Florian K.P. Sutter, Mark C. Gillies, Horst Helbig

9.1	Introduction	131
9.2	Epidemiology	131
9.3	Pathophysiology	132
9.4	Diabetic Macular Edema and Laboratory Science	132
9.5	Quality of Life	133
9.6	Diagnosis and Screening	133
9.7	Types of Diabetic Macular Edema	134
9.7.1	Clinically Significant Macular Edema	134
9.7.2	Focal Diabetic Macular Edema	134
9.7.3	Diffuse Diabetic Macular Edema	134
9.7.4	Cystoid Macular Edema	134
9.7.5	Ischemic Macular Edema	134
9.7.6	OCT Patterns of Diabetic Macular Edema	134
9.8	Treatment	135
9.8.1	Systemic Treatment	135
9.8.1.1	Glycemic Control	135
9.8.1.2	Blood Pressure Control	135
9.8.1.3	Reducing Levels of Blood Lipids	135
9.8.1.4	Treatment of Renal Dysfunction and Anemia	136
9.8.1.5	Smoking	136
9.8.2	Systemic Pharmacotherapy	136
9.8.2.1	PKC-ß Inhibitors	136
9.8.2.2	Aldose Reductase and AGE Inhibitors	136
9.8.2.3	Antioxidants	136
9.8.3	A Team Approach to the Prevention of Loss of Vision in People with Diabetes	137
9.8.4	Local Ophthalmic Treatment	138
9.8.4.1	Focal Macular Laser	138
9.8.4.2	Grid Macular Laser	138
9.8.4.3	Recent Trends in Macular Laser Therapy	138
9.8.4.4	Micropulsed, Sub-threshold "Selective" Laser Therapy	139
9.8.4.5	Vitrectomy	139
9.8.4.6	Intravitreal Steroids	139
9.8.4.7	Periocular Steroids	140
9.8.4.8	Intravitreal Anti-VEGF Antibodies	140
9.8.4.9	Cataract Surgery	141
9.9	Current Clinical Practice/ Recommendations	141

Chapter 10
Treatment of Retinal Vein Occlusions

Rajeev S. Ramchandran, R. Keith Shuler, Sharon Fekrat

10.1	Introduction	147
10.2	Pathophysiology	148
10.3	Branch and Central Vein Occlusion Studies	148
10.3.1	Background	148
10.3.2	Branch Vein Occlusion Study	149
10.3.3	Central Vein Occlusion Study	149
10.4	Systemic Pharmacologic Treatments	150
10.5	Targeting Macular Edema	151
10.6	Intravitreal Pharmacotherapy	151
10.6.1	Background	151
10.6.2	Intravitreal Triamcinolone: BRVO	153
10.6.3	Intravitreal Triamcinolone: CRVO	153
10.6.4	Fluocinolone Acetonide Intravitreal Implant	153

10.6.5	Standard of Care vs. Corticosteroid for Retinal Vein Occlusion Study	154
10.6.6	Intravitreal Anti-VEGF Therapy	155
10.7	Surgical Treatments	156
10.7.1	BRVO	156
10.7.2	CRVO	156
10.7.2.1	Laser-Induced Venous Chorioretinal Anastomosis	156
10.7.2.2	Recombinant Tissue Plasminogen Activator	156
10.7.2.3	Radial Optic Neurotomy	157
10.7.2.4	Intravitreal Triamcinolone: As Adjunctive Therapy	158
10.8	Prevention—Systemic Factor Control	158
10.9	Conclusion	158

Chapter 11
New Perspectives in Stargardt's Disease
Noemi Lois

11.1	Introduction	166
11.2	Epidemiology and Clinical Findings	166
11.3	Imaging Studies	169
11.3.1	Fluorescein Angiography	169
11.3.2	Indocyanine Green Angiography	170
11.3.3	Fundus Autofluorescence	170
11.3.4	Optical Coherence Tomography	172
11.4	Electrophysiology and Psychophysics	172
11.5	Histopathology	174
11.6	Differential Diagnosis	174
11.7	Genetics and Molecular Biology	174
11.8	Animal Models of STGD-FFM	177
11.9	Current and Future Treatments	177

Chapter 12
Idiopathic Macular Telangiectasia
Peter Charbel Issa, Hendrik P.N. Scholl, Hans-Martin Helb, Frank G. Holz

12.1	Introduction	183
12.2	Type 1 Idiopathic Macular Telangiectasia	183
12.2.1	Epidemiology	183
12.2.2	Diagnostic Approach and Clinical Findings	185
12.2.3	Functional Implications	185
12.2.4	Pathophysiological Considerations	186
12.2.5	Therapy	186
12.3	Type 2 Idiopathic Macular Telangiectasia	187
12.3.1	Epidemiology	188
12.3.2	Diagnostic Approach and Clinical Findings	188
12.3.3	Functional Implications	189
12.3.4	Associated Diseases	192
12.3.5	Pathophysiological Considerations	192
12.3.6	Therapeutic Approaches	193
12.4	Type 3: Idiopathic Macular Telangiectasia	194
12.5	Perspectives	194

Chapter 13
Artificial Vision
Peter Walter

13.1	Introduction	199
13.2	Current Concepts for Restoring Vision Using Electrical Stimulation	200
13.3	Interfacing the Neurons	200
13.3.1	Epiretinal Stimulation	201
13.3.2	Subretinal Approach	203
13.3.3	Transchoroidal, Transscleral, and Suprachoroidal Stimulation	203
13.3.4	Optic Nerve Approach	204
13.3.5	Cortical Prosthesis	204
13.4	Pixel Vision and Filters	204
13.5	Outlook	206
13.6	Conclusion	206

Subject Index ... 211

Contributors

Peter Charbel Issa, Dr.
Department of Ophthalmology
University of Bonn
Ernst-Abbe-Straße 2
53127 Bonn
Germany

Emily Y. Chew, MD
National Eye Institute/National Institutes
of Health
10 Center Drive
Bethesda, MD 20892-1204
USA

Hanna R. Coleman, MD
National Eye Institute/National Institutes
of Health
10 Center Drive
Bethesda, MD 20892-1204
USA

Sharon Fekrat, MD, FACS
Department of Ophthalmology
Duke University Medical Center
Durham, NC 27710
USA

Monika Fleckenstein, Dr.
Department of Ophthalmology
University of Bonn
Ernst-Abbe-Straße 2
53127 Bonn
Germany

Mark C. Gillies, MD
Save Sight Institute
P. O. Box 4337
Sydney NSW 2001
Australia

Heinrich Heimann, Priv.-Doz. Dr.
Consultant Ophthalmic Surgeon
St. Paul's Eye Unit, Royal Liverpool University
Hospital
Prescot Street
Liverpool, L7 8XP
UK

Hans-Martin Helb, Dr.
Department of Ophthalmology
University of Bonn
Ernst-Abbe-Straße 2
53127 Bonn
Germany

Horst Helbig, Prof. Dr.
Department of Ophthalmology
University of Regensburg
Franz-Josef-Strauß-Allee 11
93042 Regensburg
Germany

Frank G. Holz, Prof. Dr.
Department of Ophthalmology
University of Bonn
Ernst-Abbe-Straße 2
53127 Bonn
Germany

Claudia Keilhauer, Dr.
Department of Ophthalmology
University of Würzburg
Josef-Schneider-Straße 11
97080 Würzburg
Germany

Todd R. Klesert, MD, PhD
Doheny Retina Institute
of the Doheny Eye Institute
USC Keck School of Medicine
1450 San Pablo Street
Los Angeles, CA 90027
USA

Contributors

Grazia Levi, MD
II Scuola di Specialità in Oftalmologia
Università degli studi di Milano
Facoltà di Medicina e Chirurgia
Dipartimento di Scienze Cliniche Luigi Sacco
Via G.B. Grassi, 74
20157 Milano
Italy

Jennifer I. Lim, MD
Doheny Eye Institute
USC Keck School of Medicine
1450 San Pablo Street
Los Angeles, CA 90033
USA

Noemi Lois, MD, PhD
Aberdeen Royal Infirmary
University Hospital
Foresterhill
Aberdeen AB25 2ZN
UK

Silvia Pedenovi, MD
II Scuola di Specialità in Oftalmologia
Università degli studi di Milano
Facoltà di Medicina e Chirurgia
Dipartimento di Scienze Cliniche Luigi Sacco
Via G.B. Grassi, 74
20157 Milano
Italy

Rajeev S. Ramchandran, MD
Department of Ophthalmology
Duke University Medical Center
Durham, NC 27710
USA

Klaus Rohrschneider, Prof. Dr.
Department of Ophthalmology
University of Heidelberg
Im Neuenheimer Feld 400
69120 Heidelberg
Germany

Steffen Schmitz-Valckenberg, Dr.
Department of Ophthalmology
University of Bonn
Ernst-Abbe-Straße 2
53127 Bonn
Germany

Hendrik P.N. Scholl, Priv.-Doz. Dr.
Department of Ophthalmology
University of Bonn
Ernst-Abbe-Straße 2
53127 Bonn
Germany

R. Keith Shuler, MD
Department of Ophthalmology
Duke University Medical Center
Durham, NC 27710
USA

Richard F. Spaide, MD, Prof.
Vitreous, Retina, and Macula Consultants
of New York,
and LuEsther T. Mertz Retinal Research Center,
Manhattan Eye, Ear, and Throat Hospital
460 Park Avenue
New York, NY 10022
USA

Giovanni Staurenghi, MD, Prof.
Cattedra di Clinica Oculistica
II Scuola di Specialità in Oftalmologia
Università degli studi di Milano
Facoltà di Medicina e Chirurgia
Dipartimento di Scienze Cliniche Luigi Sacco
Via G.B. Grassi, 74
20157 Milano
Italy

Florian K.P. Sutter, Priv.-Doz. Dr.
Department of Ophthalmology
University of Zurich
Rämistraße 100
8049 Zurich
Switzerland

Chiara Veronese, MD
II Scuola di Specialità in Oftalmologia
Università degli studi di Milano
Facoltà di Medicina e Chirurgia
Dipartimento di Scienze Cliniche Luigi Sacco
Via G.B. Grassi, 74
20157 Milano
Italy

Peter Walter, Prof. Dr.
Department of Ophthalmology
RWTH Aachen University
Pauwelsstraße 30
52074 Aachen
Germany

Bernhard H.F. Weber, Prof. Dr.
Institute for Human Genetics
University of Regensburg
Franz-Josef-Strauß-Allee 11
93053 Regensburg
Germany

Chapter 1

Microperimetry in Macular Disease

Klaus Rohrschneider

Core Messages

- Macular diseases typically result in the deterioration of visual function. For accurate evaluation of macular disorders, conventional visual field determination has proven to be insufficient, because the accuracy of the conventional visual field relies on the assumption that fixation happens at the fovea and remains stable.
- Fundus perimetry is the only reliable method of visual field testing in patients with instable or eccentric fixation due to macular pathologies. While static threshold perimetry may be preferred in eyes with diffuse functional deterioration or irregular scotoma, kinetic test strategies allow for exact delineation of the border of the deep scotoma.
- In eyes with macular holes exact delineation of size of functional deterioration is very helpful, even in surgery.
- Counseling patients with choroidal neovascularization (CNV) due to age-related macular degeneration is much easier with the help of microperimetry due to knowledge of the paracentral scotoma influencing visual function and reading ability.
- In central serous chorioretinopathy the symptoms are often difficult to understand because visual acuity is normal. Fundus perimetry demonstrates a deep paracentral scotoma that is often very concordant with the increase in retinal thickness, explaining visual disturbance.
- Patients with Stargardt's disease exhibit a characteristic behavior of fixation, which can be documented only via fundus examination.
- Fundus perimetry provides a more complete assessment of macular function for diagnostic purposes as well as for evaluation of new treatment methods and expertise in simulation or aggravation in patients with macular diseases.

1.1 Introduction

Macular diseases typically result in the deterioration of visual function. While central visual acuity represents a parameter of this function, difficulties in daily life, such as reduced reading performance frequently caused by (para)central scotomas, are often missed. As far back as 1856, the famous German ophthalmologist Albrecht von Graefe remarked that central visual acuity is only one aspect of visual function and additional knowledge of the visual field is of equal importance. In the meantime, lots of different methods for visual field measurement have been developed. Especially in glaucoma management, in neuro-ophthalmological disorders, and in retinal diseases such as retinitis pigmentosa, perimetry is extremely important. Conventional methods of visual field testing, such as Goldmann kinetic perimetry and Humphrey or Octopus static perimetry, serve well for these applications. However, for accurate evaluation of macular disorders, conventional visual field determination has proven to be insufficient, because the accuracy of the conventional visual field relies on the assumption that fixation happens at the fovea and remains stable.

Seeking an exact correlation between retinal pathology and functional alteration, different instruments have been invented to perform perimetry under simultaneous fundus control [8, 19]. With the implication of infrared light sources, the major problem of the very high light levels necessary for retinal illumination in fundus observation could be overcome. After the invention of the scanning laser ophthalmoscope (SLO), it was possible to simultaneously visualize the fundus and perform fundus-correlated functional tests. As a result, fundus perimetry, or microperimetry, has been implemented in a clinical setting, providing simultaneous observation of the fundus and correction of eye movements during the perimetric examination. By achieving precise examination conditions for patients with small retinal or choroidal lesions and poor fixation, an exact correlation between retinal pathologies and functional defects has become possible. After the initial presentation of fundus perimetry with a SLO by Timberlake and coworkers more than 20 years ago, the value of this technique and other fundus-related function tests used in the diagnosis and follow-up of patients with macular diseases has been documented [34, 54, 56].

Although the new technique has often been named "microperimetry," neither the stimulus size nor the test grid is appropriately covered by this term. Therefore, fundus-correlated perimetry or even fundus perimetry may represent the more appropriate term for perimetry with simultaneous visualization of the fundus.

As a consequence of expanding surgical options and an increasing number of therapeutic approaches for macular diseases, accurate functional testing of the macular region has become more and more important. With the advantage of exact documentation of the actual test location on the retina and a real-time correction for eye movements, fundus perimetry is the only reliable method of visual field testing in patients with unstable or eccentric fixation due to macular pathologies.

While the scanning laser ophthalmoscope (Rodenstock Instruments, Ottobrunn, Germany) is no longer available on the market, and even maintenance of the existing instruments is becoming more and more difficult, another comparable instrument has recently been developed: the Micro Perimeter 1 (MP 1), designed and manufactured by Nidek Instruments, Padova, Italy.

This chapter describes the possibilities of fundus-controlled function testing in macular diseases with the SLO 101 and the MP-1, beginning with the technical options and followed by a selection of typical findings of specific macular diseases or pathologies.

1.2 Instruments

1.2.1 Scanning Laser Ophthalmoscope

The principle of the SLO was described in detail earlier. In brief, the SLO projects a helium neon laser beam (632.8 nm) and an infrared diode laser (780 nm) simultaneously onto the fundus with an image size of 33×21°. The amount of light projected onto the retina is well below the limits set by the ANSI (American National Standards Institute) for lasers [3]. The HeNe laser used for generation of the background and stimulus illumination is adjusted via an acousto-optic modulator in 256 steps. The image of the retina is acquired simultaneously by illumination with infrared laser light through a set of nearly confocal apertures. This makes it possible to project any desired image onto the fundus, simultaneously capture the actual fundus image and therefore perform fundus perimetry, fixation tasks or different reading tests.

While the original Rodenstock software, especially in Europe, only supported the manual detection of a light threshold for single-stimulus locations, we developed more advanced software that offers examination by automated static threshold fundus perimetry and manual or automated kinetic perimetry comparable to the options of conventional cupola perimetry [31, 33, 34, 36].

1.2.1.1 Fundus Perimetry (Microperimetry)

1.2.1.1.1 Static Threshold Fundus Perimetry

Using Heidelberg perimetry software, any stimulus can be projected exactly onto the predefined fundus position by the help of a landmark setting superimposed on the real-time image [33, 34, 36]. During each stimulus presentation, the fundus image is digitized and a correction for eye movements is performed. Background illumination is typically set at 10 cd/m². The fixation target is a cross, measuring 1.5×1.5°, with a central opening of 0.5°, which allows a stimulus to be projected into the center of fixation. Stimulus presentation time can be chosen to be either 120 or 200 ms. Stimulus intensity can be varied by 0.1 log steps from 0 to 21 dB. Here, 0 dB represented the brightest luminance of 71 cd/cm². In addition, stimulus intensities of 23.6 and 26 dB can be projected.

Stimulus diameters can be varied between Goldmann size I and V. Differential light threshold is measured with a 4-2-1 or 4-2 staircase strategy at randomly selected stimulus locations. To reduce examination time, starting luminance for the first four stimulus locations is 2 dB higher than the normal threshold. Following complete light increment threshold testing in these locations, all following start-off values may be adapted relatively to the surrounding threshold.

For the clinical application of this new technique, it was important to sample a normative database. Based on 152 eyes in 99 healthy participants, aged 16 to 77 years, a mean decrease in light sensitivity of 0.275 dB per decade was found starting with 16.6 dB at the age of 10 years [36].

Summary for the Clinician

- Static fundus perimetry allows morphologic alteration to exactly correlate with congruous functional impairment.
- Different test grids and the option to add additional test points allows specific examinations to be performed.
- A normative data base enables defect values to be calculated.

1.2.1.1.2 Kinetic Fundus Perimetry

In addition to static threshold fundus perimetry, there is an option to perform either manual or automated kinetic fundus perimetry. This allows a more precise delineation of the scotomas, i.e., accurate definition of the border of a scotoma. In manual mode, the investigator targets the stimulus with the help of a computer mouse and when the patient reacts by pressing a button, the fundus image is digitized. Using the landmark setting mentioned above, the actual location of fixation and therefore of the stimulus is calculated and stored [31].

In addition, an automated procedure can be performed. Here up to 16 directions of the stimulus, either from the center to the periphery (centrifugal) or from the periphery to the center (centripetal), will be tested one after another. The velocity and maximum distance to a predefined center may be varied. However, it should be mentioned that there is no correction for any eye movements during the test procedure, i.e., in eyes with markedly decreased stability of fixation this technique may give unexpected and artificial results.

Summary for the Clinician

- Kinetic fundus perimetry allows the border of a deep and sharply demarcated scotoma to be precisely delineated.
- The examination time of kinetic fundus perimetry is very short.

> **Summary for the Clinician**
>
> ■ In eyes with decreased stability of fixation unexpected and artificial results may be obtained.

1.2.1.1.3 Evaluation of Fixation Behavior

Examination of fixation has been of enormous interest not only in macular disease, but also in strabismus or for the detection of malingering and simulation. In the past, modified fundus cameras or special TV cameras were used, but, due to the high illumination levels, there was no physiologic rationale of fixation behavior [7, 49, 57]. In clinical practice, the star figure of the direct ophthalmoscope may be used, especially in strabismic children, even without pupil dilation. However, as a subjective test, the examiner may wish for an option of documentation. Observation of fixation into a laser light is a comparable technique, which may be documented with a fundus camera simultaneously attached to the slit-lamp.

The SLO offers the possibility of receiving information concerning the behavior of fixation with mesopic light levels, even over time. This means that stability and the area of fixation can be observed. Specific macular diseases may lead to typical changes in fixation with nearly pathognomonic movement and variation as in Stargardt's disease [29]. Patients with deep or absolute central scotoma will shift the location of fixation and develop a new, so-called preferred retinal locus (PRL). During the development of an extrafoveal PRL, alternating fixation between two or more distinct locations may be observed [35, 52]. For adequate counseling and rehabilitation, the knowledge of these changes is very important, as well as in age-related macular degeneration (AMD; Fig. 1.1).

A specific fixation task documents the stability of fixation as the patient is asked to press a button while actually looking at the fixation object. Repeating this 30 to 50 times allows a measurement of the fixation stability around the PRL to be calculated [32].

During fundus-related perimetry, the actual location of the fixation is stored for each stimulus presentation. Thus, the time course of the fixation can be monitored and even documented in a video sequence.

1.2.2 Micro Perimeter 1

The MP 1 is not a SLO. Rather, the fundus image is observed using an infrared fundus camera with a 45° field of view. Perimetry is performed using a liquid crystal display controlled by special software. The major advantage over the Rodenstock SLO, and even over our software, is the automatic eye tracking, which compensates for eye movements under real-time conditions and therefore presents any stimulus exactly at the predefined location.

In the meantime, its software has been further developed and now allows automated static threshold fundus perimetry, automated kinetic fundus perimetry, as well as specific fixation and reading tasks to be performed.

1.2.2.1 Static Threshold Fundus Perimetry

Static fundus perimetry with the MP 1 can be performed with different predefined test grids, comparable to conventional cupola perimetry or any grid defined by the investigator. Stimulus size can be varied between Goldmann sizes I and V, background illumination is either white or red with background luminance of 4 asb, presentation time either 100 or 200 ms. The offset luminance for each test point location can be defined at will, but usually will have an identical setting for all locations of 10 dB.

For exact eye tracking, a region of interest on the infrared fundus image has to be defined prior to examination. Best alignment will be achieved when clearly visible vessels or prominent structures around the optic disc are selected.

Examination time is comparable to our SLO software, but about twice as long compared with conventional perimetry. Further development of an adaptive test strategy has decreased this time.

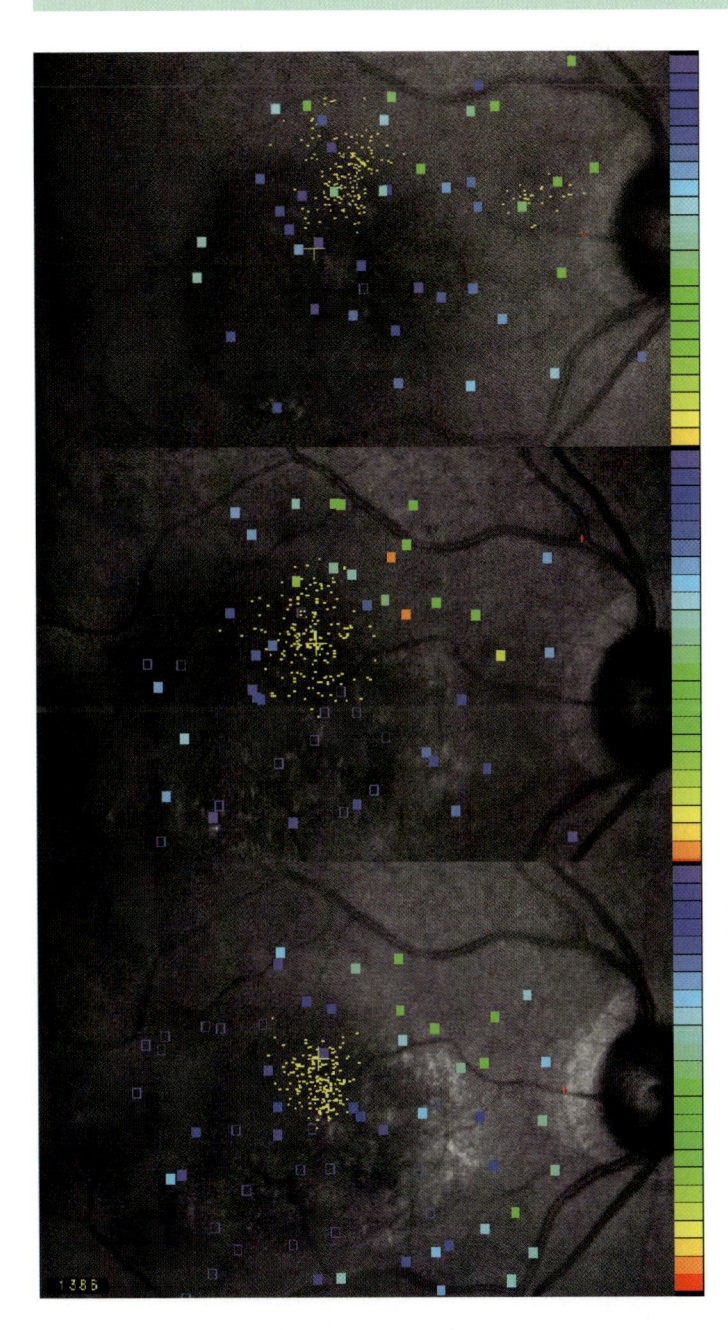

Fig. 1.1 Right eye of a 67-year-old female patient with central choroidal neovascularization (CNV). Initially, she presented with alternating preferred retinal loci (PRL), the more central one being dominant (*top*). Six weeks following laser treatment, the PRL has stabilized, and another 6 weeks later, the stability of fixation is better, as seen by the *yellow dots* representing single fixations during perimetry (*bottom*). Threshold values for static perimetry are presented according to the right-hand scale in 1-dB steps with the highest illumination at the top (*blue*). *Open rectangles* demonstrate absolute defects (from [28] with permission)

Meanwhile, a normative database has been added to the actual software. While maximum light sensitivity is 20 dB according to the maximum differential light threshold, a multicenter study group in Italy found normal values of 20 dB [22]. Therefore, the sensitivity for detecting early field defects might be lower in comparison to SLO perimetry or even conventional cupola perimetry.

> **Summary for the Clinician**
>
> - Static fundus perimetry allows morphologic alteration to exactly correlate with congruous functional impairment.
> - Different test grids and the option to add additional test points allow specific examinations to be performed.
> - A normative database enables defect values to be calculated.

1.2.2.2 Kinetic Fundus Perimetry

In addition to static threshold fundus perimetry, there is an option to perform automated kinetic perimetry. After defining stimulus size, velocity and direction, i.e., either centrifugal or centripetal relative to a defined centre, the instrument automatically performs up to six different measurements. Each stimulus movement is finished either when the patient ascertains to have seen the stimulus or when the maximum extent of the movement up to 20° eccentricity is reached. Because there is no correction for eye movements during stimulus presentation with this technique, there may be false stimulus perception. Therefore, it is possible to retest specific movements after finishing the whole procedure.

> **Summary for the Clinician**
>
> - Kinetic fundus perimetry allows the border of a deep and sharply demarcated scotoma to be precisely delineated.
> - The examination time of kinetic fundus perimetry is very short.
> - Automated kinetic test strategies enhance reliability.
> - In eyes with decreased stability of fixation unexpected and artificial results may be obtained.

1.2.3 Comparison Between SLO Perimetry and MP 1

Fundus-related perimetry has been established as an important technique for evaluating visual function in macular disease. However, using the SLO with different set-ups of the instrument itself and different software options, ranging from the original Rodenstock software to advanced solutions like those from Sunness and coworkers or our own software, led to results that were not comparable among different instruments and investigators [33, 51]. This drawback has been overcome by the invention of the MP 1. Nevertheless, veering away from the use of laser scanning optics has resulted in reduced quality of the infrared image.

Comparison between the size and depths of field defects observed with both instruments demonstrated that the MP 1 will typically enlarge the scotoma. However, there was good concordance between SLO and MP 1, even in eyes with field defects [41].

1.2.4 Accuracy of Fundus Perimetry

In addition, normal values for differential light threshold, as well as data on reliability for single locations or accuracy of determination of scotoma borders are important to judge the value of any perimeter. Even in cupola perimetry, few data exist. It has been shown in static perimetry that as the depth of any scotoma increases or as the mean defect (MD) rises variation and short-term fluctuation increase as well [11, 12].

Comparable to these findings in static perimetry, the precision of determination of any scotoma border during kinetic testing will be reduced as scotoma steepness decreases.

1.2.4.1 Static Threshold Perimetry

For both methods mentioned above, a normative database for differential light threshold values has been established [22, 36].

In addition, results concerning fluctuation have been given by our group for the SLO with repeated measurements at four specific locations in a group of normals. Ninety-five percent confidence intervals were ±4 dB around each single test point. Short-term fluctuation for all 152 eyes included in this study was 2.0±0.8 dB [36].

Mean reliability for three independent examinations in 10 eyes was 1.5±0.7 dB (range 1.1 to 3.9 dB). As expected the largest differences were observed at the border of the optic disc. For the most sensitive detection of early field defects in glaucomatous patients we found that two single defects of 7 dB or more in a small grid of 30 peripapillary points result in a pathologic examination [38].

For examination with the MP 1, the standard deviation of mean differential light thresholds varied between 0.8 dB in the center and 4.1 dB around the blind spot [47]. Most locations showed a standard deviation of less than 2 dB.

While fundus-related perimetry was mostly performed using static perimetry, measurement of scotoma size has been another issue. When examining the area of the blind spot with stimuli of different sizes, different groups have shown the influence of reflection of prominent structures [6, 21]. However, accuracy of the definition of the border largely depends on the number and distance of different stimuli.

1.2.4.2 Kinetic Perimetry

With the use of the SLO it has been found that the accuracy of measuring the blind spot as a physiologic scotoma with a kinetic procedure also depends on the morphology of the optic disc. In eyes with nasal prominent supertraction the field defect is enlarged, while in advanced cupping the border is located more closely toward the margin of the optic nerve head (Fig. 1.2). This may be explained by stray light caused by the retinal structures. Because the MP 1 does not use a scanning laser source, we expect to strengthen this effect, especially when using larger or brighter stimuli. Findings in patients with larger central scotoma demonstrated that scotoma size also varies depending on reflectivity.

Repeated measurement of the area of the blind spot with the MP 1 showed a variation of scotoma size of up to 25%. However, the software did not allow for retesting in directions with wrong results. When such findings were excluded, the accuracy was much better.

1.2.5 Fundus-related Perimetry Versus Cupola Perimetry

Since the development of automated static threshold perimetry with the SLO a number of comparisons between this technique and conventional cupola perimetry have been performed in healthy participants [4, 33]. Another study was performed comparing MP 1 and Octopus perimetry in normals [47]. All these studies demonstrated comparable results with deviation in the range of short-term fluctuation values for computerized perimetry.

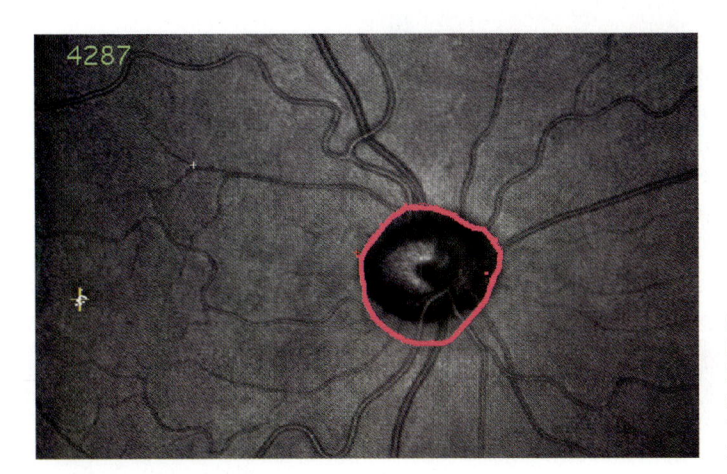

Fig. 1.2 Normal eye with large physiologic cup (CDR 0.4). Kinetic fundus perimetry (Goldmann I, 0 dB) clearly delineates the border of the disc with an inferior extension

When interpreting perimetric results one has to bear in mind that exact knowledge of the stimulus location is most important in patients with macular disease [46]. Therefore, the observation that examination time is about twice as long during fundus-related examination is of minor importance.

1.3 Clinical Implementation

While advances in medical and surgical options of retinal diseases have changed treatment modalities and therefore the prognosis of macular diseases, scientific evaluation is based upon two types of parameter: morphologic and functional. Documentation of morphological alterations of the posterior pole has been rapidly changed by new techniques such as laser scanning tomography, optical coherence tomography, and autofluorescence imaging. However, the more important measures are functional data, which are typically based on central visual acuity. Since the invention of fundus perimetry in the late 1980s, an enormous number of studies have proven the value of this method for the diagnosis and especially follow-up of macular disease [14, 16, 25, 26, 27, 34, 37, 39, 44, 58]. Another typical indication is small scotomas that are not detected by other test methods (Fig. 1.3).

Clinical examples can be summarized best according to specific diseases, for example, defined macular dystrophies or definite stages of AMD such as geographic atrophy (GA) of the retinal pigment epithelium (RPE). Most clinical studies have also focused on such groups of patients.

1.3.1 Macular Holes

One of the first exertions of microperimetry in follow-up studies was macular hole surgery. Acosta and coworkers, as early as 1991, described dense scotoma over all macular holes and movement of the preferred retinal locus (PRL) to the top of the retina. Comparable results were obtained by others [1, 10, 15, 45].

In addition, the correct diagnosis of macular holes versus pseudoholes or epiretinal membranes, which may be difficult in the early stages, is simplified by differentiation of the amount of functional impairment. Eyes suffering from macular holes develop an absolute scotoma (Fig. 1.4). Consecutively, a movement of fixation occurs outside this area, mostly toward the left margin at the retina, i.e., temporal in right eyes [40]. In

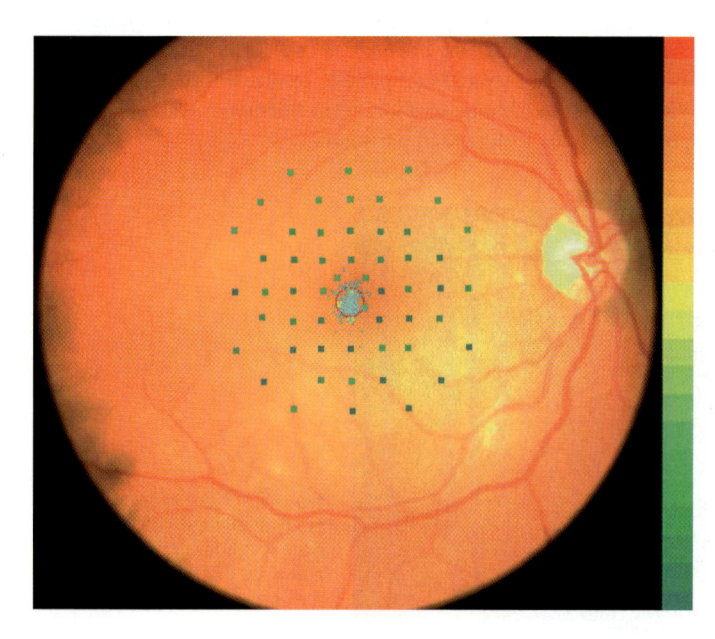

Fig. 1.3 Fundus-related perimetry with the MP 1 demarcates a small paracentral scotoma, which was not detected with conventional perimetry

contrast, patients with impending holes still had a PRL located inside the hole area (Fig. 1.5). Stability of fixation shows no significant correlation with visual acuity [20, 40].

Because surgical repair of advanced macular holes has become the treatment of choice, additional data concerning functional development over time have been added. Haritoglou and co-workers described the occurrence of paracentral scotomata in patients after vitrectomy for a macular hole. They had observed that some patients complained of small paracentral field defects despite good postoperative results in reading and visual acuity [13].

Summary for the Clinician

- Use of microperimety in macular holes has been well established for years and allows differentiation from pseudoholes.
- Accurate determination of preferred retinal locus and retinal sensitivity, especially in the area surrounding the hole, is helpful in macular hole surgery.

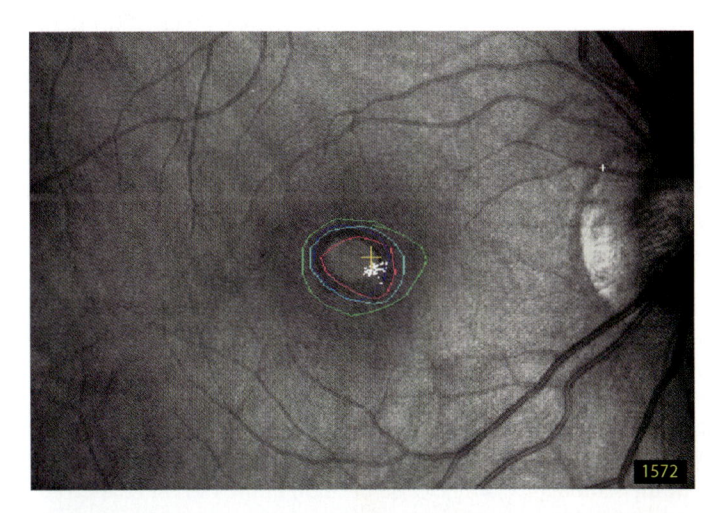

Fig. 1.4 Kinetic fundus perimetry in a right eye with macular hole stage 3. While fixation has moved towards the nasal border, there is an absolute central scotoma (Goldmann II stimuli: 0, 5, 10, 15 dB)

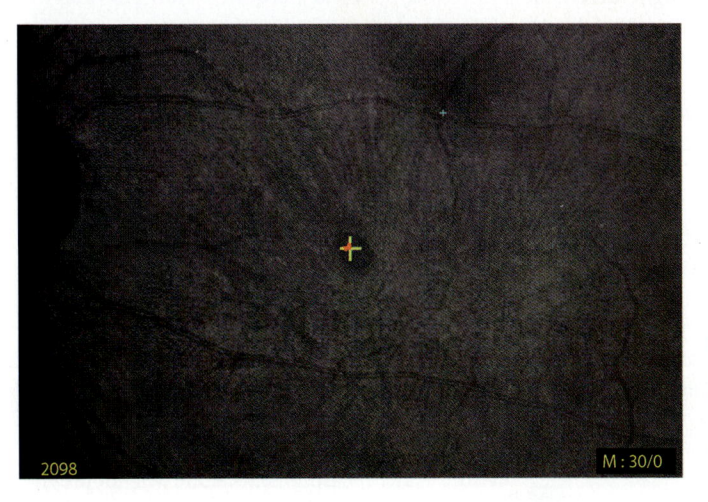

Fig. 1.5 Isolated fixation test with the scanning laser ophthalmoscope (SLO) in a left eye with epiretinal membrane and pseudohole; fixation is still stable inside the hole

1.3.2 Age-related Macular Degeneration

According to earlier findings in patients with central scotomata due to AMD, it would be expected that the location of paracentral scotomata might influence visual function [9, 34].

1.3.2.1 Geographic Atrophy of the RPE

The typical end-stage form of AMD is the development of GA of the RPE, which may result in an absolute scotoma overlying the atrophic zone and markedly diminished reading capability. It has been shown that involvement of the fovea will lead to a movement of the fixation, i.e., the PRL will change. The new PRL is typically located superior to or to the left (i.e., temporally in right eyes) of the atrophy, but sometimes the movement can be documented over time (Fig. 1.6). While it is indisputable that GA will result in an absolute scotoma, this change offers the option to evaluate the value of kinetic perimetry for exact delineation of scotoma borders. Nevertheless, there may be artificially wrong results as documented at the nasal border, where recognition has occurred beyond the blind spot for 2 isopters (Fig. 1.6). While the exact location of the stimuli allows differentiation between normal and pathologic function (Fig. 1.7), sometimes the border of the scotoma may not show a steep increase in light increment threshold values, but an mild slope [30, 50, 53]. At the moment it is not clear whether hypo- or hyperfluorescent areas during autofluorescence in the junctional zone will develop typical functional pathology [43].

Summary for the Clinician

- Fundus perimetry allows the size of the absolute scotoma overlying the GA to be exactly delineated, thereby allowing growth to be documented during follow-up.
- Development of a new eccentric PRL can be documented.

1.3.2.2 Choroidal Neovascularization in AMD

The typical appearance of wet AMD is the development of choroidal neovascularization (CNV). While advanced treatment modalities have been introduced, particularly most recently, only fundus perimetry allows changes in pericentral light sensitivity to be precisely documented.

Some years ago, when laser treatment of well-defined juxtafoveal or extrafoveal CNV was the treatment of choice, we were able to demonstrate that the option of exact delineation of the PRL in relation to the central border of the CNV may simplify counseling of patients due to better prediction of functional outcome, particularly reading ability [34].

In the meantime, the surgical stripping off of the neovascular membrane has been introduced into treatment modalities and functional results can be followed using fundus perimetry [23, 59]. In addition, follow-up examinations during photodynamic therapy (PDT) have been performed [42]. Exact documentation of functional results in more recent options like autologous RPE-choroid sheet transplantation also requires fundus perimetry (Fig. 1.8) [18, 55].

Summary for the Clinician

- Exact delineation of the PRL in relation to the central border of the CNV may simplify counseling of patients.
- Comprehensive examination of visual function is achieved using microperimetry in eyes with CNV.

1.3.3 Diabetic Retinopathy

The management of diabetic retinopathy is defined by the morphologic situation and needs either adequate laser photocoagulation or even surgical treatment of tractive structures. In contrast, for the patient only the functional options are of interest. In diabetic macular edema in particular, visual acuity measurements alone will not provide sufficient data. While light sensitivity was reduced

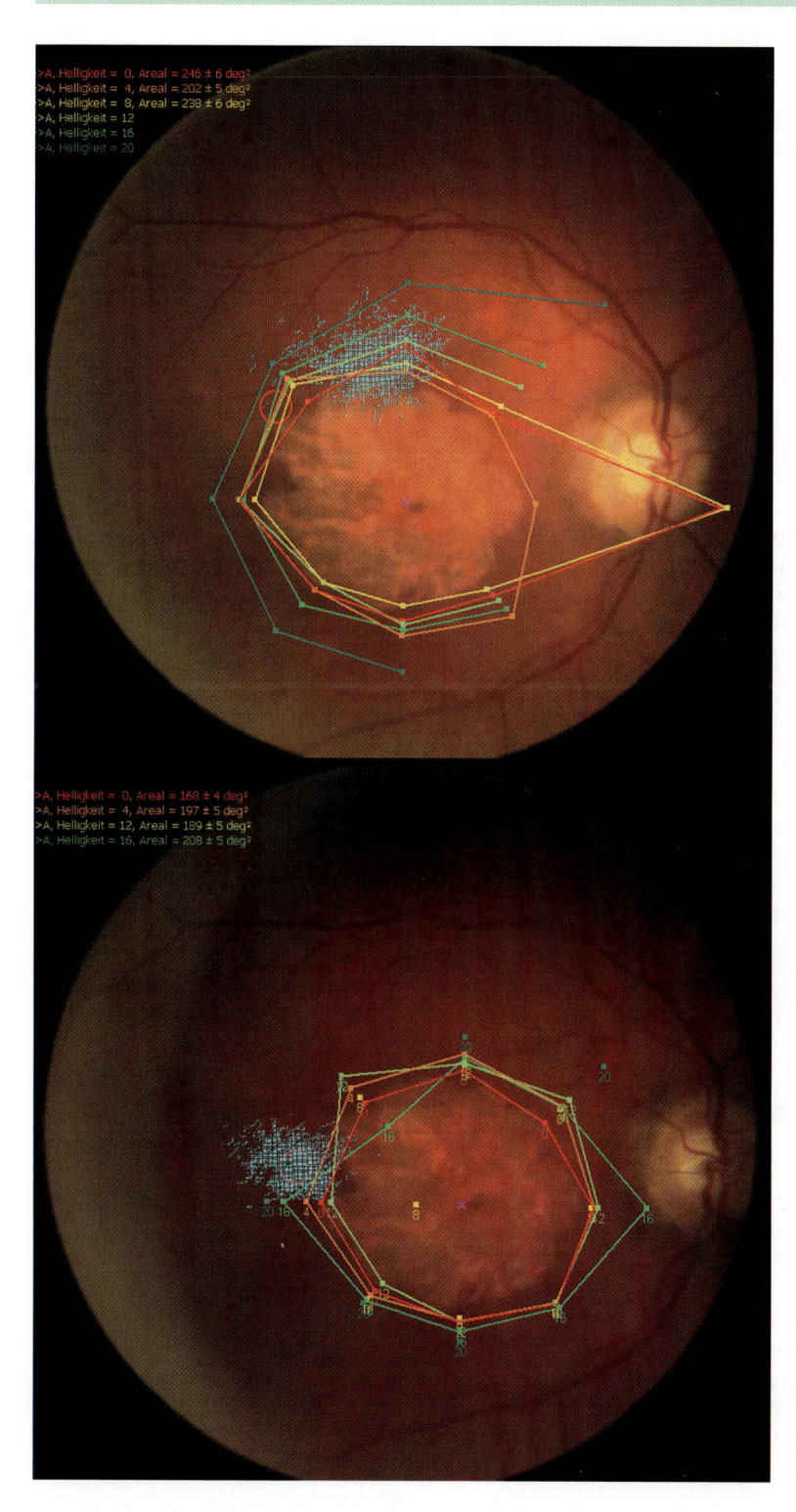

Fig. 1.6 Kinetic fundus perimetry of a right eye with geographic atrophy (GA) using the MP 1 shows instable fixation located at the superior retinal border. While perimetry delineates the morphologic pathology for most directions, the nasal border is artifactually wrong beside the optic disc (*top*). *Bottom*: 3 weeks later, fixation has moved toward the temporal (*left*) border, while the perimetry is much more exact

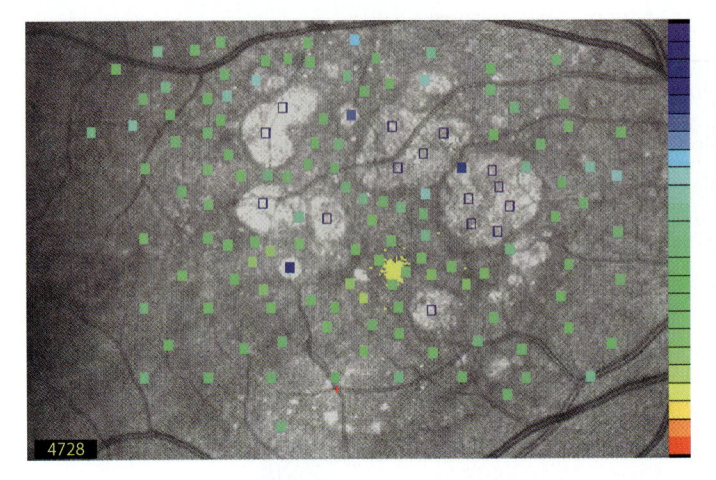

Fig. 1.7 Static fundus perimetry in a right eye with several small atrophic zones in AMD and stable central fixation (VA 0.6). While there are absolute scotomas overlying the GA areas, the surrounding is roughly normal. Threshold values for static perimetry are presented according to the right-hand scale in 1-dB steps with highest illumination at the top (*blue*). *Open rectangles* demonstrate absolute defects

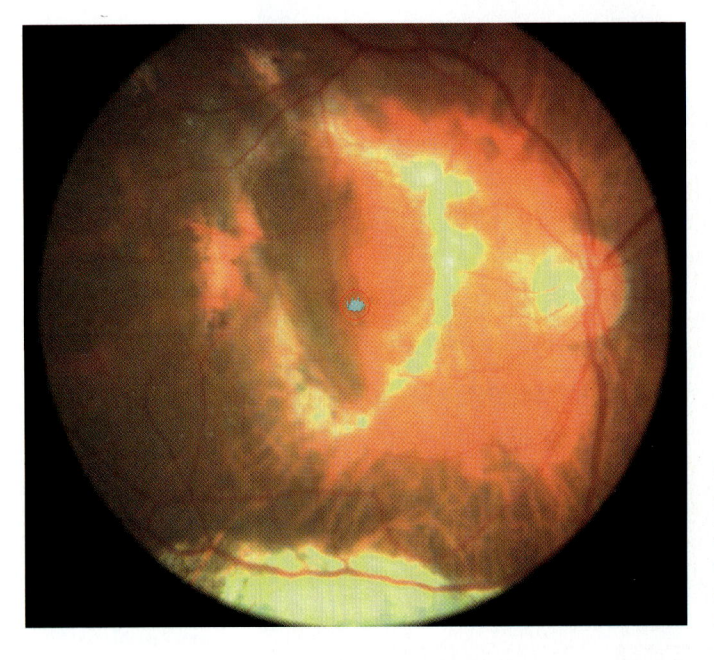

Fig. 1.8 Fixation task with the MP 1 in a right eye following RPE-choroid sheet transplantation with stable fixation in the transplanted area and reading ability preserved (patient from B. Kirchhof, Cologne)

in areas of macular edema there was no correlation between the amount of edema and visual function [39]. Different studies showed various results concerning the correlation between macular edema and light sensitivity threshold values [25, 39, 58]. Therefore, macular sensitivity, as obtained during fundus perimetry, is a valuable tool in addition to topographic data like optical coherence tomography (OCT) measurements. Moreover, fundus perimetry may be of value in predicting the outcome of diabetic macular edema.

The high accuracy is well documented as the retina overlying laser scars shows markedly decreased function (mean defect >13 dB), similar to the reduced function over blood vessels (angioscotomata) or over circinata rings (Fig. 1.9) [39].

Using the MP 1 we found similar results, with a negative correlation between retinal thickness and light sensitivity values (Fig. 1.10).

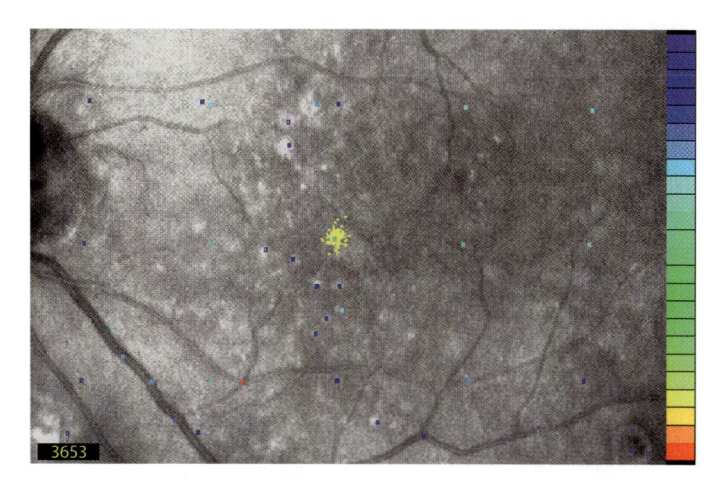

Fig. 1.9 Static fundus perimetry with the SLO in a left eye with nonproliferative diabetic retinopathy. Testing with Goldmann II stimuli offers the option to exactly delineate function loss over laser scars or small vessels. Threshold values for static perimetry are presented according to the right-hand scale in 1-dB steps with highest illumination at the top (*blue*). *Open rectangles* demonstrate absolute defects

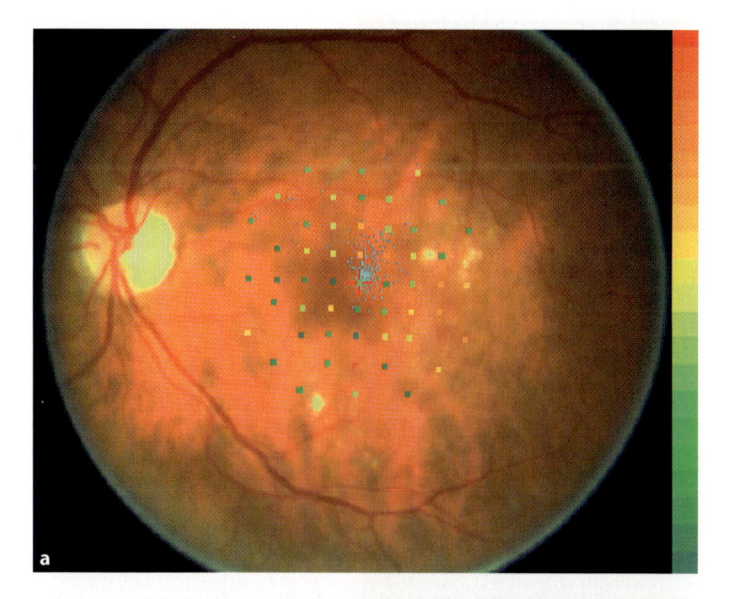

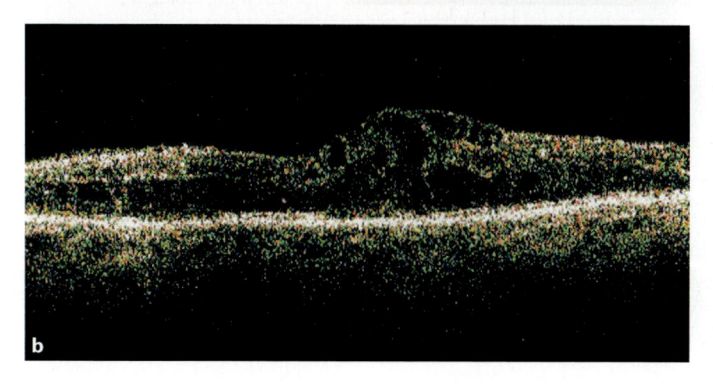

Fig. 1.10 a Fundus perimetry with the MP 1 in macular edema shows a scotoma located nasally to the fixation point; threshold values are given according to the color-coded scale on the right with high luminance in *red* and high contrast in *green*. **b** Optical coherence tomography (OCT) shows inhomogeneous edema with the majority in the nasal superior part

> **Summary for the Clinician**
> - In diabetic macular edema in particular, visual acuity measurements alone will not provide sufficient data on visual function.
> - While the concordance between morphologic and functional deterioration in macular edema may be low, functional results are of higher value to the patient.
> - Microperimetry is able to document the markedly decreased function of the retina overlying laser scars.

1.3.4 Central Serous Chorioretinopathy

Central serous chorioretinopathy is another typical disease involving the macula, leading to subjective symptoms that are not always accompanied by deterioration of visual acuity. Most of these male patients are markedly disturbed by the sudden occurrence of a (para)central retinal edema and consecutive visual field defect (Fig. 1.11). There has been a good concordance between the amount of edema and the decrease in differential light threshold, but no correlation with visual acuity [48]. Even months after resolution of macular edema and recovery of visual acuity, fundus perimetry might show diminished

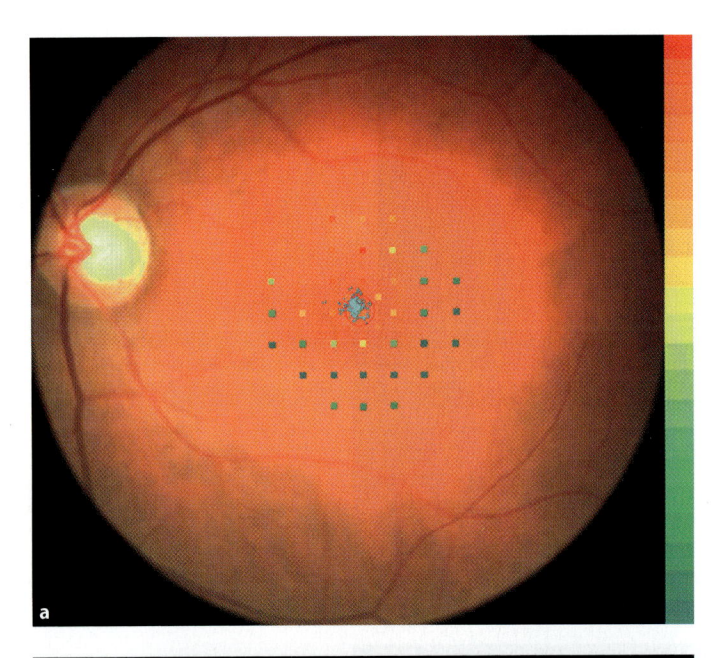

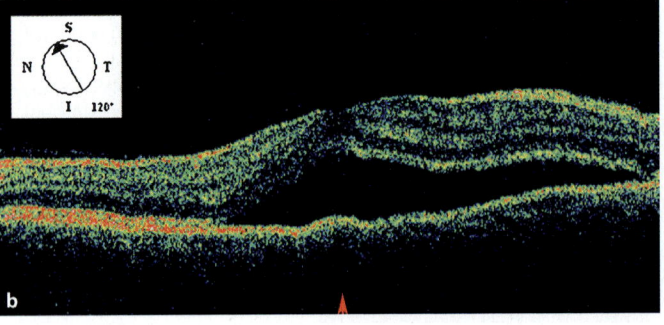

Fig. 1.11 Left eye of a patient with first occurrence of central serous chorioretinopathy (visual acuity 0.8). **a** Markedly reduced differential light sensitivity values nasally and superior to the fovea. **b** Serous retinal detachment in the OCT with maximum thickness of 532 μm (from [48] with permission)

1.3 Clinical Implementation

differential light threshold [27]. Therefore, thorough perimetry is mandatory for adequate documentation of functional impairment in these patients.

1.3.5 Stargardt's Disease

This juvenile macular dystrophy is one of the most frequent types of macular dystrophy and usually starts in the second decade of life. This autosomal recessive inherited disorder often shows a mutation of the ABCA4 gene [2]. The typical clinical appearance demonstrates macular changes, while cases with additional white flecks at the posterior pole—fundus flavimaculatus—may be differentiated [24].

The functional changes lead to pericentral and paracentral isolated small defects with remaining central fixation over a long period of time. Loss of central fixation typically leads to a PRL located at the top of the scotomatous retina, i.e., movement of the scotoma upward [35]. In addition, the center of fixation changes for different fixation targets, i.e., various letter sizes, with increasing distance to the fovea for larger letter sizes (Fig. 1.12). In more advanced stages fixation is always located outside the deep central scotoma and typically shows a much more pronounced vertical variation [32, 35]. This fixation behavior may allow these patients to be differentiated from those with cone rod dystrophy or other forms of macular dystrophy simulating Stargardt's disease.

During the late stages of Stargardt's disease fundus perimetry typically demonstrates a deep central scotoma with movement of the PRL at the retina to the upper border of the visual field defect, which means movement of the scotoma upward in the visual field (Fig. 1.13). Kinetic fundus perimetry also demonstrates an absolute central scotoma. Using the automated kinetic software implemented in the MP 1, artificial irregular borders will sometimes be found due to the remaining functional islands. Very seldom it is possible to document the remaining central island with pericentral scotomas that nearly touch at the fovea.

Summary for the Clinician

- Patients with Stargardt's disease exhibit an almost pathognomonic fixation behavior with strong vertical variation around a new PRL located superior to the macula.
- During development of the new PRL different stages may be observed.
- Fundus controlled reading tasks demonstrate that the location of the PRL is dependent on character size.

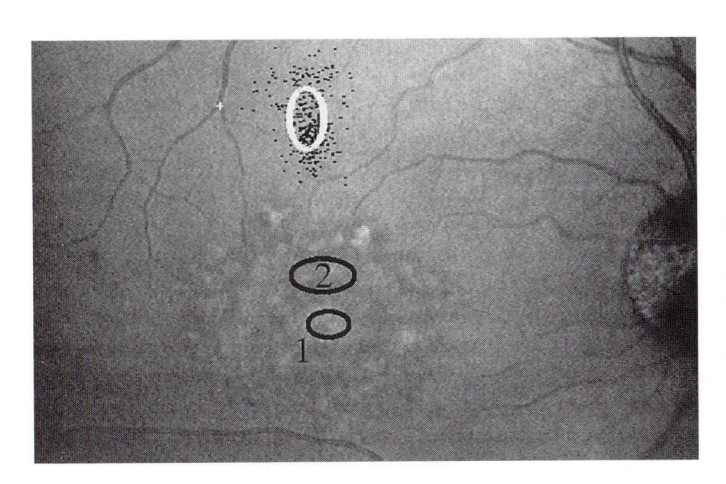

Fig. 1.12 While fixation has moved far upward at the retina (*white circle*) in this right eye with Stargardt's disease, fixation is much more central for different reading tasks: small characters were fixated centrally (*area 1*) and larger characters with *area 2*. (from [35] with permission)

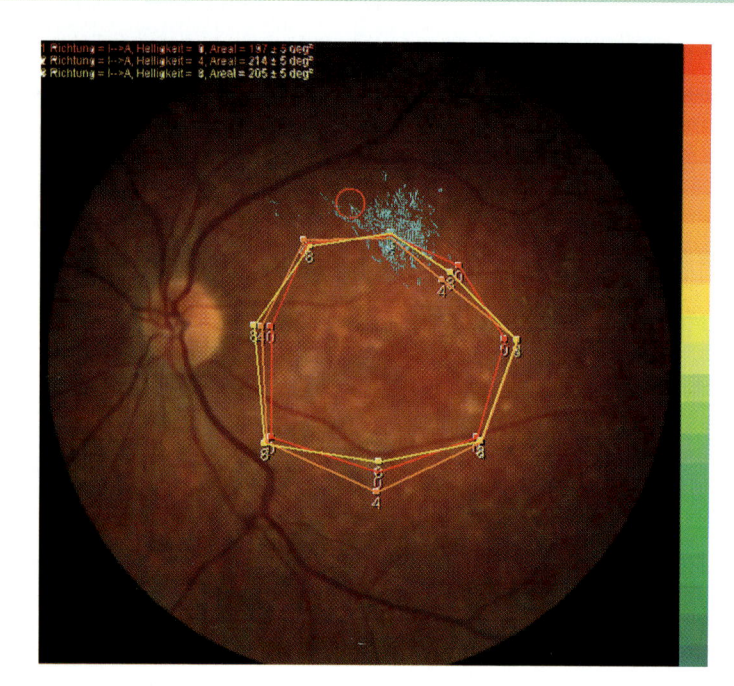

Fig. 1.13 Kinetic fundus perimetry with the MP 1 in a right eye with Stargardt's disease reveals fixation located at the superior retina, while the absolute central scotoma is outlined in good concordance with the retinal pathology. Threshold values are given according to the color-coded scale on the right, with high luminance in *red* and high contrast in *green*

1.3.6 Vitelliform Macular Dystrophy (Best's Disease)

Vitelliform macular dystrophy is another type of macular dystrophy with a typical clinical appearance and onset in childhood, and was first described by Best in 1905 [5]. This autosomal dominant inherited disease is caused by mutations in the VMD2 gene. Visual acuity in most patients is maintained in the 20/20 to 20/50 range for many decades.

The typical vitelliform or "egg yolk" lesion, composed of a round, homogeneous, opaque yellow lesion with discrete margins and measuring approximately one disc diameter in size, is not present in all patients. When the yellow material within the vitelliform cyst develops a fluid level, resulting in the appearance of a pseudohypopyon, function is often markedly lost. Late stages may include atrophic scar formation or subretinal neovascularization comparable to changes in AMD.

During fundus perimetry the vitelliform lesion may be demarcated by a deep central visual field defect, and the scrambled egg formation even more (Fig. 1.14). Because there is no correlation between different stages and remaining visual function, it is impossible to forecast findings during fundus perimetry caused by the morphologic appearance. In eyes with normal or only slightly diminished visual acuity, only small relative or absolute scotomas may be present, with fixation close to the edge of the scotoma [17].

Summary for the Clinician

- Microperimetry may show an increase in steepness of the central or paracentral scotoma during different stages of vitelliform macular dystrophy.
- While subjective deterioration of visual function in these patients may be incongruent with morphologic alteration, fundus perimetry allows the influence of paracentral scotomas to be better understood.

1.4 Conclusion

Since the development of fundus perimetry with the help of the SLO more than 25 years ago, reengineering has led to an instrument capable of performing complete fundus-related perimetry

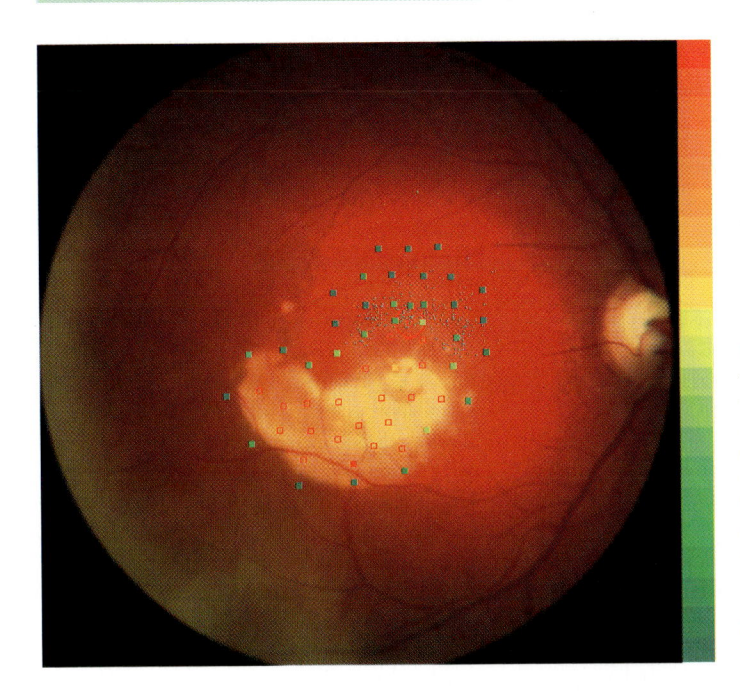

Fig. 1.14 Fundus perimetry with the MP 1 in a right eye with advanced stage Best's disease shows instable fixation (*blue dots*) and an absolute scotoma over the scrambled egg formation. The retina surrounding this shows normal threshold values. Threshold values are given according to the color-coded scale on the right, with high luminance in *red* and high contrast in *green*

with automatic correction for eye movements. This allows ophthalmologists to accurately examine patients suffering from macular disease with unstable fixation or even loss of fixation, in whom conventional computerized cupola perimetry would give artificially wrong results. Further improvement of the optical pathway, most suitably by incorporation of a scanning laser ophthalmoscope, would enhance this method further. In addition, fundus-related techniques may improve low vision rehabilitation by training of PRL and reading [28].

Acknowledgement

I greatly acknowledge the help of Stefan Bültmann, M.D., and Christina Springer, M.D., in proofreading this chapter. Supported in part by the Deutsche Forschungsgemeinschaft (DFG Ro 973/11-1 and Ro 973/11-2).

References

1. Acosta F, Lashkari K, Reynaud X et al (1991) Characterization of functional changes in macular holes and cysts. Ophthalmology 98:1820–1823
2. Allikmets R, Singh N, Sun H et al (1997) A photoreceptor cell-specific ATP-binding transporter gene (ABCR) is mutated in recessive Stargardt macular dystrophy. Nat Genet 15:236–246
3. American National Standards Institute (2000) American National Standard for the Safe Use of Lasers, Laser Institute of America, Orlando, FL
4. Andersen MVN (1996) Scanning laser ophthalmoscope microperimetry compared with Octopus in normal subjects. Acta Ophthalmol Scand 74:135–139
5. Best F (1905) Über eine hereditäre Maculaaffektion. Beiträge zur Vererbungslehre. Z Augenheilkd 13:199–212
6. Bültmann S, Rohrschneider K, Glück R et al (1998) The influence of stimulus size on fundus perimetric detection of small scotomata. Ophthalmic Research 30:79
7. Crone RA (1975) Fundus television in the study of fixation disturbances. Ophthalmologica 171:51–52
8. Enoch JM (1978) Quantitative layer-by-layer perimetry. Proctor lecture. Invest Ophthalmol Vis Sci 17:208–257
9. Fletcher DC, Schuchard RA (1997) Preferred retinal loci. Relationship to macular scotomas in a low-vision population. Ophthalmology 104:632–638

10. Guez JE, Le Gargasson JF, Massin P et al (1998) Functional assessment of macular hole surgery by scanning laser ophthalmoscopy. Ophthalmology 105:694–699
11. Haefliger IO, Flammer J (1989) Increase of the short-term fluctuation of the differential light threshold around a physiologic scotoma. Am J Ophthalmol 107:417–420
12. Haefliger IO, Flammer J (1991) Fluctuation of the differential light threshold at the border of absolute scotomas. Comparison between glaucomatous visual field defects and blind spots. Ophthalmology 98:1529–1532
13. Haritoglou C, Ehrt O, Gass CA et al (2001) Paracentral scotomata: a new finding after vitrectomy for idiopathic macular hole. Br J Ophthalmol 85:231–233
14. Haritoglou C, Gass CA, Schaumberger M et al (2002) Long-term follow-up after macular hole surgery with internal limiting membrane peeling. Am J Ophthalmol 134:661–666
15. Hikichi T, Ishiko S, Takamiya A et al (2000) Scanning laser ophthalmoscope correlations with biomicroscopic findings and foveal function after macular hole closure. Arch Ophthalmol 118:193–197
16. Hoerauf H, Kluter H, Joachimmeyer E et al (2001) Results of vitrectomy and the no-touch-technique using autologous adjuvants in macular hole treatment. Int Ophthalmol 24:151–159
17. Jarc-Vidmar M, Popovic P, Hawlina M (2006) Mapping of central visual function by microperimetry and autofluorescence in patients with Best's vitelliform dystrophy. Eye 20:688–696
18. Joussen A, Heussen F, Joeres S et al (2006) Autologous translocation of the choroid and retinal pigment epithelium in age-related macular degeneration. Am J Ophthalmol 142:17–30
19. Kani K, Ogita Y (1978) Fundus controlled perimetry. Doc Ophthalmol Proc Ser 19:341–350
20. Kristin N, Ehrt O, Gass CA et al (2001) [Preoperative scanning laser ophthalmoscopy: findings in idiopathic macular foramen]. Ophthalmologe 98:1060–1064
21. Meyer JH, Guhlmann M, Funk J (1997) Blind spot size depends on the optic disc topography: a study using SLO controlled scotometry and the Heidelberg retina tomograph. Br J Ophthalmol 81:355–359
22. Midena E, Cavarzeran F, Microperimetry Study Group (2006) Normal age-related values for fundus-related perimetry. Invest Ophthalmol Vis Sci 47:E-Abstract 5349
23. Müller S, Ehrt O, Gundisch O et al (2000) Funktionelle Ergebnisse nach CNV-Extraktion oder Photokoagulation bei alterskorrelierter Makuladegeneration. Ophthalmologe 97:142–146
24. Noble KG, Carr RE (1979) Stargardt's disease and fundus flavimaculatus. Arch Ophthalmol 97:1281–1285
25. Okada K, Yamamoto S, Mizunoya S et al (2006) Correlation of retinal sensitivity measured with fundus-related microperimetry to visual acuity and retinal thickness in eyes with diabetic macular edema. Eye 20:805–809
26. Oshima Y, Harino S, Tano Y (1998) Scanning laser ophthalmoscope microperimetric assessment in patients with successful laser treatment for juxtafoveal choroidal neovascularization. Retina 18:109–117
27. Ozdemir H, Karacorlu SA, Senturk F et al (2006) Assessment of macular function by microperimetry in unilateral resolved central serous chorioretinopathy. Eye (in press)
28. Rohrschneider K (2006) Low vision: the morphofunctional approach. In: Midena E (ed) Perimetry and the fundus: an introduction to microperimetry. Slack, Thorofare, pp 215–223
29. Rohrschneider K, Springer C (2006) Macular dystrophies. In: Midena E (ed) Perimetry and the fundus: an introduction to microperimetry. Slack, Thorofare, pp 159–168
30. Rohrschneider K, Becker M, Fendrich T et al (1995) Fundus-controlled testing of retinal sensitivity and fixation in geographic atrophy associated with age-related macular degeneration. Invest Ophthalmol Vis Sci 36:S232
31. Rohrschneider K, Becker M, Fendrich T et al (1995) Kinetische funduskontrollierte Perimetrie mit dem Scanning-Laser-Ophthalmoskop. Klin Monatsbl Augenheilkd 207:102–110
32. Rohrschneider K, Becker M, Kruse FE et al (1995) Stability of fixation—results of fundus-controlled examination using the Scanning Laser Ophthalmoscope. Ger J Ophthalmol 4:197–202
33. Rohrschneider K, Fendrich T, Becker M et al (1995) Static fundus perimetry using the scanning laser ophthalmoscope with an automated threshold strategy. Graefe's Arch Clin Exp Ophthalmol 233:743–749

34. Rohrschneider K, Glück R, Becker M et al (1997) Scanning laser fundus perimetry before laser photocoagulation of well-defined choroidal neovascularisation. Br J Ophthalmol 81:568–573
35. Rohrschneider K, Glück R, Kruse FE et al (1997) Fixationsverhalten bei Morbus Stargardt. Funduskontrollierte Untersuchungen. Ophthalmologe 94:624–628
36. Rohrschneider K, Becker M, Schumacher N et al (1998) Normal values for fundus perimetry with the scanning laser ophthalmoscope. Am J Ophthalmol 126:52–58
37. Rohrschneider K, Blankenagel A, Kruse FE et al (1998) Macular function testing in a German pedigree with North Carolina macular dystrophy. Retina 18:453–459
38. Rohrschneider K, Glück R, Kruse FE et al (1999) Automatic static fundus perimetry for precise detection of early glaucomatous function loss. In: Wall M, Wild J (eds) Perimetry update 1998/1999. Proceedings of the XIII International Perimetric Society Meeting Gardone Riviera, Italy, September 6–9 1998, Kugler, Amsterdam, New York, pp 453–462
39. Rohrschneider K, Bültmann S, Glück R et al (2000) Scanning laser ophthalmoscope fundus perimetry before and after laser photocoagulation for clinically significant diabetic macular edema. Am J Ophthalmol 129:27–32
40. Rohrschneider K, Bultmann S, Kruse FE et al (2001) Functional changes measured with SLO in idiopathic macular holes and in macular changes secondary to premacular fibrosis. Function in macular holes. Int Ophthalmol 24:177–184
41. Rohrschneider K, Springer C, Bültmann S et al (2005) Microperimetry—comparison between the Micro Perimeter 1 and Scanning Laser Ophthalmoscope—fundus perimetry. Am J Ophthalmol 139:125–134
42. Schmidt-Erfurth UM, Elsner H, Terai N et al (2004) Effects of verteporfin therapy on central visual field function. Ophthalmology 111:931–939
43. Schmitz-Valckenberg S, Bültmann S, Dreyhaupt J et al (2004) Fundus autofluorescence and fundus perimetry in the junctional zone of geographic atrophy in patients with age-related macular degeneration. Invest Ophthalmol Vis Sci 45:4470–4476
44. Sjaarda RN, Frank DA, Glaser BM et al (1993) Assessment of vision in idiopathic macular holes with macular microperimetry using the scanning laser ophthalmoscope. Ophthalmology 100:1513–1518
45. Sjaarda RN, Frank DA, Glaser BM et al (1993) Resolution of an absolute scotoma and improvement of relative scotoma after successful macular hole surgery. Am J Ophthalmol 116:129–139
46. Springer C, Rohrschneider K (2006) Fundus perimetry versus standard perimetry. In: Midena E (ed) Perimetry and the fundus: an introduction to microperimetry. Slack, Thorofare, pp 27–37
47. Springer C, Bültmann S, Völcker HE et al (2005) Fundus perimetry with the Micro Perimeter 1 in normal individuals. Comparison with conventional threshold perimetry. Ophthalmology 112:848–854
48. Springer C, Völcker H, Rohrschneider K (2006) Chorioretinopathia centralis serosa—Netzhautfunktion und -morphologie. Mikroperimetrie und optische Kohärenztomographie im Vergleich. Opthalmologe 103:791–797
49. Steiger RM, Würth A (1955) Die Fixationsphotographie und die Elektroenzephalographie in der Beurteilung der Schielamblyopie. Ophthalmologica 129:240–244
50. Sunness JS, Rubin GS, Bressler NM et al (1995) Visual function and SLO perimetry in eyes with the geographic atrophy form of AMD and good acuity. Invest Ophthalmol Vis Sci 36:S232
51. Sunness JS, Schuchard RA, Shan N et al (1995) Landmark-driven fundus perimetry using the Scanning Laser Ophthalmoscope. Invest Ophthalmol Vis Sci 36:1863–1874
52. Sunness JS, Applegate CA, Haselwood D et al (1996) Fixation patterns and reading rates in eyes with central scotomas from advanced atrophic age-related macular degeneration and Stargardt's disease. Ophthalmology 103:1458–1466
53. Sunness JS, Bressler NM, Tian Y et al (1999) Measuring geographic atrophy in advanced age-related macular degeneration. Invest Ophthalmol Vis Sci 40:1761–1769
54. Timberlake GT, Mainster MA, Webb RH et al (1982) Retinal localization of scotomata by scanning laser ophthalmoscopy. Invest Ophthalmol Vis Sci 22:91–97

55. Treumer F, Bunse A, Klatt C et al (2006) Autologous RPE-choroid sheet transplantation in AMD. Morphological and functional results. Br J Ophthalmol (in press)
56. Van de Velde FJ, Jalkh AE, McMeel JW et al (1995) Fixation characteristics and potential acuity measurements in macular disease. Invest Ophthalmol Vis Sci 36:S232
57. Von Noorden GK, Allen L, Burian HM (1959) A photographic method for the determination of the behavior of fixation. Am J Ophthalmol 48:511–514
58. Vujosevic S, Midena E, Pilotto E et al (2006) Diabetic macular edema: correlation between microperimetry and optical coherence tomography findings. Invest Ophthalmol Vis Sci 47:3044–3051
59. Wolf S, Lappas A, Weinberger AW et al (1999) Macular translocation for surgical management of subfoveal choroidal neovascularizations in patients with AMD: first results. Graefes Arch Clin Exp Ophthalmol 237:51–57

Chapter 2

New Developments in cSLO Fundus Imaging

Giovanni Staurenghi, Grazia Levi, Silvia Pedenovi, Chiara Veronese

Core Messages

- cSLO recordings provide high resolution topographic images of the living human retina. Images are rapidly produced at low monochromatic light levels with specific wavelengths.
- A near infrared laser is suitable to image subretinal structures including choroidal vessels, and subretinal deposits.
- Fundus autofluorescence (FAF) imaging allows for topographic detection of lipofuscin in the retinal pigment epithelial monolayer. This imaging mode has been used for refined classification of early and late AMD stages. In the context of atrophic AMD patterns of abnormal FAF have been identified, which confer an increased risk of disease progression.
- Distinct FAF patterns have also been identified in central serous chorioretinopathy (CSC) and give clues to distinguishing acute from chronic disease.
- Fundus autofluorescence imaging is also a rapid and noninvasive method of making differential diagnoses of macular holes.
- The development of a wide-field contact lens system has increased the imaging field of cSLO up to 150°, which is especially useful in combined fluorescein and indocyanine green angiography of large or peripheral chorioretinal alterations. The system was also successfully applied in the detection of diabetic retinopathy, retinal vascular disorders and detachment, chorioretinal tumors, and uveitis.

2.1 Introduction

Scanning laser ophthalmoscopes (SLO) were introduced into clinical practice in 1989. The SLO technologies were developed in Boston by Webb and Hughes [64] and introduced into clinical practice by Rodenstock with a nonconfocal scanning laser ophthalmoscope.

In 1995, Heidelberg Engineering introduced a confocal SLO (Heidelberg retina angiograph [HRA]), first of all with only the possibility of fluorescein angiography (FA). In 1997 this instrument was upgraded to provide the possibility of performing simultaneous FA and indocyanine green angiography (ICGA).

The principal difference between conventional ophthalmoscopy and scanning laser ophthalmoscopy is in the nature of illuminating the retina. In scanning laser technology, a laser beam scans across the retina, and all the light energy is focused onto a small spot for a short time. Light reflected or emitted from the illuminated spot is detected and electronically coded for subsequent image composition on a computer screen. The point-by-point illumination with efficient detection of the reflected light allows imaging with relatively low levels of light, the ability to image through a small pupil and through cloudy media. Confocal imaging is obtained by introducing a small pinhole aperture in a plane conjugate to the focus plane. This causes rejection of light originating from the plane of interest in the eye. These two characteristics lead to a sharp image with good contrast. Objects outside the plane of interest are not imaged very well, so a proper imaging technique involves surveying the fundus to make sure the correct plane is imaged. However, because of the real-time acquisition of images afforded by the scanning laser and the rejection of light that does not originate from the plane of interest it is possible to obtain images with additional lenses, such as wide-field lenses, or to perform gonioangiography.

Scanning laser ophthalmoscope allows different imaging modalities:
1. Near infrared imaging
2. Blue AF imaging
3. Near infrared AF imaging
4. Dynamic fluorescein angiography
5. Dynamic ICGA
6. Wide field imaging

2.2 Near Infrared Imaging

2.2.1 Introduction

Infrared (IR) imaging is commonly used to improve visualization and diagnosis of vascular diseases of the eye. In particular, it provides better visibility for subretinal features.

Subretinal pathology is a hallmark AMD, one of the chief causes of visual loss in elderly adults in industrialized countries [34].

Histopathological studies of human eyes indicate that there is a deposition of material in the layers beneath the retina. There is a diffuse thickening within Bruch's membrane or between the RPE and the basement membrane, as well as focal deposits (drusen) within Bruch's membrane. There is also a redistribution of the melanin in the RPE, as sick cells shed their melanin and neighboring cells take it up [6]. Potential pathological fundus structures can be quantified using an SLO [65].

Infrared imaging is used to acquire digital images of the human fundus. Near infrared imaging is well-suited to investigating subretinal structures [17, 18].

With an SLO, initial IR images (790 nm) reveal details of most fundus features [66]. Contemporary IR images with a fundus camera reveal only large or highly pigmented structures [5]. IR images detected pathology [20], despite the presence of hemorrhage or cataract [22].

Infrared illumination may improve the imaging of subretinal features, because increased penetration through the fundus could provide information from deeper layers and differential absorption of IR light compared with visible light may provide additional clinical information.

2.2.2 The Effect of Wavelength on Imaging in the Human Fundus

The layers of the human fundus contain a variety of absorbing, reflecting, and scattering materials, which differ significantly among individuals [11, 59]. Absorbing substances, such as blood and melanin, greatly influence the information in fundus images in visible wavelength illumination [12]. Macular pigment, which masks the underlying fundus layers in the foveal region to a variable extent across individuals, also has peak absorption in the short wavelengths with much less absorption at other wavelengths including infrared light [52, 69]. The absolute absorptions of the pigments cannot be compared with one another, since they depend upon the concentration of each pigment. Several studies [12, 16] have demonstrated that the four primary ocular pigments have different absorption wavelengths:
1. At about 500–650 nm, there are the major absorbing components of blood.
2. At 700–900 nm, oxygenated hemoglobin (choroidal blood) increases in absorption monotonically, whereas melanin continues to decrease in absorption in this spectral range.
3. At about 950–1,050 nm, there is a large decrease that corresponds to the increase in water absorption.

2.2.3 Comparison of Light Tissue Interactions for Visible and Near Infrared Wavelengths Using SLO

The SLO provides several ways to improve contrast over fundus camera imaging, it illuminates only a small region of the fundus at a time (the fundus camera illuminates the entire field of view), it captures the light returning to the detector, and a section of aperture permits the spatial sampling of the light returning from the fundus [19].

2.2.4 Mode of Imaging

There are two modes of imaging, direct and indirect, and the mode of imaging is determined by the selection of aperture in a confocal imaging system.

In direct mode imaging, there is a smaller circular aperture, and the image is determined from direct reflection or backscattered light from the plane of focus [5, 66].

In indirect mode imaging, there is an annular aperture; light is more laterally scattered [21]. At longer wavelengths light that can penetrate deeply, structures in the RPE or choroids may be back- or side-illuminated.

2.2.5 Contrast of the Fundus

The contrast of the fundus features varies both with wavelength and imaging mode. In the direct mode good contrast images arere obtained at all wavelengths, including IR wavelengths not previously used for imaging.

The light levels needed to acquire IR images are comfortable, even for children, and invisible to most patients.

2.2.6 Fundus Features

Choroidal vessels are seen in the normal eye with near IR imaging and less well at other wavelengths. The choroidal vessel contrast for IR is usually dark on a light fundus background. Retinal vessels appear dark or have dark borders at all wavelengths in direct mode imaging. The optic disc rim appears dark at all wavelengths in confocal mode. The optic disc in pathological eyes can appear pale, especially in patients with dark pigmentation or pathology near the disc, such as a retinal detachment or staphyloma. The lamina cribrosa appears light and is often well visualized in older patients.

2.2.7 Imaging of Pathological Features in Direct and Indirect Mode

Subretinal pathology is seen to a much greater extent with infrared imaging than with routine clinical techniques. In direct mode subretinal deposits appear light, partially blocking the view of choroidal vessels. These deposits are never seen in patients under the age of 20 years and are usually small (<25 μm in diameter) in patients aged 20–50 years. These are always seen in patients with AMD.

In patients with exudative AMD and pigment epithelial detachment, drusen were clearly seen. The drusen seen in IR light were not seen to the same extent at 594 nm.

Subretinal hemorrhage appears as a dark region. Scars, such as those following resolution of choroidal new vessels or laser photocoagulation, appear bright. These scars, atrophic regions, and some types of deposits are so highly reflective that to obtain an image, the light level must be reduced beyond that useful for the surrounding fundus.

In indirect mode deeper layers must be imaged differently, such by retroillumination.

Topographical changes are emphasized in the deeper layer, such as thickness changes due to areas of atrophy, fluid accumulation, or choroidal new vessels, ore subretinal deposits.

The clinical hallmark of the nonexudative form of AMD is drusen [8]. Determining who is at risk of visual loss due to AMD is difficult for several reasons.

First, drusen are often obscured in an aging population by media changes. Small drusen are not resolved and contrast is reduced for the borders of soft drusen. Second, there are large individual differences in fundus appearance and drusen visibility due to the variation in the concentration of ocular pigments, such as melanin, across individuals [12, 67].

> **Summary for the Clinician**
> - Infrared light is used to improve imaging of subretinal structures, which passed readily into and out of the deeper fundus layers [20].
> - It can be used in adults and children.
> - Subretinal deposits appear light and thickened.
> - The optic nerve head, retinal vessels, and choroidal vessels appear dark.

2.3 Blue Autofluorescence Imaging

Fluorescence is luminescence characterized by an emission of light on a short time scale after excitation. Light is absorbed by the fluorophores, causing electrons to become excited to a higher electronic state. The electrons remain in the excited state for a nanosecond, and then energy is emitted as they return to their ground state. The whole process is frequently illustrated using the Jablonnski diagram, which illustrates the basic mechanism of fluorescence [48].

2.3.1 Autofluorescence and the Eye

Most ocular media and tissue exhibit fluorescence emission upon excitation by suitable wavelengths of light [48]. A large variety of these ocular fluorophores exhibit marked changes in their fluorescence properties with regard to age and pathology. Thus, the biological and functional properties of many ocular media and tissues and their modifications are indicators of aging or disease and can be used as diagnostic tools. The accumulation of natural fluorescent proteins in ocular tissue can result from exposure to ambient light [33, 58] or to ocular pathologies [35]. Ocular endogenous fluorophores are visible in the cornea, lens, and RPE.

2.3.1.1 Fluorescence of the Retinal Pigment Epithelium

Fluorescence of the RPE is mainly related to lipofuscin. It is a fluorescent pigment that is absent in fetal and newborn RPE| and continuously accumulates in the RPE as a result of incomplete digestion of spent rod outer segment disks. Lipofuscin is potentially noxious, for it acts as a photosensitizer in blue light, generating free radicals both in isolated granules and within RPE cells. Lipofuscin contains several distinct fluorescent components, one of which is A2E, a red-emitting fluorophore of lipofuscin. It has noxious effects on RPE cells in vitro, inhibiting lysosomal digestion of proteins and causing blue light-mediated disruption of lysosomal membranes and RPE apoptosis [7, 28, 49]. An increase of about 40% in the fluorescence intensity of lipofuscin is commonly considered an indicator of aging [48]. Similarly, it has been demonstrated that the RPE contains abnormally high levels of lipofuscin in a number of inherited retinal disorders, such as Best's disease and Stargardt's fundus flavimaculatus [36], and is likely to be a crucial event in the development of AMD [36]. Thus, the study of the lipofuscin content in the RPE may give us more insight into the pathogenesis of a number of retinal diseases. Intact human lipofuscin granules exhibit a broadband excitation spectrum from 300 to about 620 nm, and an emission spectrum that peaks in the yellow-orange region. Both excitation and emission spectra are age-related [15]. Melanin is the other main chromophore of RPE; it is generally considered to be nonfluorescent. However, studies on melanin granules in vitro showed age-related fluorescence properties, probably due to some combination with lipofuscin. The excitation maximum of melano-lipofuscin fluorescence is 364 nm, with an emission maximum at 540 nm [48].

2.3.1.2 How to Evaluate RPE Autofluorescence

The confocal imaging fluorometer is used as a diagnostic method to investigate RPE autofluorescence. The excitation light is focused in a small area and the collection optics image this area on the sensitive area of the photodetector. A complete characterization of the collection optics can be performed by replacing the detector with an appropriate light source and defining the observation beam in this way. The volume under test is defined by the overlap between the excitation and the observation beam in the focus position. To obtain fluorescence images, the illuminated area and the observation beam scan the region of interest. For confocal fluorometry, laser light is used to achieve a higher spatial resolution. Recently, several confocal fluorescence measurements have been performed using scanning laser ophthalmoscope (SLO) [48]. Using a confocal scanning laser ophthalmoscope, characteristic patterns of fundus AF in normal participants and in patients with different retinal disorders have been described. Similarly, AF measurements can be obtained by this method [60, 61, 62].

2.3.2 Fundus Autofluorescence Changes in Early AMD

Areas with abnormally increased or decreased FAF signals may or may not correspond to funduscopically visible alterations. To develop a classification system of abnormal FAF patterns in early AMD a workshop was organized by the FAM Study group (fundus AF in AMD) in Frankfurt, Germany, on 30 July 2003, which was funded by the German Research Council (Deutsche Forschungsgemeinschaft—DFG). Alterations in FAF can be classified into nine phenotypic patterns including normal, minimal change, focally increased, focally plaque-like, patchy, linear, lace-like, reticular, and speckled.

The *normal* FAF pattern is characterized by a homogeneous background AF with a gradual decrease in the inner macula toward the foveola due to the masking effect of yellow macular pigment. Absence of abnormal alterations on FAF images may be seen even in the presence of soft or hard drusen.

Minimal change pattern describes eyes presenting with only minimal variations from the normal pattern; appearance showed very limited irregular increase or decrease in background FAF with no obvious topographic pattern.

The *focally increased* pattern is defined by the presence of at least one spot (<200 μm in diameter) of markedly increased FAF that is much brighter than the surrounding background fluorescence. The borders are well defined with no gradual decrease in FAF observed between the background and the area with focally increased FAF. Some areas of focally increased FAF may be surrounded by a darker looking halo. These areas of focally increased FAF may or may not correspond to visible alterations on color fundus photographs such as focal hyperpigmentation or drusen.

The *patchy* pattern is characterized by the presence of at least one larger area (>200 μm in diameter) of markedly increased FAF. These areas are brighter than the surrounding background fluorescence. The borders of these areas are typically less well-defined than the previous pattern and there is a gradual increase in FAF from the background to the patchy area. Again, these areas of increased FAF may or may not correspond to large soft drusen and areas of hyperpigmentation.

The *linear* pattern is defined by the presence of at least one linear area with markedly increased FAF. The borders of these areas of increased FAF are typically well demarcated with no gradual decrease of FAF observed between the background and the linear structure. These linear structures of increased FAF usually correspond to hyperpigmented lines on the color fundus photograph.

The *lace-like* pattern shows multiple branching linear structures of increased FAF forming a lacy pattern. The borders may be difficult to define as a gradual decrease of FAF is occasionally observed from the center of the linear areas toward the surrounding background. This lace-like pattern of increased FAF may correspond to hyperpigmentation on the color image or to no visible abnormality.

The *reticular* pattern is defined by the presence of multiple small areas (<200 μm in diameter) of decreased FAF. The borders of these areas of decreased FAF are typically difficult to determine since there is a decrease in FAF from the center of the lesions toward the surrounding background fluorescence. The reticular pattern was found to occur not only in the macular area, but also more typically in a supero-temporal location. This pattern of decreased FAF may be associated with funduscopically visible numerous small soft drusen, hard drusen, areas with pigmentary changes or with no visible abnormality in the fundus photograph.

The *speckled* FAF pattern is characterized by the simultaneous presence of a variety of FAF abnormalities in a larger area of the FAF image. The changes extend beyond the macular area and may cover the entire posterior fundus. Typically, these abnormalities include multiple small areas of irregularly increased and decreased FAF. The small areas of focally increased FAF may be punctuate or resemble linear structures. The corresponding abnormalities visible on color fundus photographs include hyper- and hypopigmentation, multiple subconfluent, and confluent drusen [22].

An international FAF classification system may be useful for other groups performing FAF imaging in the context of AMD research. It may help to perform meta-analyses of similar studies in the future. In addition, if certain FAF patterns turn out to represent high-risk characteristics for disease progression, predictive factors may be identified that may help to target future prophylactic interventions. Furthermore, refined phenotypic classification may potentially facilitate identification of genetic risk factors in AMD [56]. Preliminary data suggest that there is a correlation between FAF changes and risk of progression to AMD with visual loss, especially for the patchy pattern.

2.3.3 Fundus Autofluorescence Changes in Choroidal Neovascularization in AMD

In the clinical setting, fundus fluorescein angiography (FFA) is routinely used to assess the location, extent, and nature of lesions in AMD. Neovascular complexes are classified as classic or occult lesions based on the definitions by the Macular Photocoagulation Group. Autofluorescence imaging has been developed as a tool to evaluate RPE during aging and in ocular disease. It allows the assessment of AF derived from lipofuscin in RPE [13, 60, 61]. Excessive accumulation of this compound precedes photoreceptor degeneration [37, 63, 68]. The ability to assess the integrity of RPE is important because it may affect the behavior of new choroidal vessels. Also, visual outcome may be determined by whether the RPE maintains its physiological function. Patients with neovascular membrane of recent onset show areas of hyperfluorescence on fundus fluorescein angiography corresponding to areas of normal AF with adjacent areas of increased AF [10]. Preserved AF indicates viable RPE initially, which has implications for treatment interventions and long-term visual prognosis. Patients with a diagnosis of neovascular membrane made within 1–6 months, or with late-stage neovascular membrane, showed areas of decreased AF corresponding in the first group to areas of previous leakage on fundus fluorescein angiography and in the second group to atrophy. Decreased AF indicates loss of RPE and photoreceptors.

2.3.4 Fundus Autofluorescence Changes in Geographic Atrophy in AMD

Geographic atrophy of the RPE is a frequent cause of severe visual loss in patients with AMD, and it is responsible for approximately 20% of legal blindness [32]. The pathophysiologic mechanisms underlying the atrophic process, which involves not only the RPE but also the outer neurosensory retina and choriocapillaris, are poorly understood at present. Holz and colleagues recorded a diffuse, irregular, increased AF at the posterior pole at baseline in the presence of unifocal or multifocal patches of geographic atrophy. Within these areas of elevated AF, new atrophic areas developed, and existing patches of atrophy enlarged during the review period, whereas this was not observed in areas with normal background AF. The total area of abnormal AF also showed enlargement over time. Thus, preliminary findings suggest that areas of increased AF precede the development and enlargement of outer retinal atrophy in eyes with AMD. Preliminary observation using FAF images suggested that there may be distinct phenotypes with regard to change in FAF in the junctional zone of GA [31]. The Fundus Autofluorescence in Age-related Macular Disease Study Group classified four patterns of abnormal FAF in the junctional zone of geographic atrophy: focal, banded, patchy, and diffuse patterns.

Focally increased AF describes the presence of single or multiple small spots of markedly focally increased FAF at the margin of the atrophic patch.

Banded increased AF is characterized by the presence of a continuous stippled band of increased FAF surrounding the entire atrophic area.

Patchy increased AF involves the presence of larger areas of patchy increased FAF outside the area of GA. Their intensity tends to be to a lesser degree compared with the focal pattern.

Diffusely increased AF is the most frequent pattern of increased FAF that is not confined to the margin of the atrophic areas, but shows a larger spread at the posterior pole. These diffuse changes are classified into four subtypes: reticular, branching, fine granular, and fine granular with peripheral punctate spots.

The *reticular* pattern is characterized by various lines of increased FAF with a preferential radial orientation and *branching* by a diffusely increased FAF with a fine branching pattern of increased FAF signal. The *fine granular* pattern is characterized by a larger area of increased FAF with a granular-like appearance surrounding the GA. *Fine granular changes with peripheral punctate spots* indicates the presence of diffuse FAF change surrounding the atrophic area with elongated small lesions with increased FAF signal. These distinct patterns may reflect heterogeneity at a cellular and molecular level in contrast to a nonspecific ageing process. A refined phenotypic classification may be helpful to identify prognostic determinants for the spread of atrophy and visual loss, for the identification of genetic risk factors, and for the design of future interventional trials [4].

2.3.5 Fundus Autofluorescence in Acute and Chronic Recurrent Central Serous Chorioretinopathy

Central serous chorioretinopathy (CSC) is characterized by a shallow, round, and serous detachment of the neurosensory retina, although small detachments of the RPE may also occur. It is a disease of the RPE, leading to pathological breaks within the RPE layer and to consecutive subretinal leakage; however, the choroid also seems to be affected. Thus, reverse pumping of fluid into the subretinal space due to choroidal and RPE changes might also lead to neuroretinal detachment. This supports the generally adopted opinion that RPE plays a crucial role in the development of CSC. Distinct AF patterns of CSC can be observed in both acute and chronic recurrent disease. AF is therefore an interesting tool for use in differentiating between acute and chronic recurrent stages. In acute CSC, decreased AF is presumably due to a blockage caused by edema, whereas in chronic recurrent forms, irregular and increased AF is observed, possibly reflecting reactive RPE changes secondary to RPE defects and neurosensory detachment. Anther AF change is decreased AF at the point of leakage, which could be explained by the subretinal fluid blocking the AF, or RPE atrophy at the leakage point itself, as is presumed in chronic recurrent cases [24].

2.3.6 Fundus Autofluorescence in Stargardt's Macular Dystrophy-Fundus Flavimaculatus

Stargardt's macular dystrophy-fundus flavimaculatus (STGD-FFM) is inherited retinal dystrophy characterized by the presence of white-yellow deep retinal lesions, the so-called flecks, in the posterior pole exclusively or extending to the midperipheral retina. Most patients will develop overt atrophic macular lesions. Functional abnormalities in STGD-FFM include loss of macular function with or without loss of generalized cone, or cone and rod function [25, 26, 37]. The disease is inherited as an autosomal recessive trait and it is caused by mutations in the ABCA4 gene. Using a noninvasive fundus spectrophotometer, Delori and associates demonstrated abnormally high fluorescence intensity, with the spectral characteristic of lipofuscin, in 5 patients with STGD-FFM and dark choroids. Although previous reports [14, 61] found high levels of AF in all patients with STGD-FFM, some may have normal or even low levels of AF. These findings could be explained as the result of the wider variety of STGD-FFM phenotypes included. Some patients with STGD-FFM had normal levels of AF across the entire area studied. In these cases, however, there was an abnormal distribution of AF on cSLO images, and abnormal macular function, as demonstrated by pattern electroretinography (PERG). This may suggest that the threshold for RPE damage caused by lipofuscin may vary among patients and, thus, in some cases, RPE damage could occur with normal levels of lipofuscin within the cell. Alternatively, normal levels of AF could be the result of loss of photoreceptors or RPE cells without marked atrophy. Loss of photoreceptor cells would decrease the amount of photoreceptor outer segments shed, which would subsequently decrease the amount of lipofuscin formed by the RPE cells. Lastly, it would be still possible that these patients with normal AF levels may represent a different phenotype within STGD-FFM, or even a different disease that simulates STGD-FFM. There seemed to be a relationship between patterns of AF and peripheral functional abnormalities. All patients tested with low levels of AF at the center of the macula, including the fovea, and normal or low levels of AF temporally and nasally, had peripheral cone and rod dysfunction. Thus, it appears that this pattern of AF may be associated with more widespread disease. Most patients with normal or high levels of AF at the center of the macula, including the fovea, and high levels of AF temporally and nasally, and those with normal levels of AF across the entire area studied, had normal peripheral cone and rod function. However, there appeared to be no relationship between levels of AF and macular dysfunction, as detected by PERG, since all patients had marked PERG abnormalities independently of levels of AF. Levels of AF, however, were measured only within a rectangular band across the macula, and not throughout the entire macular region. Thus, it is possible that a closer relationship between levels of AF and electrophysiologic abnormalities might be found if levels of AF were measured in a larger area of the retina. A relative peripapillary sparing is characterized by a lack of flecks and atrophy in this region, even in those cases of diffuse RPE abnormalities and atrophy. It is unclear why the peripapillary area may remain relatively "protected" from the damage caused by lipofuscin [38].

2.3.7 Fundus Autofluorescence in Patients with Macular Holes

Autofluorescence imaging is useful for the diagnosis and staging of macular holes and is comparable with the results of fluorescein angiography. AF imaging demonstrates the bright fluorescence of macular holes with an appearance similar to that obtained by fluorescein angiography. In contrast, macular pseudoholes showed no such AF. The attached operculum in stage 2 macular holes and the preretinal operculum in stage 3 macular holes showed focally decreased AF. The associated retinal elevation and the cuff of subretinal fluid were less fluorescent compared with the background AF of the normal fellow eyes. Following successful surgical treatment the AF of the macular holes was no longer visible. Being noninvasive and rapid, AF imaging may become a useful alternative to fluorescein angiography in the assessment and differential diagnosis of full thickness macular holes [63].

Summary for the Clinician

- Fluorescence is characterized by an emission of light after excitation.
- Fluorophores absorb light with excitation of electrons; energy is produced as they return to their ground state.
- There are nine phenotypic patterns: normal, minimal change, focally increased, focally plaque-like, patchy, linear, lace-like, reticular, and speckled.
- Decreased AF indicates loss of RPE and photoreceptors
- There are four patterns of abnormal FAF in the junctional zone of geographic atrophy: focal, banded, patchy, and diffuse.
- Fundus AF may also be used in cases of Stargardt's macular dystrophy-fundus flavimaculatus and in patients with macular holes.

2.4 Wide-Field Contact Lens System

2.4.1 Introduction

Modern confocal laser scanning ophthalmoscopy (SLO) is used to perform simultaneous fluorescein and ICGA (HRA; Heidelberg Engineering GmbH, Dossenheim, Germany) [2, 27]. With this instrument, the field of view is variable at 10°, 20°, and 30°. Typical 30° SLO images are excellent for most retinal applications, but inadequate for recording chorioretinal findings that are large or located well anterior to the ocular equator. The development of a wide-field contact lens system that increases the imaging field of a confocal SLO up to 150°, providing a 5-fold increase in the field of view, allowed this limitation to be exceeded [55].

2.4.2 Materials and Methods

2.4.2.1 Structure of a Wide-Field Contact Lens System

The lens used to explore the periphery of the retina is an integrated, multielement, wide-field contact lens system. (Ocular Staurenghi 230 SLO Retina Lens; Ocular Instruments, Bellevue, WA, USA). It consists of two biconvex aspheric lenses and a two-element convex–concave contact lens. It has ×0.23 magnification and is afocal when used with gonioscopic gel. Antireflection coatings reduce reflections to less than 0.1% for 514-nm red-free and 835-nm IR reflectance. The wide-field contact lens system was designed and constructed to increase the 10°, 20°, and 30° imaging fields of the SLO to 50°, 100°, and 150° respectively. All design calculations for the lens system were performed with the OSLO ray tracing program (release 6.1; Lambda Research Corporation, Littleton, MA, USA), using a modified Le Grand–El Hage unaccommodated theoretical eye model [55].

2.4.2.2 Limit and Advantage of a Wide-Field Contact Lens System

The wide-field lens complements other previously documented advantages of SLO [2, 23, 27, 29, 30, 54]. Structures well anterior to the chorioretinal equator are imaged readily. Even more peripheral structures are detectable and recordable with changes in patient fixation. The extended imaging field provided by the lens obviates the need for photomontages, avoiding their potential limitations, which include skipped areas and local variations in contrast and magnification. The peripheral retina and choroid are imaged readily through a small patient pupil (although field size is not as large as with dilated pupils), and iris neovascularization can be documented easily. The good vascular detail afforded by confocal SLO IR reflectance imaging is unimpaired. The wide-field SLO lens can be used with adults or children, although the contact element is too large for infants. It is also useful for patients with aphakic and pseudophakic eyes, and for patients with cataracts of low to moderate opacity. Placement of the wide-field SLO lens on a patient's cornea requires a few seconds. On account of the insufficient overall optical transmission of the wide-field SLO lens, it is not possible to perform AF imaging. Reflections during fluorescein and ICGA are negligible because of the excellent angiography filters of the SLO, but lens reflections can be seen in the IR fundus. Good resolution is preserved in late angiogram frames [55].

2.4.2.3 Technique for Performing the Examination

Each patient requires topical pharmacologic dilation and is positioned for imaging using a standard chin rest. Patients viewed a fixation target with their contralateral eye when feasible. After topical anesthesia, a wide-field SLO lens is placed with gonioscopic gel on the cornea of the eye to be examined. The examiner views the monitor of the SLO, which displays an inverted image of the patient's fundus produced by the wide-field contact lens system. Modified HRA Eye Explorer software, version 1.3 (Heidelberg Engineering) permits image inversion to facilitate ophthalmoscopy and angioscopy. The SLO focus is adjusted for maximum retinal vessel contrast. Alignment between the optical axes of the lens and the axis of the HRA SLO is required to optimize image quality. Retinal angiography is performed by injecting a 5-ml solution of 25 mg of ICG diluted with 5 ml of 20% sodium fluorescein. Although these are normal doses for conventional fundus cameras, they are higher than typical SLO doses, which are inadequate for wide-field imaging. Angiographic dye injection is followed by a 5-ml isotonic sodium chloride solution flush. Dynamic, simultaneous fluorescein and ICGA movies are recorded at 6 frames per second at 256×256-pixel resolution. Recording begins when ICG fluorescence first appears on the SLO monitor and lasts for approximately 20 s. A series of fluorescein and ICGA images (512×512 pixels, 1-mm scan depth) are then recorded at different focal planes. Image collection typically required less than 2 min per eye. Patients with conditions such as diabetic retinopathy or central retinal vein occlusion received only sodium fluorescein

(5 ml of 20% sodium fluorescein dye followed by a 5-ml isotonic sodium chloride solution flush).

The "compute mean" and "compute composite" software functions of the HRA SLO are used to average and process images from different focal planes respectively. The 512×512-pixel image files required 288 KB of computer disk storage space. Local and global chorioretinal features can be documented with the wide-field SLO lens system by zooming in on selected structures using smaller SLO field settings. Higher SLO resolutions are available when needed by removing the contact lens, irrigating the cornea (ideally with a 5% glucose solution), and using the 30°, 20°, or 10° image field sizes of the SLO [55].

2.4.3 Other Techniques of Execution of Wide-field Fluorescein Angiograms

Wide-field fluorescein angiograms can be created by:
1. Using a dedicated wide-field camera system
2. Using an accessory lens to expand the imaging field of a standard noncontact fundus camera or SLO
3. Producing a photomontage from a conventional fundus camera or SLO images

Each method has its advantages and disadvantages.

Photomontages of static images can be produced manually or by computer automation. Manual photomontages are created by cutting and pasting photographic prints or by overlapping and blending their digitized images with photo-editing software [9, 39, 51]. Higher resolution is achievable with wide-field manual photomontages [42, 50], but their preparation is lengthy and laborious. The HRA Eye Explorer software automates photomontage preparation, producing photomontages that range from 100 to 140° [47]. The software takes approximately 5 min to identify and align retinal vascular patterns in adjacent images. The additional photography required to produce a photomontage requires only a few minutes for an experienced photographer.

Manual and automated photomontages have excellent image detail in their individual small-field images, but neither is useful for dynamic angiography. Both techniques introduce inaccuracies in judging the extent of or changes in a large peripheral chorioretinal structure because:
1. Contrast and brightness can vary across photomontages
2. Magnification and distortion can vary within and between photomontage elements that represent different two-dimensional projections of the highly curved peripheral retina
3. Automated processes can produce skipped areas

Dynamic angioscopy, changes in patient fixation, and the broad 150° SLO imaging field provided by a wide-field SLO contact lens system obviate the need for manual or computer-automated photomontages.

Several dedicated wide-field camera systems are available currently. A two-color, very wide-field SLO has been developed for retinal examination (Panoramic200; Optos, Dunfermline, UK) with lower resolution than angiographic SLOs. Non-SLO wide-field camera systems use a contact ophthalmoscopic lens and either transscleral illumination primarily for adult patients (Panoret 1000; Medibell, Haifa, Israel) or transpupillary illumination primarily for pediatric patients (Retcam 120; Massie Research Laboratories, Dublin, CA, USA). The original Equator-plus camera used either type of illumination [45] and produced static, low-magnification, 148° film images.

Contemporary wide-field contact cameras are independent, computer-automated imaging systems that offer dynamic, 90° to 110° digital images with higher resolution than the original Equator-plus camera. They produce excellent wide-field images, but since all available retinal detail is in the ophthalmoscopic image produced by their contact ophthalmoscopy lens [41, 46] magnifying that image optically and/or digitally cannot provide the additional detail available in high-resolution, smaller-field fundus cameras or SLO images.

Accessory contact and noncontact lenses have been used to increase the field of view of conventional fundus cameras [43, 44, 53]. The feasibility of increasing the imaging field of the first nonconfocal SLO was demonstrated using the contact lens element of an Equator-plus camera.

A handheld, noncontact 30-D ophthalmoscopy lens was used to increase the imaging field of a confocal SLO (Rodenstock, Munich, Germany) from 40 to 70° to study the watershed zone of the peripheral choroid [57].

2.4.4 Clinical Application

Angiography with a wide-field contact lens system is useful in different pathologies such as diabetic retinopathy, chorioretinal tumors, uveitis, retinal vascular disorders (central and branch retinal vein occlusion), retinal detachment, and other peripheral chorioretinal disorders.

> **Summary for the Clinician**
>
> - Wide-field fluorescein angiograms can be created by using a dedicated wide-field camera system, by using an accessory lens to expand the imaging field of a standard noncontact fundus camera or SLO, or by producing a photomontage from a conventional fundus camera or SLO images
> - Manual and automated photomontages have excellent image detail in their individual small-field images.
> - Both techniques introduce inaccuracies because: contrast and brightness can vary across photomontages, magnification and distortion can vary within and between photomontage elements, and automated processes can produce skipped areas.
> - Wide-field contact lens systems are useful in diabetic retinopathy, chorioretinal tumors, uveitis, retinal vascular disorders, retinal detachment, etc.

References

1. Allikmets R, Singh N, Sun H et al (1997) A photoreceptor cell-specific ATP-binding transporter gene (ABCR) is mutated in recessive Stargardt macular dystrophy. Nat Genet 15:236–246
2. Bartsch DU, Weinreb RN, Zinser G et al (1995) Confocal scanning infrared laser ophthalmoscopy for indocyanine green angiography. Am J Ophthalmol 120:642–651
3. Bindewald A, Bird AC, Dandekar S, Dollar-Szczasny J, Fitzke FW, Einbock W, Holz FG, Jorzig JJ, Kleinhauer C, Lois N, Mlynsky J, Pauleikhoff D, Staurenghi G, Wolf S (2005) Classification of fundus autofluorescence patterns in early age related macular disease. Invest Ophthalmol Vis Sci 46(9):3309–3314
4. Bindewald A, Schmitz-Valckenberg S, Jorzik JJ, Dolar-Szczasny J, Sieber H, Keilhauer C, Weinberger AW, Dithmar S, Pauleikhoff D, Mansmann U, Wolf S, Holz FG (2005) Classification of abnormal fundus autofluorescence patterns in the junctional zone of geographic atrophy in patients with age related macular degeneration. Br J Ophthalmol 89(7):874–878
5. Bonin P, Faunay F, Fauconnier T (1990) Notre experience de l'étude clinique de l'œil dans le domaine du proche infrarouge. Ophtalmologie 4:33–39
6. Boulton M, Docchio F, Dayhaw-Barker P, Ramponi R, Cubeddu R (1990) Age-related changes in the morphology, absorption, and fluorescence of melanosomes and lipofuscin granules of the retinal pigment epithelium. Vision Res 9:1291–1303
7. Boulton M, Dontsov A, Jarvis-Evans J, Ostrvsky M, Svistunenko D (1993) Lipofuscin is a photoinducible free radical generator. J Photochem Photobiol B 19:201–204
8. Bressler NM, Bressler SB, Seddon JM, Gragoudas ES, Jacobsen LP (1988) Drusen characteristics in patients with exudative versus non-exudative age-related macular degeneration. Retina 8:109–114
9. Clark TM, Freeman WR, Goldbaum MH et al (1992) Digital overlay of fluorescein angiograms and fundus images for treatment of subretinal neovascularisation. Retina 12:118–126
10. Dandekar SS, Jenkins SA, Peto T, Scholl HP, Sehmi KS, Fitzke FW, Bird AC, Webster AR (2005) Autofluorescence imaging of choroidal neovascularization due to age-related macular degeneration. Arch Ophthalmol 123(11):1507–1513
11. Delori FC, Pflibsen KP (1989) Spectral reflectance of the human ocular fundus. Appl Opt 28:1061–1077

12. Delori FC, Gragoudas ES, Francisco R, Pruett RC (1977) Monochromatic ophthalmoscopy and fundus photography: the normal fundus. Arch Ophthalmol 95:861–868
13. Delori FC, Dorey CK, Staurenghi G, Arend O, Goger DG, Weiter JJ (1995) In vivo fluorescence of the ocular fundus exhibits retinal pigment epithelium lipofuscin characteristics. Invest Ophthalmol Vis Sci 36:718–729
14. Delori FC, Staurenghi G, Arend O, Dorey CK, Goger DG, Weiter JJ (1995) In vivo measurement of lipofuscin in Stargardt's disease-fundus flavimaculatus. Invest Ophthalmol Vis Sci 36:2327–2333
15. Dorey CK, Wu G, Ebenstein D, Garsd A, Weiter JJ (1989) Cell loss in the aging retina: relationship to lipofuscin accumulation and macular degeneration. Invest Ophthalmol Vis Sci 30:1691–1699
16. Ducrey NM, Delori FC, Gragoudas ES (1979) Monochromatic ophthalmoscopy and fundus photography. II. The pathological fundus. Arch Ophthalmol 97:288–293
17. Elsner AE, Burns SA, Webb RH (1988) Photopigment densitometry with a scanning laser ophthalmoscope. Opt Soc Am Tech Digest 11:WY3
18. Elsner AE, Burns SA, Delori FC, Webb RH (1990) Quantitative reflectometry with the SLO. In: Naseman JE, Burk RO (eds) Laser scanning ophthalmoscopy and tomography. Quintessenz, New York, pp 109–121
19. Elsner AE, Burns SA, Hughes GW, Webb RH (1990) Evaluating the photoreceptor/RPE complex with an SLO. Non invasive assessment of the visual system. Opt Soc Am Tech Dig 3:40–43
20. Elsner AE, Burns SA, Kreitz MR, Weiter JJ (1991) New views of the retina/RPE complex: quantifying sub-retinal pathology. Noninvasive assessment of the visual system. Opt Soc Am Tech Dig 1:150–153
21. Elsner AE, Burns SA, Hughes GW, Webb RH (1992) Reflectometry with a scanning laser ophthalmoscope. Appl Opt 31:3697–3710
22. Elsner AE, Jalkh AE, Weiter JJ (1993) New devices in retinal imaging and functional evaluation. In: Freeman W (ed) Practical atlas of retinal disease and therapy (pp. 19-35). Raven, New York, pp 19–35
23. Elsner AE, Burns SA, Weiter JJ et al (1996) Infrared imaging of sub-retinal structures in the human ocular fundus. Vis Res 36:191–205
24. Framme C, Walter A, Gabler B, Roider J, Sachs HG, Gabel VP (2005) Fundus autofluorescence in acute and chronic-recurrent central serous chorioretinopathy. Acta Ophthalmol Scand 83(2):161–167
25. Franceschetti A (1963) Über tapeto-retinale Degenerationen im Kindesalter. Dritter Fortbildungskurs der Deutschen Ophthalmologischen Gesellschaft, Hamburg 1962. In: Sautter H (ed) Entwicklung und Fortschritt in der Augenhielkunde. Enke, Stuttgart, pp 107–120
26. Franceschetti A (1965) A special form of tapetoretinal degeneration—fundus flavimaculatus. Trans Am Acad Ophthalmol Otolaryngol 69:1048–1053
27. Freeman WR, Bartsch DU, Mueller AJ et al (1998) Simultaneous indocyanine green and fluorescein angiography using a confocal scanning laser ophthalmoscope. Arch Ophthalmol 116:455–463
28. Gaillard RR, Atherton SJ, Eldred G, Dillon J (1995) Photophysical studies on human retinal lipofuscin. Photochem Photobiol 61:448–453
29. Holz FG, Bellmann C, Dithmar S et al (1997) Simultaneous fluorescein and indocyanine green angiography with a confocal scanning laser ophthalmoscope. Ophthalmologe 94:348–353
30. Holz FG, Bellmann C, Rohrschneider K et al (1998) Simultaneous confocal scanning laser fluorescein and indocyanine green angiography. Am J Ophthalmol 125:227–236
31. Holz FG, Bellmann C, Margaritidis M, Schutt F, Otto TP, Volcker HE (1999) Patterns of increased in vivo fundus autofluorescence in the junctional zone of geographic atrophy of the retinal pigment epithelium associated with age-related macular degeneration. Graefes Arch Clin Exp Ophthalmol 237(2):145–152
32. Hyman LG, Lilienfeld AM, Ferris FL III, Fine SL (1983) Senile macular degeneration: a case-control study. Am J Epidemiol 118(2):213–227
33. Kurzel RB, Wolbarsht ML, Tamanashi BS (1973) Spectral studies on normal and cataractous intact human lenses. Exp Eye Res 17:65–71
34. Leibowitz H, Kruger DE, Maunder LR, Milton RC, Kini MM, Kahn HA, Mickerson RJ, Pool J, Colton TL, Ganley JP, Loewenstein J (1980) The Framingham Eye Study Monograph: an ophthalmological and epidemiological study of cataract, glaucoma, diabetic retinopathy, macular degen-

eration, and visual acuity in a general population of 2631 adults, 1973–1975. Surv Ophthalmol 24 [Suppl]:335–610
35. Lerman S, Kuck JF, Borkman JF, Saker E (1976) Introduction, acceleration and prevention (in vitro) of a parameter in the ocular lens. Ophthalmic Res 8:213–226
36. Lois N, Halfyard AS, Bunce C, Bird A, Fitzke FW (1999) Reproducibility of fundus autofluorescence measurements obtained using a confocal scanning laser ophthalmoscope. Br J Ophthalmol 83:276–279
37. Lois N, Holder GE, Bunce C, Fitzke F, Bird AC (2001) Phenotypic subtypes of Stargardt macular dystrophy—fundus flavimaculatus. Arch Ophthalmol 119:359–369
38. Lois N, Halfyard AS, Bird AC, Holder GE, Fitzke FW (2004) Fundus autofluorescence in Stargardt macular dystrophy-fundus flavimaculatus. Am J Ophthalmol 138(1):55–63
39. Mahurkar AA, Vivino MA, Trus BL et al (1996) Constructing retinal fundus photomontages: a new computer based method. Invest Ophthalmol Vis Sci 37:1675–1683
40. Mainster MA, Timberlake GT, Webb RH et al (1982) Scanning laser ophthalmoscopy: clinical application. Ophthalmology 89:852–857
41. Mainster MA, Reichel E, Harrington PG et al (2001) Ophthalmoscopic contact lenses for transpupillary thermotherapy. Semin Ophthalmol 16:60–65
42. Niki T, Muraoka K, Shimizu K (1984) Distribution of capillary nonperfusion in early-stage diabetic retinopathy. Ophthalmology 91:1431–1439
43. Noyory KS, Chino K, Deguchi T (1983) Wide field fluorescein angiography by use of contact lens. Retina 3:131–134
44. Ozerdem U, Freeman WR, Bartsch DU et al (2001) A simple noncontact wide-angle fundus photography procedure for clinical and research use. Retina 21:189–190
45. Pomerantzeff O (1975) Equator-plus camera. Invest Ophthalmol 14:401–406
46. Pomerantzeff O, Webb RH, Delori FC (1979) Image formation in fundus camera. Invest Ophthalmol Vis Sci 18:630–637
47. Rivero ME, Bartsch DU, Otto T et al (1999) Automated scanning laser ophthalmoscope image montages of retinal diseases. Ophthalmology 106:2296–2300
48. Rovati L, Docchio F (2004) Autofluorescence methods in ophthalmology. J Biomed Opt 9(1):9–21
49. Rozanowska M, Jarvis-Evans J, Korytowsky W, Boulton ME, Burke JM, Sarna T (1995) Blue light-induced reactivity of retinal age pigment. In vitro generation of oxygen-reactive species. J Biol Chem 270:18825–18830
50. Shimizu K, Kobayashi Y, Muraoka K (1981) Midperipheral fundus involvement in diabetic retinopathy. Ophthalmology 88:601–612
51. Sleightholm MA, Arnold J, Aldington SJ et al (1984) Computer-aided digitisation of fundus photographs. Clin Phys Physiol Meas 5:295–301
52. Snoddlery DM, Brown PL, Delori FC, Auran JD (1984) The macular pigment. I. Absorbance spectra, localization and discrimination from other yellow pigments in primate retinas. Invest Ophthalmol Vis Sci 25:660–673
53. Spaide RF, Orlock DA, Hermann-Delemazure B et al (1998) Wide-angle indocyanine green angiography. Retina 18:44–49
54. Staurenghi G, Aschero M, La Capria A et al (1996) Visualization of neovascular membranes with infrared light without dye injection by means of a scanning laser ophthalmoscope. Arch Ophthalmol 114:365
55. Staurenghi G, Viola F, Mainster MA et al (2005) Scanning laser ophthalmoscopy and angiography with a wide-field contact lens system. Arch Ophthalmol 123:244–252
56. Stöhr H, Weber BHF (2004) Genetics of AMD. In: Holz FG, Pauleikhoff D, Spaide RF, Bird AC (eds) Age-related macular degeneration. Springer, Berlin, pp 23–30
57. Takahshi K, Muraoka K, Kishi S et al (1996) Watershed zone in the human peripheral choroid. Ophthalmology 103:336–342
58. Van Best JA, Delft JL, Keunen JE (1998) Long term follow-up of lenticular autofluorescence and transmittance in healthy volunteers. Exp Eye Res 66:117–123
59. Van Norren D, Tiemeijer LF (1986) Spectral reflectance of the human eye. Vis Res 26:313–320
60. Von Ruckmann A, Fitzke FW, Bierd AC (1995) Distribution of fundus autofluorescence with scanning laser ophthalmoscope. Br J Ophthalmol 79:407–412

61. Von Ruckmann A, Fitzke FW, Bierd AC (1997) In vivo fundus autofluorescence in macular dystrophies. Arch Ophthalmol 115:609–615
62. Von Ruckmann A, Fitzke FW, Bierd AC (1997) Fundus autofluorescence in age related macular disease with a laser scanning ophthalmoscope. Invest Ophthalmol Vis Sci 38:478–486
63. Von Ruckmann A, Fitzke FW, Gregor ZJ (1998) Fundus autofluorescence in patients with macular holes imaged with a laser scanning ophthalmoscope. Br J Ophthalmol 82(4):346–351
64. Webb RH, Hughes GW (1981) Scanning laser ophthalmoscope. IEEE Trans Biomed Eng 28:488–492
65. Webb RH, Hughes GL, Delori FC (1987) Confocal scanning laser ophthalmoscope. Appl Opt 26:1492–1499
66. Webb RH, Delori FC (1988) How we see the retina. In: Marshall J (ed) Laser technology in ophthalmology. Kugler and Ghedini, Amsterdam, pp 3–14
67. Weiter JJ, Delori FC, Wing GL, Fitch KF (1986) Retinal pigment epithelium lipofuscin and melanin and choroidal melanin in human eyes. Invest Ophthalmol Vis Sci 27:145–152
68. Wing GL, Blanchard GC, Weiter JJ. The topography and age relationship of lipofuscin concentration in the retinal pigment epithelium. Invest Ophthalmol Vis Sci 17:601–607
69. Wyszecki G, Stiles WS (1982) Color science. Wiley, New York, pp 101–102

Chapter 3

Genetics of Age-Related Macular Degeneration: Update

Hendrik P.N. Scholl, Monika Fleckenstein, Peter Charbel Issa, Claudia Keilhauer, Frank G. Holz, Bernhard H.F. Weber

Core Messages

- Age-related macular degeneration (AMD) is a genetically complex disorder of the photoreceptor–retinal pigment epithelium–Bruch's membrane–choriocapillaris complex.
- Susceptibility to disease is genetically influenced. The heritability has been estimated to be 71%.
- Linkage and association studies found strongest evidence for AMD susceptibility loci on chromosome 1q31 and 10q26.
- Variants in the complement factor H gene on chromosome 1q31 have been shown to be associated with an increased risk of AMD in the Caucasian population. These findings suggest that the innate immune system plays a central role in AMD pathogenesis.
- The LOC387715/HTRA1 locus on 10q26 has been identified as an independent major locus contributing to AMD pathogenesis.
- Considering variants at CFH, LOC387715/HTRA1, and C2-BF, homozygosity for risk alleles at all three loci account for an approximately 250-fold greater risk of AMD compared with baseline.

3.1 Introduction: Genetic Influence on AMD

Age-related macular degeneration (AMD) is a genetically complex disorder of the photoreceptor-retinal pigment epithelium–Bruch's membrane–choriocapillaris complex [7, 14, 34, 84]. Late AMD is now the most common cause of legal blindness in the western world, with a prevalence of 0.05% before the age of 50 years and 11.8% after 80 years of age [21]. Unless effective methods of prevention and treatment are found, the prevalence of AMD is expected to double in the coming decades due to an expected demographic shift toward an aging population [21].

A genetic influence on AMD pathology is well known from family and twin studies [15, 23, 25, 32, 37, 40, 62, 83]. First-degree relatives of patients with AMD, compared with first-degree relatives in families without the disorder, are at increased risk (odds ratio, 2.4) of the condition [62], are affected at a younger age [9, 40], and have an increased lifetime risk of late AMD (risk ratio, 4.2) [40].

In order to determine the relative contribution of heredity and environment to the etiology of AMD, Seddon and co-workers performed a population-based twin study of AMD including both concordant/discordant and monozygotic/dizygotic sibling pairs [65]. Heritability estimates for AMD were significant and ranged from 46 to 71%. These results underscored the need to pursue the search for AMD-related genes, despite the initial difficulties encountered with genetic analyses of a complex disease with late onset.

> **Summary for the Clinician**
>
> - Family and twin studies have shown that susceptibility to disease is genetically influenced.
> - Heritability is significant and is estimated to be approximately 71%.

3.2 Analysis of Candidate Genes for AMD

The progress made within the last decade by studying hereditary monogenic macular and retinal dystrophies has offered some investigative leads to the further study of AMD genetics. The similarities that exist between the phenotypic expression in the hereditary early onset diseases and some of the later onset complex traits as seen in AMD suggested the potential involvement of such candidate genes in AMD-related pathology. In addition, candidate genes were identified based on linkage study results (positional criteria) and knowledge about gene function (functional criteria). However, this approach has not led to a breakthrough. Table 3.1 summarizes such candidate genes with negative (i.e., no involvement in AMD pathogenesis) results to date [29].

For other genes, some evidence of an association with AMD was shown. Genes with at least one result of positive association to date include: *ABCA4*, *HEMICENTIN* (*Fibulin6*), *CX3CR1*, *HLA* genes, *VEGF*, *ELOVL4*, *SOD2*, *PON1*, *VLDLR*, *TLR4*, *LRP6*, *Fibulin5*, *ACE*, *APOE*, *CST3*, and *MMP9* (for a comprehensive review of these genes including references, see Haddad et al. [29]). If verified, variations in these genes likely account for only a small fraction of AMD susceptibility.

Fibulin5 represents an example of these genes. Stone and colleagues found that the disruption of a gene of the same gene family, *EFEMP1* (*Fibulin3*), is linked to Malattia leventinese/Doyne honeycomb retinal dystrophy [74]. This disorder is characterized by confluent drusen accumulation beneath the retinal pigment epithelium (RPE), an early hallmark of AMD. EFEMP1 is an extracellular matrix protein. The interaction with other extracellular matrix proteins, such as adhesion molecules, collagens, elastins, fibronectins, laminins, tenascins, hemicentins, and vitronectins, suggests that an entire group of genes might be possible candidates for involvement in drusen

Table 3.1 Candidate gene studies for age-related macular degeneration: genes with negative results to date. For references, see Haddad et al. [29]

Chromosome	Gene
1	ADPRT1, EPHX1, GLRX2, LAMC1, LamC2, LAMB3, OCLM, PRELP, RGS16, TGFB2
2	EFEMP1 (Fibulin 3), GPR75, IL1A, Fibulin 2, GPX1
3	IMPG2
6	RDS
7	AhR
8	NAT2
10	CYP2E1
11	CAT, Fibulin 4, VMD2
12	A2M, MGST1
14	CKB
15	CYP1A1, CYP1A2
17	APOH, ITGB4
22	CYP2D6, Fibulin 1, TIMP3

formation [74]. Later, Stone et al. systematically evaluated five fibulin genes in a large series of patients with AMD. They demonstrated a significant association between sequence variations in *fibulin5* and AMD. However, missense mutations in *fibulin5* were estimated to account for only 1.7% of patients with AMD [75].

The photoreceptor cell-specific ATP-binding cassette transporter (*ABCA4*) gene was identified in 1997 and found to be mutated in patients with Stargardt's macular dystrophy [6]. *ABCA4* has been evaluated as being a possible cause of other diseases with similar pathology in the macula, including AMD. Two studies by Allikmets and co-workers have shown evidence of an association between *ABCA4* polymorphisms and AMD [4, 5]. While other studies have provided support [10, 69], a number of reports have failed to confirm an association of *ABCA4* with AMD [22, 28, 43, 52, 57, 71, 73, 81]. The number of patients and controls included in the latter studies appears large enough to rule out a major contribution of mutant *ABCA4* alleles in the predisposition to AMD; however, they may not be sufficient to allow minor effects to be discerned. This makes it extremely difficult to determine the significance of individual mutant *ABCA4* alleles for predisposition to AMD, particularly those that are present at very low frequency in the general population. The phenotypic similarities between typical juvenile Stargardt macular dystrophy and some forms of late atrophic AMD suggest that refined phenotyping may be of value in discerning between the two conditions. Figure 3.1 shows fundus autofluorescence images of a patient with Stargardt's macular dystrophy (age, 17 years) and a patient with geographic atrophy due to AMD (age, 71 years).

Recently, it has been shown that by means of fundus autofluorescence imaging different phenotypic patterns of abnormal fundus autofluorescence in the junctional zone of late atrophic AMD can be identified [11]. Moreover, there was a high degree of intra-individual symmetry in the fundus autofluorescence pattern in the two eyes in individual patients, but a high degree of inter-individual variability, which may suggest genetic heterogeneity. In a preliminary analysis, 7 AMD patients exhibiting the fundus autofluorescence pattern "diffuse-fine granular with peripheral punctate spots" (resembling Stargardt's macular dystrophy; age of onset, 50–84 years) and 14 geographic atrophy patients exhibiting other fundus autofluorescence patterns were screened

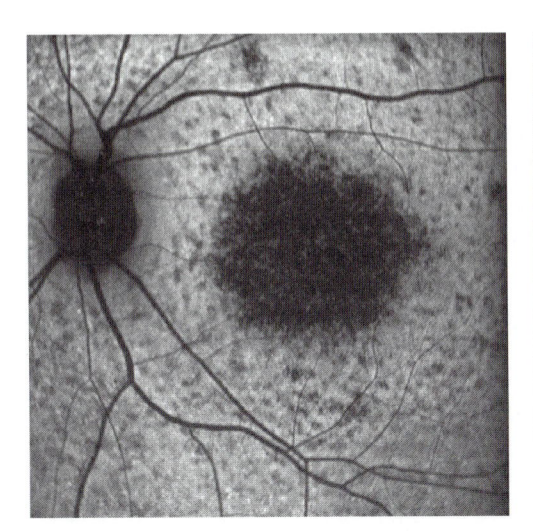

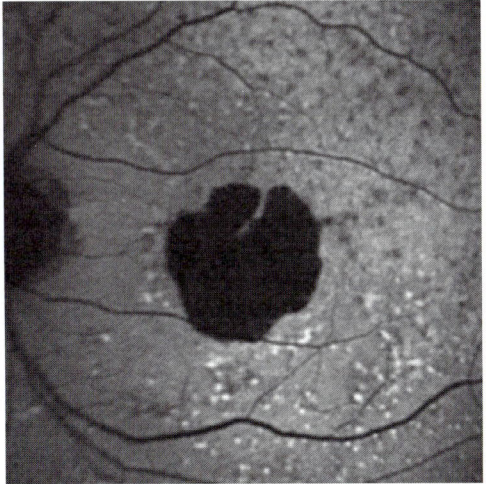

Fig. 3.1 Fundus autofluorescence images obtained with a confocal scanning laser ophthalmoscope (cSLO; Heidelberg retina angiograph, HRA 2; Heidelberg Engineering, Dossenheim, Germany) according to a standard operating procedure. *Left*: patient diagnosed with Stargardt's macular dystrophy (age, 17 years). *Right*: patient diagnosed with atrophic age-related macular degeneration (AMD) and a fundus autofluorescence pattern "diffuse-fine granular with peripheral punctate spots" according to Bindewald et al. [11] (age: 71 years)

for *ABCA4* mutations. In the first group, all patients showed at least one mutated allele, and in 2 patients, two mutated alleles were detected. In the control group of 14 AMD patients exhibiting geographic atrophy, but a different pattern of abnormal fundus autofluorescence, only 2 patients showed one mutated allele [19]. We suggest that this distinct AMD phenotype exhibiting "diffuse-fine granular with peripheral punctate spots" reflects genetic alterations in *ABCA4* and we speculate that this distinct phenotype might represent late onset Stargardt's macular dystrophy mimicking atrophic AMD. These preliminary data suggest that refined phenotyping is paramount in dissecting the role of candidate genes.

Summary for the Clinician

- AMD shares phenotypic similarities with some of the monogenic macular dystrophies. However, the responsible genes underlying those dystrophies do not appear to substantially contribute to AMD susceptibility.
- Specifically, the role of *ABCA4* is controversial and, more comprehensive phenotyping may help to better understand the role of these individual genes in AMD pathology.

3.3 Linkage and Association Studies in AMD

Over the past few years, researchers have carried out both linkage studies and association studies in an attempt to identify the genomic regions containing susceptibility loci for AMD. While linkage studies search for genetic markers that segregate with the disease in a familial constellation, association analyses identify genetic marker alleles that either cause disease or are in strong linkage disequilibrium (LD) with the disease-causing alleles.

Fisher and colleagues used the genome-scan meta-analysis (GSMA) method, which allows linkage results from several studies to be combined, providing greater power to identify regions that show only weak evidence of linkage in individual studies [18]. This method has been successful in a number of complex diseases and was applied to six published AMD genome-wide linkage scans: Abecasis et al. [1], Iyengar et al. [38], Majewski et al. [47], Schick et al. [56], Seddon et al. [64], and Weeks et al. [82]. For each study, 120 genomic bins of 30 cM were defined and ranked according to maximum evidence of linkage within each bin. Bin ranks were weighted according to study size and summed across all studies. A high summed rank indicates a region with consistent evidence of linkage across studies (Fig. 3.2).

The strongest evidence for an AMD susceptibility locus was found on chromosome 10q26 (Fig. 3.2), where genome-wide significant linkage was observed ($p=0.00025$). Several other regions met the empirical significance criteria for bins likely to contain linked loci including adjacent pairs of bins on chromosomes 1q, 2p, 3p, and 16. Several of the regions identified here showed only weak evidence of linkage in the individual studies. The analysis performed by Fisher and colleagues may help prioritize regions for future positional and functional candidate gene studies in AMD.

Summary for the Clinician

- Linkage and association studies have identified several chromosomal regions that are likely to contain AMD susceptibility loci.
- The strongest evidence of an AMD susceptibility locus was found in chromosomal regions 1q31 and 10q26.

3.4 Complement Factor H Gene

Several genome-wide linkage analyses and the genome-scan meta-analysis of Fisher and colleagues had pointed to a locus on 1q25-q31 [1, 38, 41, 47, 64, 82]. Case-control studies recently identified complement factor H (*CFH*) as the responsible gene [17, 30, 31, 42]. The *CFH* Y402H variant, located within a binding site for C-reactive protein

3.4 Complement Factor H Gene

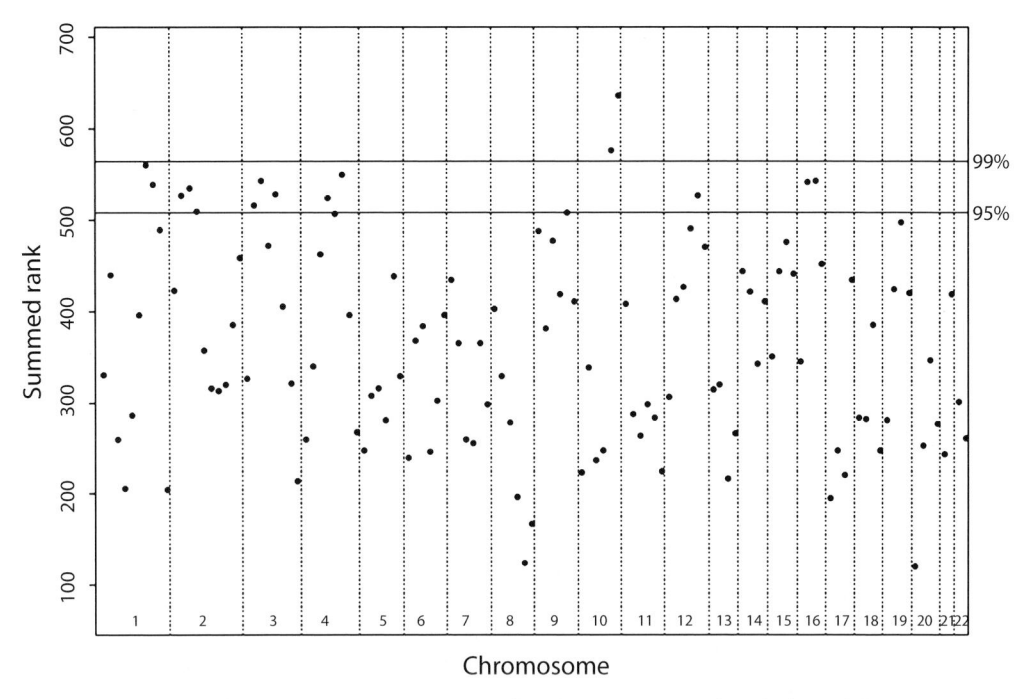

Fig. 3.2 Results from the AMD genome-scan meta-analysis (GSMA). Summed ranks for each bin (weighted by the square root of the number of affected individuals in each study); 95 and 99% confidence limits are shown. From Fisher et al. Fig. 1A [18], used with permission

(CRP), has consistently been shown to reveal a strong association with AMD [46, 72, 85].

In a population-based prospective study design with a total of 5,681 individuals, investigators of the Rotterdam Eye Study have shown that *CFH* is implicated in all stages of AMD from early hallmarks such as drusen to vision-disabling late AMD [16]. The risk increased with each successive stage to a final odds ratio of 11.0 for late AMD. It was calculated that individuals homozygous for the *CFH* Y402H polymorphism had a 48% risk of developing late AMD by the age of 95 years while this risk did not exceed 22% for noncarriers. Interestingly, complement factor H was associated with both late AMD subtypes (choroidal neovascularization [CNV] and geographic atrophy) in this study. Homozygous *CFH* Y402H carriers were at higher risk of bilateral than of unilateral late AMD, and risks of geographic atrophy and mixed AMD were slightly but not significantly higher than of neovascular AMD. This is in agreement with other studies that reported higher frequencies of CFH Y402H carriers in patients with geographic atrophy [53, 85] and one study that suggested a lower risk of geographic atrophy for a *CFH* haplotype containing the nonrisk allele [30]. In a comprehensive survey including variants from three gene loci (*CFH*, *LOC387715I*, and *C2-CFB*), Maller and co-workers did not find any association among phenotypic subclassifications of advanced AMD despite substantial power of detection [48]. These findings suggest that the high risk of both subtypes of advanced AMD signifies a common pathogenesis involving the complement system.

Complement factor H is an important regulator of the complement system. Three enzyme cascades exist: the classical complement pathway, initiated by antigen–antibody complexes and surface-bound CRP; the lectin pathway, instigated by mannose groups of microbial carbohydrates; and the alternative complement pathway, activated by surface-bound C3b. The pathways converge at the point where C3 is cleaved into C3a and C3b by C3 convertase, which initiates C5 convertase, finally resulting in the formation of the membrane attack complex with the terminal components (C5b–C9). CFH specifically inhibits the alternative complement cascade, but also regulates the common pathway. It binds C3b and acts as a cofactor in the proteolysis of C3b by factor I, resulting in an inactive C3b molecule. This prevents the production of C3 convertase in the alternative cascade as well as the production of C5 convertase in the common pathway. As a result, CFH interferes with progression of the entire cascade [12, 50, 54, 86]. Indeed, Hageman and co-workers showed that CFH and C3b/iC3b co-localize within drusen, suggesting that these regions represent complement activating surfaces within drusen and Bruch's membrane (Fig. 3.3) [12, 30].

A recent study suggests that there may be multiple susceptibility alleles in the *CFH* genomic region with noncoding *CFH* variants possibly playing a role in disease susceptibility [44]. In 544 unrelated affected individuals and 268 unrelated controls, Li and co-workers examined the impact of 84 polymorphisms on disease susceptibility located in a region of 123 kb overlapping the *CFH* gene. As expected, strong association was observed between disease status and the Y402H-encoding variant (rs1061170). Unexpectedly, 20 other variants showed even stronger association. The strongly associated single nucleotide polymorphisms (SNPs) fell into two LD groups (colored in purple and green in Fig. 3.4). The Y402H-encoding variant was included in one of

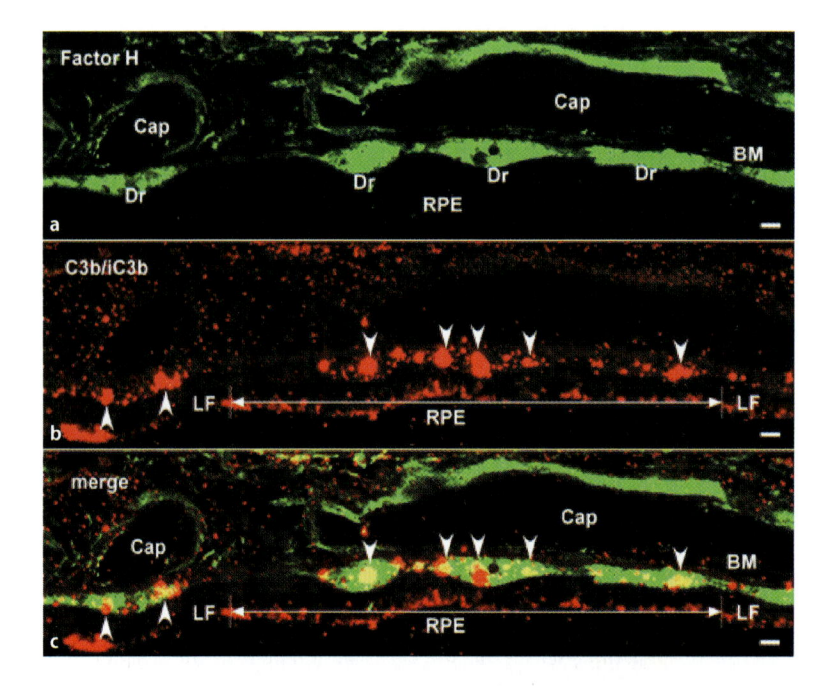

Fig. 3.3a,b Immunohistochemical co-localization of complement factor H (CFH) and C3b/iC3b within drusen. Immunolocalization of **a** CFH and **b** C3b/iC3b, and **c** a corresponding merged image of **a** and **b**, along the retinal pigment epithelium (RPE)–choroid complex of an 83-year-old donor with a clinical diagnosis of atrophic AMD. Anti-HF1 antibody labels drusen and regions of vasculature within the choroid (Cy2/fluorescein; *green*). Anti-C3b/iC3b antibody reacts with distinct spherical substructural elements within drusen (*arrowheads*; Cy3/Texas Red channel). The immunoreactive CFH and C3b/iC3b domains co-localize (*yellow*) in many instances (*arrowheads* in **c**), suggesting that these regions represent complement activating surfaces within drusen and in the sub-RPE space. *BM* Bruch's membrane, *Dr* drusen, *Cap* choriocapillaris. A region of nonspecific autofluorescent RPE lipofuscin granules (*LF*) is bracketed (*solid line*; Cy3/Texas Red channel) in **b**. (Scale bars, 10 mm.) From Hageman et al., supplementary Fig. 6 [30], used with permission

the LD groups (the purple group in Fig. 3.4). The three SNPs showing strongest association were a synonymous SNP in exon 10, rs2274700, and two intronic SNPs, rs1410996 and rs7535263.

The authors conclude that multiple haplotypes in the genomic region seem to modulate the AMD disease risk and that there are multiple disease-predisposing variants. Because the polymorphisms showing the strongest association with AMD susceptibility appear not to affect the primary CFH protein sequence, the authors speculate that these variants may be important in regulating the expression of *CFH*, or other nearby complement genes, or both [44].

The region that includes the *CFH* gene cluster also contains numerous CFH-like genes (e.g., *CFHR1*, *CFHR2*, *CFHR3*, *CFHR4*, and *CFHR5*), which reveal high sequence conservation, making any analysis difficult. Hughes and colleagues genotyped polymorphisms spanning the *CFH* gene cluster in 173 individuals with severe neovascular AMD and 170 controls and found a common haplotype, GTATAAAG, associated with decreased risk of AMD, which was present on 8% of chromosomes in AMD patients and 20% of chromosomes in controls (Fig. 3.5).

They found that this haplotype carried a deletion of *CFHR1* and *CFHR3*. Protein blot analysis of serum samples from individuals homozygous for each haplotype confirmed the absence of CFHR1 and CFHR3 protein in haplotype 5 homozygotes. CFHR1 and CFHR3 proteins are usually present in the circulation and have the potential to compete with CFH for C3 binding. Possibly, CFH produced from full-length transcripts is beneficial in terms of AMD risk and other CFH-related proteins interfere with regulation of complement activity [36].

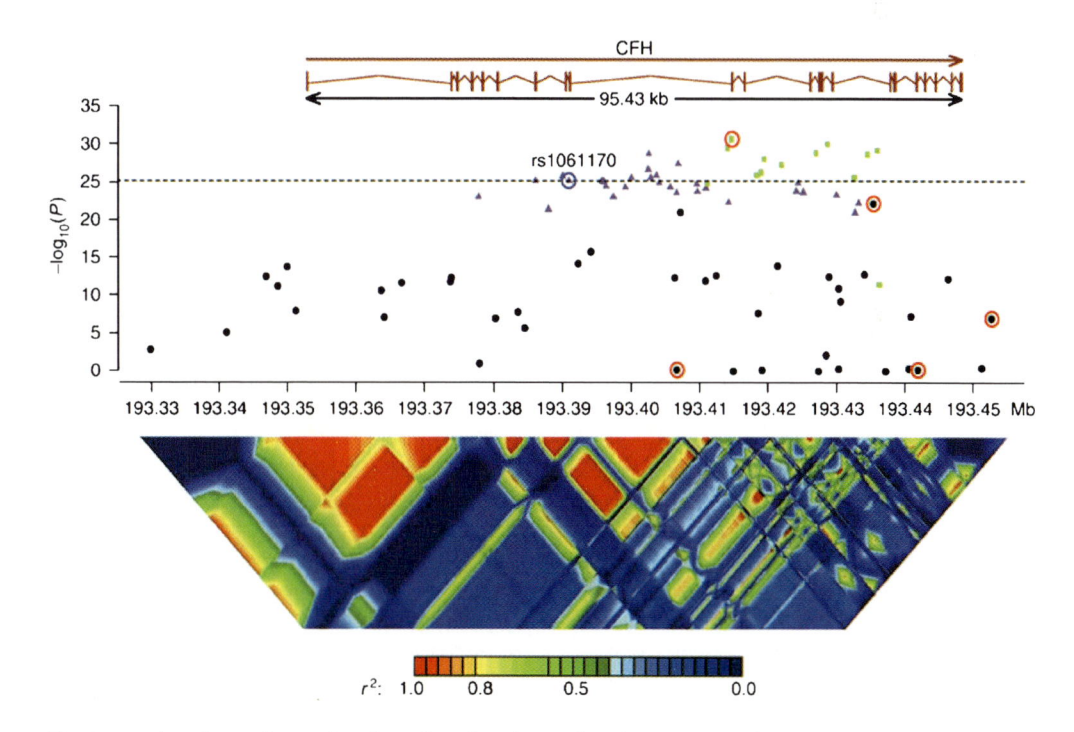

Fig. 3.4 *P* values for single SNP (single nucleotide polymorphism) association, when comparing unrelated affected individuals (cases) and controls. The *dotted horizontal line* is −log10(P) of the original Y402H variant (*circled in blue*). Strongly associated SNPs fall into one of two linkage disequilibrium (LD) groups (SNPs in one of these groups are colored in *green*; SNPs in the other group are colored in *purple*; SNPs outside either group are in *black*). SNPs selected from the stepwise haplotype association analysis are *circled in red*. Linkage disequilibrium across the CFH region is shown below, plotted as pairwise r2 values. From Li et al. Fig. 1 [44], used with permission

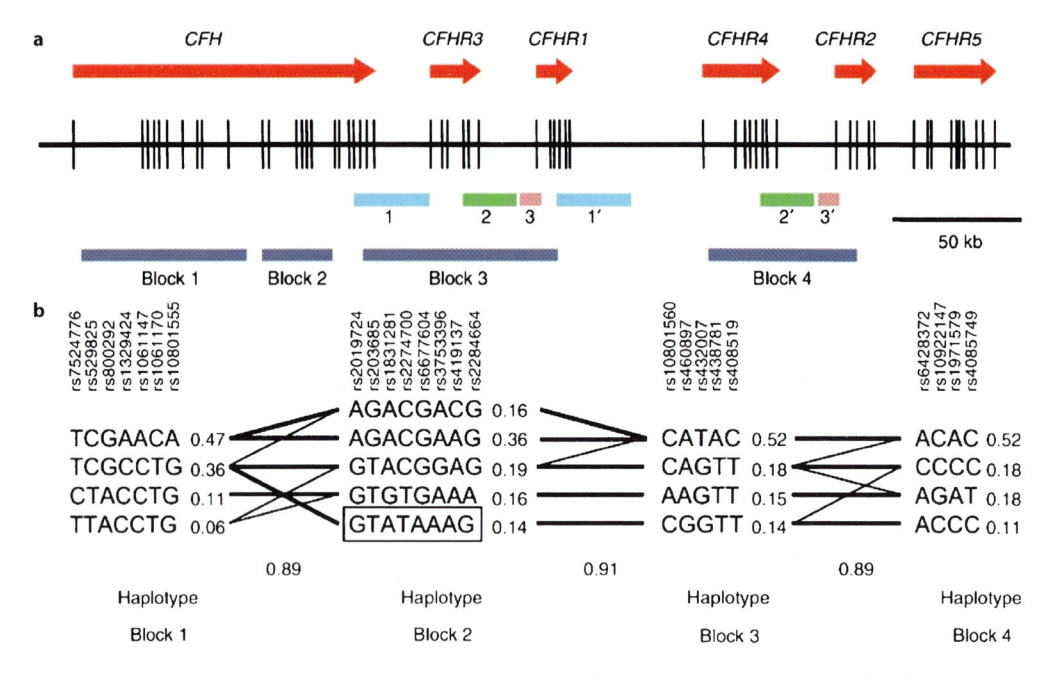

Fig. 3.5a,b Haplotype block structure in CFH and CFH-related genes. **a** Duplicated regions that share orientation and greater than 96% homology are shown below the genomic structure of genes. The haplote block structure of markers is shown in *blue*. **b** Haplotypes of SNPs are shown in blocks with overall frequencies (in affected individuals and controls) and connections from one block to the next. In the crossing areas, a value of multiallelic D' is shown. This reflects the level of recombination between two adjacent blocks. The *black box* outlines the protective haplotype 5 in this block. From Hughes et al., Fig. 1 [36], used with permission

It has long been known that the prevalence of AMD varies widely among different ethnicities [20, 27, 35, 49, 51, 80]. Moreover, the phenotypic spectrum of AMD among these groups is quite heterogeneous [8, 45, 55, 68, 78]. For example, in the Japanese, soft drusen are only a moderate risk indicator (18%) for developing CNV compared with Caucasians, whereas serous pigment epithelial detachments are a very common high risk indicator (58%) for developing CNV in Japanese patients [78]. To explore the ethnic variation of the frequency of the *CFH* Y402H sequence variant, Grassi and co-workers analyzed the frequency of the risk (C) allele in populations from five different ethnicities. Widely divergent frequencies were noted between some of these populations (7–35%; Table 3.2).

These data suggest that there are other as yet unidentified genetic factors important in the pathogenesis of AMD. These factors may operate independently or mitigate the effects of the *CFH* Y402H sequence variant. Specifically, the findings suggest the presence of additional genetic risk factors for AMD in Japanese individuals.

Summary for the Clinician

- Variants in the *CFH* gene at 1q31 have been shown by several independent studies to be associated with a significantly increased risk of AMD in the Caucasian population.
- These findings imply that the innate immune system might be implicated in AMD pathogenesis.
- The findings may not simply be transferable to other, non-Caucasian populations.

Table 3.2 Prevalence of the histidine alteration in five different populations of different ethnicities. Values are frequency (standard error) [26]

	Caucasian	African-American	Hispanic	Japanese	Somali
C	0.34 (0.03)	0.35 (0.04)	0.17 (0.03)	0.07 (0.02)	0.34 (0.03)
T	0.66 (0.03)	0.65 (0.04)	0.83 (0.03)	0.93 (0.02)	0.66 (0.03)
CC	0.07 (0.02)	0.11 (0.03)	0.05 (0.02)	0.02 (0.02)	0.07 (0.02)
CT	0.54 (0.04)	0.48 (0.06)	0.25 (0.05)	0.09 (0.03)	0.55 (0.04)
TT	0.39 (0.04)	0.41 (0.06)	0.70 (0.05)	0.89 (0.03)	0.38 (0.04)
Total patients	148	75	81	82	128

3.5 LOC387715

Two recent reports have highlighted the *LOC387715/HTRA1* locus within 10q26 as a second major locus contributing to AMD pathogenesis [39, 53]. Rivera and co-workers found the strongest association over the *LOC387715* gene conferring a 7.6-fold increased risk for individuals homozygous for a nonsynonymous coding SNP, Ala69Ser. These findings were fully replicated in an independent case–control cohort. Furthermore, Rivera et al. replicated the strong association of AMD with the Y402H coding variant of *CFH*. The results indicated the independent contribution of the effects of risk alleles at the *LOC387715* (Ala69Ser) and *CFH* (Tyr402His) gene locus to the overall disease risk (Fig. 3.6). Very recently, the findings have been independently replicated by others [13, 48, 58, 67].

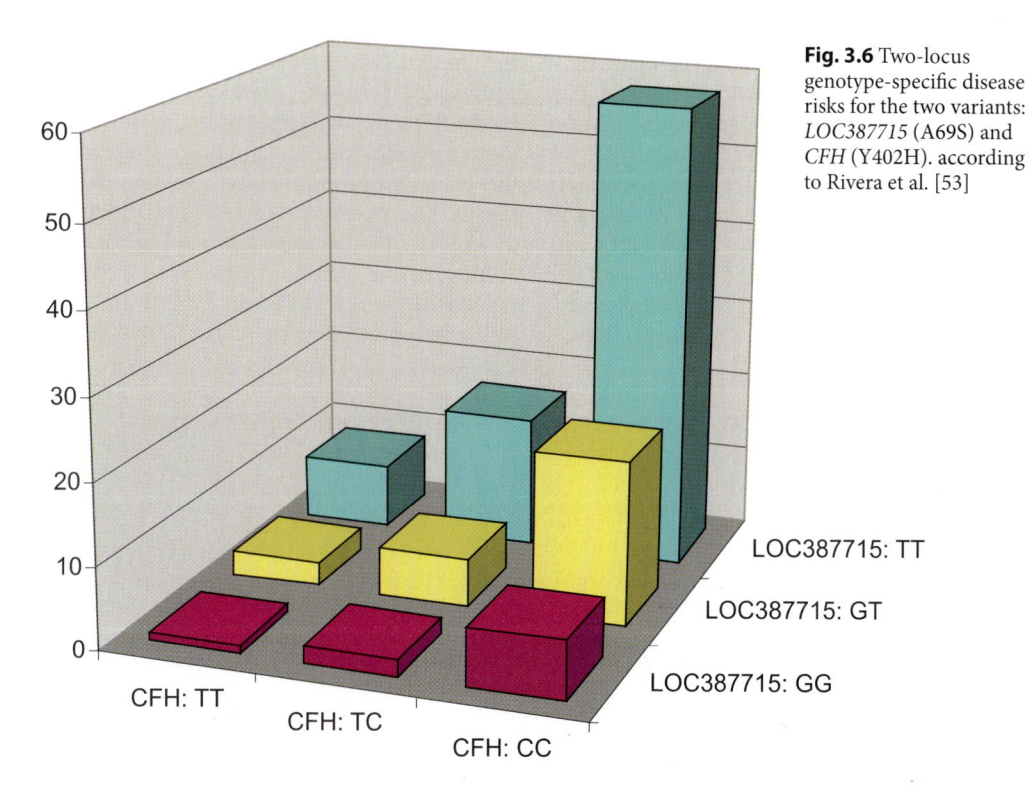

Fig. 3.6 Two-locus genotype-specific disease risks for the two variants: *LOC387715* (A69S) and *CFH* (Y402H). according to Rivera et al. [53]

Patient groups of early high-risk AMD and late AMD were not different with regard to risk allele distribution in *LOC387715*. This was also true for geographic atrophy and neovascular AMD. So far, it is unknown whether risk alleles at *LOC387715* and/or *CFH* correlate with severity stage of AMD with a clinical outcome measure that would be a target of therapeutic intervention. Based on longitudinal data of serial fundus autofluorescence images from patients with late atrophic AMD, it has become feasible to determine the progression of geographic atrophy in individual patients (Fig. 3.7) [33, 59].

This progression rate represents both a biologically based quantitative phenotype of late AMD and the most relevant target for future treatment strategy. In a preliminary analysis, we determined whether the risk alleles of both *CFH* and *LOC387715* are correlated with the progression of geographic atrophy in 207 AMD patients with geographic atrophy (with no signs of CNV). We found that the risk allele distribution of Y402H in *CFH* and A69S in *LOC387715* for patients with geographic atrophy is similar to those previously reported for pooled AMD samples. However, no correlation was found between the rate of progression of geographic atrophy and *CFH* and/or *LOC387715* genotype [60]. These data suggest that both genes contribute to the increased risk of advanced AMD largely or entirely through their impact on early disease events (such as drusen and/or other RPE/Bruch's membrane changes). This may have implications for therapeutic interventions in patients with late AMD, because the attempt to modify the respective gene products may not be promising [60].

Summary for the Clinician

- The *LOC387715/HTRA1* locus within 10q26 has been identified as a second major locus contributing to AMD pathogenesis.
- The two late forms of AMD, CNV and geographic atrophy, have not been found to be different in risk allele distribution.
- Variants within *CFH* and *LOC387715* may contribute to the increased risk of advanced AMD largely or entirely through their impact on precursors, such as drusen and/or other RPE/Bruch's membrane changes.

3.6 Factor B

A recent study has demonstrated that a candidate gene approach can be successful given the pre-existing knowledge that the complement system plays a significant role in AMD pathogenesis. In this study, Gold and colleagues reported an association with two other genes that encode regulatory proteins, which act along the same biological pathway as *CFH* [24]. These two genes are factor B (*BF*) and complement component 2 (*C2*), located 500 bp apart on chromosome 6p within the major histocompatibility complex class III region. The reported association was found in a sample of 898 patients with various forms of AMD and 389 controls. There was a common risk haplotype across *BF* and *C2* (OR, 1.32), as well as two protective haplotypes (OR, 0.36, and

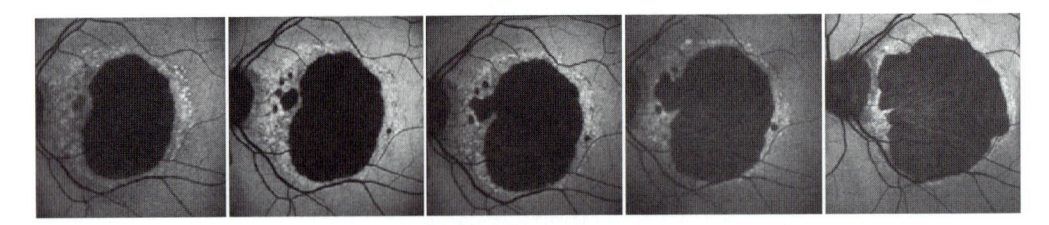

Fig. 3.7 Fundus autofluorescence images obtained in 12-month intervals in an AMD patient with a cSLO (Heidelberg retina angiograph, HRA classic and HRA 2; Heidelberg Engineering, Dossenheim, Germany). A large kidney-shaped area of geographic atrophy (GA) was present at baseline (*left*) corresponding to decreased fundus autofluorescence (*dark area*). Recovered in yearly intervals, the area of the central atrophic area increased [33]

0.45 respectively) [24]. These data were independently replicated [48].

Backing the statistical data, BF and C2 expression was found in the neural retina, RPE, and choroid. BF protein was present in ocular drusen and Bruch's membrane, and less prominently in the choroidal stroma. The distribution of BF was similar to that of C3, both of which are similar to that of CFH and C5b-9 [24].

3.7 Gene–Gene and Gene–Environment Interaction in AMD

In a comprehensive survey of variants at *CFH*, *LOC387715*, and *C2-BF* in 2,172 unrelated individuals (1,238 affected individuals and 934 controls), Maller and co-workers developed a risk model for AMD based on five validated common variants. In contrast to the modest elevation in overall risk to siblings (two- to six-fold [32, 40, 62]), the predictive value of specific genotype combinations was notable. For example, approximately 10% of the population are at a 40-fold greater risk and 1% (high-risk homozygotes at all three loci) are at a more than 250-fold greater risk compared with the baseline risk, which is observed in individuals carrying the lowest risk genotypes at all three loci (approximately 2% of the population; Fig. 3.8) [48].

When evaluating the role of gene–gene interaction (epistasis) among the five common variants at the three loci (*CFH*, *LOC387715*, and *C2-BF*), statistically significant nonadditive interactions were not found, despite excellent powers of detecting epistasis. Specifically, a model in which the risk alleles at the three gene loci act independently (individual risks are multiplied to generate a combined risk profile) provided a better fit of the observed data than the same model with the inclusion of interlocus interference [48]. Similarly, the study of Rivera et al. had indicated that the two risk alleles, *CFH* Y402H and *LOC387715* A69S, independently contribute to disease risk. Fitting an interaction model

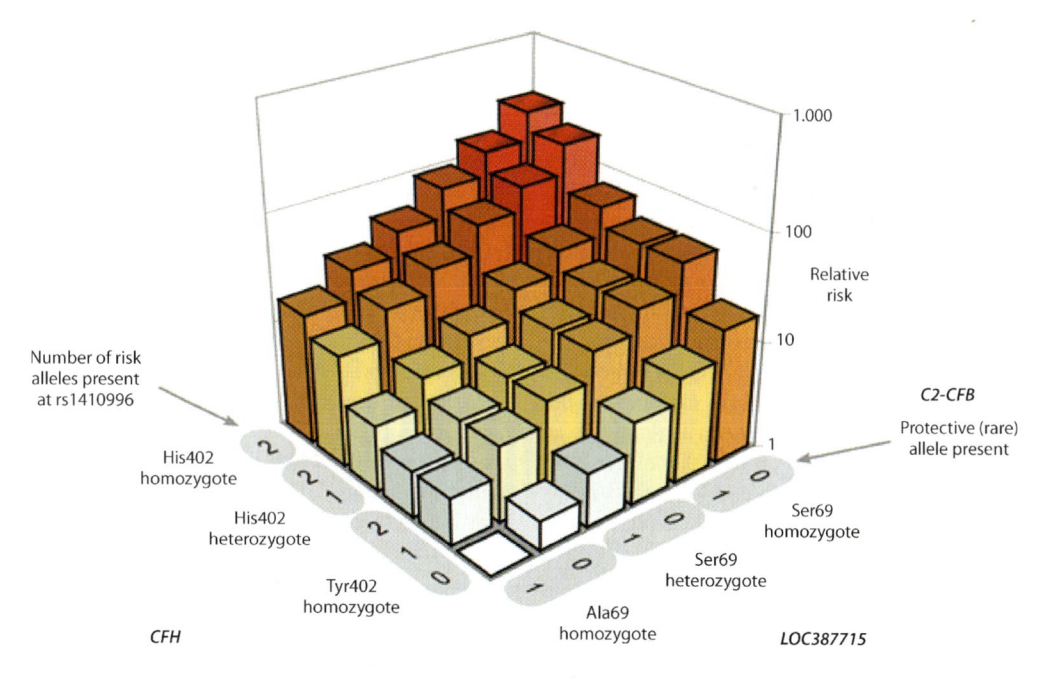

Fig. 3.8 Relative risk plotted as a function of the genetic load of the five variants that influence risk of AMD. Two variants are in *CFH*: Y402H and rs1410996. Another common variant (A69S) is *LOC387715*. Two relatively rare variants are observed in the C2 and factor B (BF) genes. From Maller et al., Fig. 1 [48], used with permission

between *CFH* and *LOC387715*, no evidence of epistasis was found [53]. Conley et al. also found an independent multiplicative effect of *CFH* and *LOC387715* without significant interaction in two independent cohorts [13].

Several environmental factors have been identified over the past decade including cigarette smoking [61, 70, 76, 77], higher body mass index (BMI) [2, 63], and nutritional factors [3, 79], with smoking being the most consistent in several population-based studies worldwide [70, 77]. So far, however, there are inconclusive data on gene–environment interactions. In an extended collection of 848 AMD cases, Rivera et al. [53] did not detect any significant differences in risk allele frequency for either *CFH* or *LOC387715* between smokers and nonsmokers, despite substantial power, whereas Schmidt and co-workers observed significant evidence of a statistical interaction between the *LOC387715* A69S variant and a history of cigarette smoking [58]. Despriet and colleagues found that the combined effect of homozygosity for the Y402H variant in *CFH* and smoking exceeds the sum of the independent effects. Compared with no exposure, smoking increased the risk of AMD 3.3-fold, the presence of two *CFH* Y402H risk alleles increased the risk 12.5-fold, while the combination of both determinants increased this risk 34-fold [16]. In contrast, Conley and co-workers did not find any significant interaction of risk allele distribution in *CFH* or *LOC3897715* and cigarette smoking [13]. Similarly, Seddon and co-workers found no statistically significant interaction between *CFH* genotype and cigarette smoking, but the susceptibility to advanced AMD was modified by the body mass index (BMI). Compared with lean individuals with the *CFH* TT genotype, an increased risk of AMD among these lean individuals with BMI lower than 25 was found only for the CC homozygotes. For heavier persons with BMI greater than 25, the risk varied from a nonsignificant null or slightly protective association for the TT genotype, to a moderately high 2.2-fold increased risk for the heterozygotes, and a very high 5.9-fold increased risk for the CC homozygote state. This interaction between BMI and the genotype-related risk of advanced AMD was statistically significant for the CT vs. TT genotype [66].

> **Summary for the Clinician**
>
> - Considering variants at *CFH*, *LOC387715*, and *C2-BF*, approximately 10% of the population are at a 40-fold greater risk and 1% are at a >250-fold greater risk of AMD compared with baseline.
> - So far, gene–gene interaction has not been detected.
> - Data on gene–environment interaction are inconclusive so far.

3.8 Conclusions

Genetic studies have convincingly demonstrated that there are common alleles that have a substantial effect on AMD pathogenesis at at least two independent gene loci.

The finding of such common alleles with substantial effect makes predictive DNA testing a tempting option, although the biological consequences of the common risk alleles at the respective gene loci are not yet understood. Consequently, the knowledge of being a carrier of risk alleles is currently not matched by adequate options for preventive strategies or possible treatment modalities.

The finding that variants at *CFH* and factor B are responsible for a large fraction of AMD cases (at least in Caucasians) suggests the importance of the alternative complement pathway in the pathobiology of AMD and further strengthens the notion that inflammation plays a major role in this common disease [24].

So far, the identification of genetic factors has not yet resulted in therapeutic strategies to modify the disease. The data on gene–environment interactions are inconclusive and gene–gene interactions have not been observed despite the substantial statistical power of the respective studies. Other genetic factors are most likely yet to be discovered. These, in combination with environmental variables, will further stratify individual risk more accurately. A correlation between the common genetic risk variants and clinical outcome measures (e.g., the progression of geographic atrophy) has not been observed. The role of rare variants is still obscure. Especially for the latter, refined phenotyping may be paramount.

Strategies to elucidate the genetic influence on AMD may include:
1. The search for additional susceptibility genes
2. The examination of the biological role of the known common variants (especially *CFH* and *LOC387715*)
3. The investigation of the gene–environment and gene–gene interactions
4. The identification of modifying genes

To achieve these goals, large cohorts of phenotypically well-characterized subcategories will be needed. Biologically-based quantitative phenotyping is required to increase the power of linkage and association studies. Because AMD is a complex disease, individual gene effects might only be detected within subgroups of patients with specific environmental exposures. Environmental factors for stratification include cigarette smoking and BMI. Also, a given gene variant might only result in a detectable phenotype when acting in combination with additional susceptibility alleles, either additively or multiplicatively. Additional work exploring these types of interactions should bring us closer to all the genes influencing the onset and progression of AMD.

Acknowledgements

Supported by: European Union (EU) FP6, Integrated Project "EVI-GENORET" (LSHG-CT-2005-512036); Deutsche Forschungsgemeinschaft (DFG) Heisenberg Fellowship SCHO 734/2-1; Pro Retina Research Grant Pro-Re/Seed/Issa. 1; DFG WE 1259/14-3; and the Ruth and Milton Steinbach Foundation, New York.

References

1. Abecasis GR, Yashar BM, Zhao Y, Ghiasvand NM, Zareparsi S, Branham KE, Reddick AC, Trager EH, Yoshida S, Bahling J, Filippova E, Elner S, Johnson MW, Vine AK, Sieving PA, Jacobson SG, Richards JE, Swaroop A (2004) Age-related macular degeneration: a high-resolution genome scan for susceptibility loci in a population enriched for late-stage disease. Am J Hum Genet 74:482–494
2. Anonymous (2000) Risk factors associated with age-related macular degeneration. A case-control study in the age-related eye disease study: age-related eye disease study report number 3. Age-Related Eye Disease Study Research Group. Ophthalmology 107:2224–2232
3. Age-Related Eye Disease Study Research Group (2001) A randomized, placebo-controlled, clinical trial of high-dose supplementation with vitamins C and E and beta carotene for age-related cataract and vision loss: AREDS report no. 9. Arch Ophthalmol 119:1439–1452
4. Allikmets R (2000) Further evidence for an association of ABCR alleles with age-related macular degeneration. The International ABCR Screening Consortium. Am J Hum Genet 67:487–491
5. Allikmets R, Shroyer NF, Singh N, Seddon JM, Lewis RA, Bernstein PS, Peiffer A, Zabriskie NA, Li Y, Hutchinson A, Dean M, Lupski JR, Leppert M (1997) Mutation of the Stargardt's disease gene (ABCR) in age-related macular degeneration. Science 277:1805–1807
6. Allikmets R, Singh N, Sun H, Shroyer NF, Hutchinson A, Chidambaram A, Gerrard B, Baird L, Stauffer D, Peiffer A, Rattner A, Smallwood P, Li Y, Anderson KL, Lewis RA, Nathans J, Leppert M, Dean M, Lupski JR (1997) A photoreceptor cell-specific ATP-binding transporter gene (ABCR) is mutated in recessive Stargardt macular dystrophy. Nat Genet 15:236–246
7. Ambati J, Ambati BK, Yoo SH, Ianchulev S, Adamis AP (2003) Age-related macular degeneration: etiology, pathogenesis, and therapeutic strategies. Surv Ophthalmol 48:257–293
8. Andersen N (2004) Age-related macular degeneration among the Inuit in Greenland. Int J Circumpolar Health 63 Suppl 2:320–323
9. Assink JJ, Klaver CC, Houwing-Duistermaat JJ, Wolfs RC, van Duijn CM, Hofman A, de Jong PT (2005) Heterogeneity of the genetic risk in age-related macular disease: a population-based familial risk study. Ophthalmology 112:482–487
10. Baum L, Chan WM, Li WY, Lam DS, Wang PB, Pang CP (2003) ABCA4 sequence variants in Chinese patients with age-related macular degeneration or Stargardt's disease. Ophthalmologica 217:111–114

11. Bindewald A, Schmitz-Valckenberg S, Jorzik JJ, Dolar-Szczasny J, Sieber H, Keilhauer C, Weinberger AW, Dithmar S, Pauleikhoff D, Mansmann U, Wolf S, Holz FG (2005) Classification of abnormal fundus autofluorescence patterns in the junctional zone of geographic atrophy in patients with age related macular degeneration. Br J Ophthalmol 89:874–878
12. Charbel Issa P, Scholl HPN, Holz FG, Oppermann M, Knolle P, Kurts C (2005) Das Komplementsystem und dessen mögliche Beteiligung an der Pathogenese der altersabhängigen Makuladegeneration (AMD) [The complement system and its possible role in the pathogenesis of age-related macular degeneration (AMD)]. Ophthalmologe 102:1036–1042
13. Conley YP, Jakobsdottir J, Mah T, Weeks DE, Klein R, Kuller L, Ferrell RE, Gorin MB (2006) CFH, ELOVL4, PLEKHA1, and LOC387715 genes and susceptibility to Age-Related Maculopathy: AREDS and CHS cohorts and meta-analyses. Hum Mol Genet 15(21):3206–3218
14. De Jong PT (2006) Age-related macular degeneration. N Engl J Med 355:1474–1485
15. De Jong PT, Klaver CC, Wolfs RC, Assink JJ, Hofman A (1997) Familial aggregation of age-related maculopathy. Am J Ophthalmol 124:862–863
16. Despriet DD, Klaver CC, Witteman JC, Bergen AA, Kardys I, de Maat MP, Boekhoorn SS, Vingerling JR, Hofman A, Oostra BA, Uitterlinden AG, Stijnen T, van Duijn CM, de Jong PT (2006) Complement factor H polymorphism, complement activators, and risk of age-related macular degeneration. JAMA 296:301–309
17. Edwards AO, Ritter R III, Abel KJ, Manning A, Panhuysen C, Farrer LA (2005) Complement factor H polymorphism and age-related macular degeneration. Science 308:421–424
18. Fisher SA, Abecasis GR, Yashar BM, Zareparsi S, Swaroop A, Iyengar SK, Klein BE, Klein R, Lee KE, Majewski J, Schultz DW, Klein ML, Seddon JM, Santangelo SL, Weeks DE, Conley YP, Mah TS, Schmidt S, Haines JL, Pericak-Vance MA, Gorin MB, Schulz HL, Pardi F, Lewis CM, Weber BH (2005) Meta-analysis of genome scans of age-related macular degeneration. Hum Mol Genet 14:2257–2264
19. Fleckenstein M, Bindewald-Wittich A, Schmitz-Valckenberg S, Scholl HPN, Dreyhaupt J, Mansmann U, Holz FG, FAM study group. Patterns of abnormal fundus autofluorescence in advanced atrophic AMD – impact on progression and sample size calculation for interventional clinical trials. Invest Ophthalmol Vis Sci 2006;47 [Suppl]:#5687(Abstract)
20. Friedman DS, O'Colmain BJ, Munoz B, Tomany SC, McCarty C, de Jong PT, Nemesure B, Mitchell P, Kempen J (2004) Prevalence of age-related macular degeneration in the United States. Arch Ophthalmol 122:564–572
21. Friedman DS, O'Colmain BJ, Munoz B, Tomany SC, McCarty C, de Jong PT, Nemesure B, Mitchell P, Kempen J (2004) Prevalence of age-related macular degeneration in the United States. Arch Ophthalmol 122:564–572
22. Fuse N, Suzuki T, Wada Y, Yoshida M, Shimura M, Abe T, Nakazawa M, Tamai M (2000) Molecular genetic analysis of ABCR gene in Japanese dry form age-related macular degeneration. Jpn J Ophthalmol 44:245–249
23. Gass JD (1973) Drusen and disciform macular detachment and degeneration. Arch Ophthalmol 90:206–217
24. Gold B, Merriam JE, Zernant J, Hancox LS, Taiber AJ, Gehrs K, Cramer K, Neel J, Bergeron J, Barile GR, Smith RT, Hageman GS, Dean M, Allikmets R, Chang S, Yannuzzi LA, Merriam JC, Barbazetto I, Lerner LE, Russell S, Hoballah J, Hageman J, Stockman H (2006) Variation in factor B (BF) and complement component 2 (C2) genes is associated with age-related macular degeneration. Nat Genet 38:458–462
25. Gorin MB, Breitner JC, de Jong PT, Hageman GS, Klaver CC, Kuehn MH, Seddon JM (1999) The genetics of age-related macular degeneration. Mol Vis 5:29
26. Grassi MA, Fingert JH, Scheetz TE, Roos BR, Ritch R, West SK, Kawase K, Shire AM, Mullins RF, Stone EM (2006) Ethnic variation in AMD-associated complement factor H polymorphism p.Tyr402His. Hum Mutat 27:921–925
27. Gregor Z, Joffe L (1978) Senile macular changes in the black African. Br J Ophthalmol 62:547–550
28. Guymer RH, Heon E, Lotery AJ, Munier FL, Schorderet DF, Baird PN, McNeil RJ, Haines H, Sheffield VC, Stone EM (2001) Variation of codons 1961 and 2177 of the Stargardt's disease gene is not associated with age-related macular degeneration. Arch Ophthalmol 119:745–751

29. Haddad S, Chen CA, Santangelo SL, Seddon JM (2006) The genetics of age-related macular degeneration: a review of progress to date. Surv Ophthalmol 51:316–363
30. Hageman GS, Anderson DH, Johnson LV, Hancox LS, Taiber AJ, Hardisty LI, Hageman JL, Stockman HA, Borchardt JD, Gehrs KM, Smith RJ, Silvestri G, Russell SR, Klaver CC, Barbazetto I, Chang S, Yannuzzi LA, Barile GR, Merriam JC, Smith RT, Olsh AK, Bergeron J, Zernant J, Merriam JE, Gold B, Dean M, Allikmets R (2005) A common haplotype in the complement regulatory gene factor H (HF1/CFH) predisposes individuals to age-related macular degeneration. Proc Natl Acad Sci USA 102:7227–7232
31. Haines JL, Hauser MA, Schmidt S, Scott WK, Olson LM, Gallins P, Spencer KL, Kwan SY, Noureddine M, Gilbert JR, Schnetz-Boutaud N, Agarwal A, Postel EA, Pericak-Vance MA (2005) Complement factor H variant increases the risk of age-related macular degeneration. Science 308:419–421
32. Heiba IM, Elston RC, Klein BE, Klein R (1994) Sibling correlations and segregation analysis of age-related maculopathy: the Beaver Dam Eye Study. Genet Epidemiol 11:51–67
33. Holz FG, Bellmann C, Staudt S, Schütt F, Völcker HE (2001) Fundus autofluorescence and development of geographic atrophy in age-related macular degeneration. Invest Ophthalmol Vis Sci 42:1051–1056
34. Holz FG, Pauleikhoff D, Klein R, Bird AC (2004) Pathogenesis of lesions in late age-related macular disease. Am J Ophthalmol 137:504–510
35. Hsu WM, Cheng CY, Liu JH, Tsai SY, Chou P (2004) Prevalence and causes of visual impairment in an elderly Chinese population in Taiwan: the Shihpai Eye Study. Ophthalmology 111:62–69
36. Hughes AE, Orr N, Esfandiary H, az-Torres M, Goodship T, Chakravarthy U (2006) A common CFH haplotype, with deletion of CFHR1 and CFHR3, is associated with lower risk of age-related macular degeneration. Nat Genet 38:1173–1177
37. Hyman LG, Lilienfeld AM, Ferris FL, Fine SL (1983) Senile macular degeneration: a case-control study. Am J Epidemiol 118:213–227
38. Iyengar SK, Song D, Klein BE, Klein R, Schick JH, Humphrey J, Millard C, Liptak R, Russo K, Jun G, Lee KE, Fijal B, Elston RC (2004) Dissection of genomewide-scan data in extended families reveals a major locus and oligogenic susceptibility for age-related macular degeneration. Am J Hum Genet 74:20–39
39. Jakobsdottir J, Conley YP, Weeks DE, Mah TS, Ferrell RE, Gorin MB (2005) Susceptibility genes for age-related maculopathy on chromosome 10q26. Am J Hum Genet 77:389–407
40. Klaver CC, Wolfs RC, Assink JJ, van Duijn CM, Hofman A, de Jong PT (1998) Genetic risk of age-related maculopathy. Population-based familial aggregation study. Arch Ophthalmol 116:1646–1651
41. Klein ML, Schultz DW, Edwards A, Matise TC, Rust K, Berselli CB, Trzupek K, Weleber RG, Ott J, Wirtz MK, Acott TS (1998) Age-related macular degeneration. Clinical features in a large family and linkage to chromosome 1q. Arch Ophthalmol 116:1082–1088
42. Klein RJ, Zeiss C, Chew EY, Tsai JY, Sackler RS, Haynes C, Henning AK, Sangiovanni JP, Mane SM, Mayne ST, Bracken MB, Ferris FL, Ott J, Barnstable C, Hoh J (2005) Complement factor H polymorphism in age-related macular degeneration. Science 308:385–389
43. Kuroiwa S, Kojima H, Kikuchi T, Yoshimura N (1999) ATP binding cassette transporter retina genotypes and age related macular degeneration: an analysis on exudative non-familial Japanese patients. Br J Ophthalmol 83:613–615
44. Li M, tmaca-Sonmez P, Othman M, Branham KE, Khanna R, Wade MS, Li Y, Liang L, Zareparsi S, Swaroop A, Abecasis GR (2006) CFH haplotypes without the Y402H coding variant show strong association with susceptibility to age-related macular degeneration. Nat Genet 38:1049–1054
45. Lim JI, Kwok A, Wilson DK (1998) Symptomatic age-related macular degeneration in Asian patients. Retina 18:435–438
46. Magnusson KP, Duan S, Sigurdsson H, Petursson H, Yang Z, Zhao Y, Bernstein PS, Ge J, Jonasson F, Stefansson E, Helgadottir G, Zabriskie NA, Jonsson T, Bjornsson A, Thorlacius T, Jonsson PV, Thorleifsson G, Kong A, Stefansson H, Zhang K, Stefansson K, Gulcher JR (2006) CFH Y402H confers similar risk of soft drusen and both forms of advanced AMD. PLoS Med 3:e5
47. Majewski J, Schultz DW, Weleber RG, Schain MB, Edwards AO, Matise TC, Acott TS, Ott J, Klein ML (2003) Age-related macular degeneration – a genome scan in extended families. Am J Hum Genet 73:540–550

48. Maller J, George S, Purcell S, Fagerness J, Altshuler D, Daly MJ, Seddon JM (2006) Common variation in three genes, including a noncoding variant in CFH, strongly influences risk of age-related macular degeneration. Nat Genet 38:1055–1059
49. Munoz B, West SK, Rubin GS, Schein OD, Quigley HA, Bressler SB, Bandeen-Roche K (2000) Causes of blindness and visual impairment in a population of older Americans: The Salisbury Eye Evaluation Study. Arch Ophthalmol 118:819–825
50. Oppermann M, Manuelian T, Jozsi M, Brandt E, Jokiranta TS, Heinen S, Meri S, Skerka C, Gotze O, Zipfel PF (2006) The C-terminus of complement regulator Factor H mediates target recognition: evidence for a compact conformation of the native protein. Clin Exp Immunol 144:342–352
51. Oshima Y, Ishibashi T, Murata T, Tahara Y, Kiyohara Y, Kubota T (2001) Prevalence of age related maculopathy in a representative Japanese population: the Hisayama study. Br J Ophthalmol 85:1153–1157
52. Rivera A, White K, Stohr H, Steiner K, Hemmrich N, Grimm T, Jurklies B, Lorenz B, Scholl HPN, Apfelstedt-Sylla E, Weber BHF (2000) A comprehensive survey of sequence variation in the ABCA4 (ABCR) gene in Stargardt's disease and age-related macular degeneration. Am J Hum Genet 67:800–813
53. Rivera A, Fisher SA, Fritsche LG, Keilhauer CN, Lichtner P, Meitinger T, Weber BH (2005) Hypothetical LOC387715 is a second major susceptibility gene for age-related macular degeneration, contributing independently of complement factor H to disease risk. Hum Mol Genet 14:3227–3236
54. Rodriguez de Corba S, Esparza-Gordillo J, Goicoechea de JE, Lopez-Trascasa M, Sanchez-Corral P (2004) The human complement factor H: functional roles, genetic variations and disease associations. Mol Immunol 41:355–367
55. Schachat AP, Hyman L, Leske MC, Connell AM, Wu SY (1995) Features of age-related macular degeneration in a black population. The Barbados Eye Study Group. Arch Ophthalmol 113:728–735
56. Schick JH, Iyengar SK, Klein BE, Klein R, Reading K, Liptak R, Millard C, Lee KE, Tomany SC, Moore EL, Fijal BA, Elston RC (2003) A whole-genome screen of a quantitative trait of age-related maculopathy in sibships from the Beaver Dam Eye Study. Am J Hum Genet 72:1412–1424
57. Schmidt S, Postel EA, Agarwal A, Allen IC, Jr., Walters SN, De La Paz MA, Scott WK, Haines JL, Pericak-Vance MA, Gilbert JR (2003) Detailed analysis of allelic variation in the ABCA4 gene in age-related maculopathy. Invest Ophthalmol Vis Sci 44:2868–2875
58. Schmidt S, Hauser MA, Scott WK, Postel EA, Agarwal A, Gallins P, Wong F, Chen YS, Spencer K, Schnetz-Boutaud N, Haines JL, Pericak-Vance MA (2006) Cigarette smoking strongly modifies the association of LOC387715 and age-related macular degeneration. Am J Hum Genet 78:852–864
59. Schmitz-Valckenberg S, Bindewald-Wittich A, Dolar-Szczasny J, Dreyhaupt J, Wolf S, Scholl HP, Holz FG (2006) Correlation between the area of increased autofluorescence surrounding geographic atrophy and disease progression in patients with AMD. Invest Ophthalmol Vis Sci 47:2648–2654
60. Scholl HPN, Bindewald-Wittich A, Schmitz-Valckenberg S, Fleckenstein M, Rivera A, Weber BHF, Holz FG, FAM study group. Correlation of CFH Y402h allele distribution and risk of progression of geographic atrophy in patients with age-related macular degeneration (AMD). Invest Ophthalmol Vis Sci 2006;47 (Suppl):#4338 (Abstract)
61. Seddon JM, Willett WC, Speizer FE, Hankinson SE (1996) A prospective study of cigarette smoking and age-related macular degeneration in women. JAMA 276:1141–1146
62. Seddon JM, Ajani UA, Mitchell BD (1997) Familial aggregation of age-related maculopathy. Am J Ophthalmol 123:199–206
63. Seddon JM, Cote J, Davis N, Rosner B (2003) Progression of age-related macular degeneration: association with body mass index, waist circumference, and waist-hip ratio. Arch Ophthalmol 121:785–792
64. Seddon JM, Santangelo SL, Book K, Chong S, Cote J (2003) A genomewide scan for age-related macular degeneration provides evidence for linkage to several chromosomal regions. Am J Hum Genet 73:780–790
65. Seddon JM, Cote J, Page WF, Aggen SH, Neale MC (2005) The US twin study of age-related macular degeneration: relative roles of genetic and environmental influences. Arch Ophthalmol 123:321–327

66. Seddon JM, George S, Rosner B, Klein ML (2006) CFH gene variant, Y402H, and smoking, body mass index, environmental associations with advanced age-related macular degeneration. Hum Hered 61:157–165
67. Shastry BS (2006) Further support for the common variants in complement factor H (Y402H) and LOC387715 (A69S) genes as major risk factors for the exudative age-related macular degeneration. Ophthalmologica 220:291–295
68. Sho K, Takahashi K, Yamada H, Wada M, Nagai Y, Otsuji T, Nishikawa M, Mitsuma Y, Yamazaki Y, Matsumura M, Uyama M (2003) Polypoidal choroidal vasculopathy: incidence, demographic features, and clinical characteristics. Arch Ophthalmol 121:1392–1396
69. Shroyer NF, Lewis RA, Yatsenko AN, Wensel TG, Lupski JR (2001) Cosegregation and functional analysis of mutant ABCR (ABCA4) alleles in families that manifest both Stargardt's disease and age-related macular degeneration. Hum Mol Genet 10:2671–2678
70. Smith W, Assink J, Klein R, Mitchell P, Klaver CC, Klein BE, Hofman A, Jensen S, Wang JJ, de Jong PT (2001) Risk factors for age-related macular degeneration: pooled findings from three continents. Ophthalmology 108:697–704
71. Souied EH, Ducroq D, Rozet JM, Gerber S, Perrault I, Munnich A, Coscas G, Soubrane G, Kaplan J (2000) ABCR gene analysis in familial exudative age-related macular degeneration. Invest Ophthalmol Vis Sci 41:244–247
72. Souied EH, Leveziel N, Richard F, Dragon-Durey MA, Coscas G, Soubrane G, Benlian P, Fremeaux-Bacchi V (2005) Y402H complement factor H polymorphism associated with exudative age-related macular degeneration in the French population. Mol Vis 11:1135–1140
73. Stone EM, Webster AR, Vandenburgh K, Streb LM, Hockey RR, Lotery AJ, Sheffield VC (1998) Allelic variation in ABCR associated with Stargardt's disease but not age-related macular degeneration. Nat Genet 20:328–329
74. Stone EM, Lotery AJ, Munier FL, Heon E, Piguet B, Guymer RH, Vandenburgh K, Cousin P, Nishimura D, Swiderski RE, Silvestri G, Mackey DA, Hageman GS, Bird AC, Sheffield VC, Schorderet DF (1999) A single EFEMP1 mutation associated with both Malattia Leventinese and Doyne honeycomb retinal dystrophy. Nat Genet 22:199–202
75. Stone EM, Braun TA, Russell SR, Kuehn MH, Lotery AJ, Moore PA, Eastman CG, Casavant TL, Sheffield VC (2004) Missense variations in the fibulin 5 gene and age-related macular degeneration. N Engl J Med 351:346–353
76. Thornton J, Edwards R, Mitchell P, Harrison RA, Buchan I, Kelly SP (2005) Smoking and age-related macular degeneration: a review of association. Eye 19:935–944
77. Tomany SC, Wang JJ, Van LR, Klein R, Mitchell P, Vingerling JR, Klein BE, Smith W, de Jong PT (2004) Risk factors for incident age-related macular degeneration: pooled findings from 3 continents. Ophthalmology 111:1280–1287
78. Uyama M, Takahashi K, Ida N, Miyashiro M, Ando A, Takahashi A, Yamada E, Shirasu J, Nagai Y, Takeuchi M (2000) The second eye of Japanese patients with unilateral exudative age related macular degeneration. Br J Ophthalmol 84:1018–1023
79. Van LR, Boekhoorn S, Vingerling JR, Witteman JC, Klaver CC, Hofman A, de Jong PT (2005) Dietary intake of antioxidants and risk of age-related macular degeneration. JAMA 294:3101–3107
80. Varma R, Fraser-Bell S, Tan S, Klein R, Azen SP (2004) Prevalence of age-related macular degeneration in Latinos: the Los Angeles Latino eye study. Ophthalmology 111:1288–1297
81. Webster AR, Heon E, Lotery AJ, Vandenburgh K, Casavant TL, Oh KT, Beck G, Fishman GA, Lam BL, Levin A, Heckenlively JR, Jacobson SG, Weleber RG, Sheffield VC, Stone EM (2001) An analysis of allelic variation in the ABCA4 gene. Invest Ophthalmol Vis Sci 42:1179–1189
82. Weeks DE, Conley YP, Tsai HJ, Mah TS, Schmidt S, Postel EA, Agarwal A, Haines JL, Pericak-Vance MA, Rosenfeld PJ, Paul TO, Eller AW, Morse LS, Dailey JP, Ferrell RE, Gorin MB (2004) Age-related maculopathy: a genomewide scan with continued evidence of susceptibility loci within the 1q31, 10q26, and 17q25 regions. Am J Hum Genet 75:174–189
83. Yates JR, Moore AT (2000) Genetic susceptibility to age related macular degeneration. J Med Genet 37:83–87
84. Zarbin MA (2004) Current concepts in the pathogenesis of age-related macular degeneration. Arch Ophthalmol 122:598–614

85. Zareparsi S, Branham KE, Li M, Shah S, Klein RJ, Ott J, Hoh J, Abecasis GR, Swaroop A (2005) Strong association of the Y402H variant in complement factor H at 1q32 with susceptibility to age-related macular degeneration. Am J Hum Genet 77:149–153

86. Zipfel PF, Misselwitz J, Licht C, Skerka C (2006) The role of defective complement control in hemolytic uremic syndrome. Semin Thromb Hemost 32:146–154

Chapter 4

Anti-VEGF Treatment for Age-Related Macular Degeneration

Todd R. Klesert, Jennifer I. Lim

Core Messages

- VEGF (vascular endothelial growth factor) is a key central mediator of choroidal neovascularization (CNV).
- VEGF is also a potent mediator of vascular permeability.
- VEGF acts as both a mitogen and survival factor for vascular endothelial cells, and its expression is regulated by tissue oxygen tension.
- VEGF acts through three tyrosine kinase receptors: VEGFR-1, VEGFR-2, and VEGFR-3.
- The only two anti-VEGF agents currently approved by the FDA for treatment of CNV are pegaptanib (Macugen) and ranibizumab (Lucentis).
- Pegaptanib is an aptamer (short oligonucleotide) that specifically binds and inhibits the action of the VEGF-165 isoform.
- Ranibizumab is a fragment of a humanized monoclonal antibody directed against all VEGF isoforms, including active breakdown products, and is a potent inhibitor of CNV.
- Bevacizumab is a full-sized humanized monoclonal antibody directed against VEGF, and is approved by the FDA for treatment of colon cancer. Bevacizumab is used widely off-label for the treatment of CNV.
- The efficacy and safety of bevacizumab for the treatment of CNV have been demonstrated in several small case series, but have not yet been confirmed in a large, randomized, controlled clinical trial
- Several new pharmacologic approaches to VEGF inhibition are currently in development, and may provide additional treatment options in the future.

4.1 Basic Science

4.1.1 Historical Perspective

In 1948, Michaelson [32] was the first to postulate that a diffusible factor produced by the retina ("factor X") was responsible for retinal and iris neovascularization associated with conditions such as proliferative diabetic retinopathy and central retinal vein occlusion. In 1968, experiments showed that neovascularization in a host could be stimulated by transplanted tumor cells, even when those cells were separated from the host by a Millipore filter, thus confirming the presence of endogenous, soluble, pro-angiogenic factors [11, 17].

Because of its dual physiologic properties, vascular endothelial growth factor (VEGF) was discovered independently through two separate lines of research. In 1983, Senger et al. [44] identified a protein that could induce vascular leakage in skin. They named this protein "tumor vascular permeability factor" or VPF. In 1989, Ferrara and Henzel [13] isolated a diffusible protein from bovine pituitary follicular cells that showed cell-specific mitogenic activity for vascular endothelium. They named this protein vascular endothelial growth factor (VEGF). Cloning of the cDNAs for both VPF and VEGF in 1989 demonstrated that the two molecules were in fact one –and the same [22, 26].

Evidence suggesting that VPF/VEGF might be Michaelson's long sought "factor X" first came in 1992 [48], when VEGF mRNA expression was found to be inducible in cell culture by hypoxia. Miller et al. [34] then demonstrated that aqueous VEGF levels correlated with the degree of neovascularization in a primate vein occlusion model, and that VEGF mRNA levels were upregulated in ischemic retina in these animals. In a study of 210 patients undergoing ocular surgery, Aiello et al. [2] confirmed that VEGF levels in ocular fluid correlated with neovascularization secondary to diabetic retinopathy and ischemic vein occlusion. The role for VEGF in CNV was confirmed soon after [25, 52].

4.1.2 VEGF Isoforms

Since the initial discovery of the VEGF/VPF gene (now known as VEGF-A), several additional closely related genes have been identified, including VEGF-B, VEGF-C, VEGF-D, and PlGF (placental growth factor). However, the role of these genes in angiogenesis appears to be more limited. It is VEGF-A signaling that represents the critical rate-limiting step in both normal and pathologic angiogenesis [21].

The human VEGF-A gene, located on chromosome 6p21.3, consists of eight exons and seven introns. Alternative splicing produces mRNA transcripts that code for at least six different protein isoforms: 121, 145, 165, 183, 189, and 206 amino acids in length [41]. These different isoforms vary in their affinity for heparin binding, and therefore in their affinity for the extracellular matrix. The larger isoforms, such as VEGF-189 and VEGF-206, bind heparin with high affinity, and are therefore almost completely sequestered in the extracellular matrix. The smaller isoform, VEGF-121, does not bind heparin and is freely diffusible. VEGF-165 lies somewhere in the middle. Because the heparin-binding domain appears to be critical for mitogenic activity [23], VEGF-165 is thought to represent the best compromise between bioavailability and biologic potency. Indeed, VEGF-165 is the predominant isoform and the primary mediator of neovascularization in the eye [12].

All VEGF isoforms contain a plasmin cleavage site. Cleavage at this site creates a freely-diffusible, 110-kD, bioactive form of VEGF (VEGF-110). Plasmin-mediated extracellular proteolysis may therefore be an important regulator of VEGF bioavailability [23].

4.1.3 VEGF Expression

The primary trigger of VEGF-A gene expression in the eye is hypoxia [27, 28]. Like the erythropoietin gene, the VEGF-A gene contains a 5' enhancer sequence that binds to hypoxia-inducible factor 1 (HIF-1). HIF-1, a basic helix-loop-helix transcription factor, is a key player in hypoxic responses in the cell [12], and is the primary mediator of hypoxia-induced gene expression of VEGF-A.

4.1.4 VEGF Receptors

VEGF binds to three closely related receptor tyrosine kinases, VEGFR-1, VEGFR-2, and VEGFR-3. VEGFR-1 (also known as Flt-1) was the first VEGF receptor to be identified [9], but its role remains incompletely understood. VEGFR-1 is the highest affinity receptor of the three, and its main function may be to act during embryonal development as a "decoy" by sequestering VEGF, thereby preventing the activation of VEGFR-2 [12]. In adults, VEGFR-3 is expressed only in lymphatic endothelial cells and appears to play a key role in lymphangiogenesis [20].

VEGFR-2 (also known as Flk-1 or KDR) is the primary mediator of the pathologic effects of VEGF in the eye. Binding of VEGF ligand to VEGFR-2 results in dimerization and autophosphorylation of the receptor, followed by phosphorylation of numerous proteins involved in cellular signal transduction, such as phospholipase C, PI3-kinase, ras GTPase activating protein, and src family proteins [12].

All three receptors are necessary for proper mammalian development. Mice with null mutations for any of the receptors die in utero between days 8.5 and 9.5 [10, 15, 46]. These mouse knock-out models also suggest the possible role of VEGF in hematopoiesis.

4.1.5 VEGF Activity

VEGF exerts multiple effects on endothelial cells, relating to its function as a pro-angiogenic factor. These include stimulation of cell proliferation, invasion, migration, and enhancement of cell survival. The mitogenic properties of VEGF are mediated through the protein C and MAP kinase pathways. Endothelial cell survival is mediated by the PI3 kinase/Akt pathway, as well as by upregulation of anti-apoptotic proteins such as Bcl-2, A1, and XIAP. Invasion and migration are mediated through upregulation of integrin expression, alteration of the cytoskeleton, and induction of metalloproteinases [12, 19].

Of particular importance in the pathogenesis of CNV is the potent effect VEGF has on vascular permeability. Vascular leakage is thought to facilitate angiogenesis because the leakage of plasma proteins and fibrin creates a gel-like environment conducive to endothelial cell growth and migration. Increased permeability is a result of both vasodilation and an uncoupling of endothelial tight junctions. Increased vascular permeability seems to be mediated, at least in part, via the nitrous oxide synthase (NOS) pathway [51], which may explain why hypertension has been observed in some patients treated with VEGF inhibitors.

4.2 Current Anti-VEGF Therapies

4.2.1 Aptamers: Pegaptanib Sodium (Macugen)

Approved by the FDA in 2004, pegaptanib (Macugen; OSI/Eyetech Pharmaceuticals, New York, NY, USA) is the first anti-VEGF agent with proven efficacy for the treatment of CNV secondary to age-related macular degeneration. Pegaptanib is an aptamer, a short single-stranded oligonucleotide sequence that functions as a high affinity inhibitor of a specific protein target. Aptamers are created by a form of in vitro evolution called SELEX (systematic evolution of ligands by exponential enrichment) [36].

Pegaptanib is a 28-base RNA oligonucleotide that is covalently linked to two 20-kD polyethylene glycol moieties to extend the half-life. Pegaptanib selectively binds to the heparin-binding domain of VEGF165 and larger isoforms, preventing ligand receptor binding. The smaller VEGF isoforms and proteolytic fragments are therefore not inhibited by pegaptanib [36].

The safety and efficacy of pegaptanib for the treatment of neovascular age-related macular degeneration was established through the VEGF Inhibition Study in Ocular Neovascularization (VISION) [16]. VISION consisted of two phase III prospective, multicenter, randomized, controlled, double-masked trials comparing intravitreal injection of pegaptanib every 6 weeks with sham injection. Patients (1,186 in total) were randomized to receive pegaptanib (at a dose of 0.3 mg, 1.0 mg, or 3.0 mg) or sham injection, every 6 weeks for a total of 54 weeks. The primary endpoint of the study was the number of patients losing less than 15 letters of ETDRS (Early Treatment Diabetic Retinopathy Study) visual acuity at 54 weeks. The study enrolled patients with all choroidal neovascular lesion subtypes up to and including 12 disc areas in size, and permitted use of concomitant photodynamic therapy with verteporfin (Visudyne) at the physician's discretion. Twenty-five percent of the patients in the study also received photodynamic therapy during the study period.

In the pooled analysis, efficacy was demonstrated for all three doses, without a dose–response relationship, with 70% of pegaptanib-treated patients losing less than 15 letters, compared with 55% of sham-treated control patients. More pegaptanib-treated patients maintained their visual acuity or gained visual acuity (33%) at 54 weeks than sham-treated controls (23%). In addition, the sham-treated group was twice as likely to experience severe vision loss (≥30 letters) during the study period than pegaptanib-treated patients. However, only 6% of pegaptanib-treated patients in the study gained ≥15 letters at 54 weeks (compared with 2% of sham-treated controls), and as a group, the pegaptanib-treated patients lost an average of 8 letters over the study period (compared with 15 letters in the sham-treated group). Adverse ocular events in the VISION trial resulted in severe vision loss in 0.1% of patients. These adverse events included endophthalmitis (1.3%), traumatic lens injury (0.6%), and retinal detachment (0.6%). No increase in the rate of serious systemic adverse events was noted in the pegaptanib-treated patients.

For year 2 of the VISION study, patients were re-randomized to the treatment and sham arms [8]. The results indicated that those patients continuing with pegaptanib treatment for a second year did better than those reassigned to the sham control arm at 54 weeks, and better than those assigned to the control arm for the entire 2 years. The percentage of pegaptanib-treated patients who progressed to vision loss of >15 letters (from baseline) during the second year of treatment was half (7%) that of those reassigned to the control group at 54 weeks (14%), and those who continued in the control group for the second year (14%). Of note, however, patients who had benefited from their year 1 treatment assignment (defined as vision loss of ≥0 letters from baseline), and who subsequently lost ≥10 letters of vision after re-randomization at 54 weeks, were allowed to receive "salvage therapy" (a reassignment back to their original year 1 treatment arm)

Studies with pegaptanib are ongoing. The VERITAS study is a phase III prospective, multicenter, randomized, double-masked trial comparing photodynamic therapy combined with one of two doses of intravitreal triamcinolone (1 mg or 4 mg) versus photodynamic therapy combined with 0.3 mg of intravitreal pegaptanib. Approximately 100 patients have been enrolled, including cases of all choroidal neovascular lesion subtypes (Kaiser et al., *abstract*, Retina Society Meeting, Cape Town, South Africa, October 2006).

Studies are also ongoing at OSI/Eyetech to create a sustained-release form of pegaptanib, with the goal of reducing the frequency of intravitreal injections required for treatment, and thereby reducing the risk of serious adverse events associated with intravitreal injections, such as endophthalmitis and retinal detachment. Preliminary animal work with poly(lactic-co-glycolic) acid (PLGA)-based microsphere encapsulation suggests that sustained-release of pegaptanib for more than 6 months is possible after a single intravitreal injection (Adamis et al., *abstract*, Retina Society Meeting, Cape Town, South Africa, October 2006).

4.2.2 Monoclonal Antibodies: Ranibizumab (Lucentis)

In June 2006, ranibizumab (Lucentis; Genentech, South San Francisco, CA, USA) became the second VEGF inhibitor approved by the FDA for use in the treatment of CNV secondary to age-related macular degeneration. Ranibizumab is a humanized, affinity-maturated Fab fragment of a murine monoclonal antibody directed against human VEGF-A. Ranibizumab is a potent, non-selective inhibitor of all VEGF-A isoforms and bioactive proteolytic products. Ranibizumab was created from a full-sized antibody (bevacizumab – see Sect. 4.2.3) developed previously as an anti-cancer agent. It was felt that a full-sized antibody would be unable to penetrate efficiently to the inner retina and choroid, as suggested by a histologic study of the herceptin antibody [35]. More recent histologic analysis of bevacizumab in rabbits by Shahar et al. [45], however, suggests that the full-length antibody actually penetrates all layers of the retina quite effectively. Because ranibizumab is missing the Fc region, it is also felt that the molecule will be less likely to incite an immune response, as it can no longer bind to complement C1q or Fc gamma receptors [21].

Efficacy and safety of ranibizumab has thus far been established through two large prospective, multicenter, randomized, double-masked, controlled clinical trials: MARINA [43] and ANCHOR [7]. MARINA stands for Minimally Classic/Occult Trial of Anti-VEGF Antibody Ranibizumab in the Treatment of Neovascular Age-Related Macular Degeneration. As the name implies, the MARINA trial was limited to patients with subfoveal occult or minimally classic CNV, either primary or recurrent, with evidence of recent disease progression. Seven hundred and sixteen patients were randomized 1:1:1 to receive monthly intravitreal injections of ranibizumab (either 0.3 mg or 0.5 mg) or sham injections. The primary outcome measure was the proportion of patients losing less than 15 letters of ETDRS visual acuity at 12 months; 94.5% of patients assigned to the 0.3-mg group and 94.6% of patients assigned to the 0.5-mg ranibizumab treatment arms, compared with 62.2% in the sham treatment arm, met this endpoint. The percentage of patients gaining 15 or more letters of visual acuity by month 12 was likewise higher in the ranibizumab treatment arms: 24.8% in the 0.3-mg group and 33.8% in the 0.5-mg group, compared with 5.0% in the sham-treated group. Mean visual acuity at month 12 increased by 6.5 letters in the 0.3-mg group and 7.2 letters in the 0.5-mg group. In contrast, mean visual acuity dropped by 10.4 letters in the sham-treated group. In general, vision gains were maintained throughout year 2 of the MARINA trial in ranibizumab-treated patients, whereas vision continued to decline in the sham-treated patients, to a mean loss of 14.9 letters.

Measurement of choroidal neovascular lesions during the course of the study demonstrated that while lesion size on average remained stable in the ranibizumab-treated patients, lesion size increased by about 50% by the end of year 1 in the sham-treated patients. Moreover, the area of measured leakage in the lesions of ranibizumab-treated patients decreased on average by approximately half at 1 year, while the leakage area increased in the sham-treated patients.

Adverse ocular events in ranibizumab-treated patients in the MARINA trial over 24 months included presumed endophthalmitis in 1.0% of patients and serious uveitis in 1.3% of patients. No retinal detachments were observed in the ranibizumab-treated patients, although retinal tears were identified in 2 patients (0.4%). Lens damage as a result of intravitreal injection was seen in 1 patient (0.2%). No statistically significant difference in serious systemic adverse events was observed between the treatment and control arms of the study.

The ANCHOR trial—short for Anti-VEGF Antibody for the Treatment of Predominantly Classic Choroidal Neovascularization in AMD—has likewise demonstrated the efficacy of ranibizumab for the treatment of predominantly classic choroidal neovascular lesions secondary to age-related macular degeneration. ANCHOR was designed as a head-to-head comparison between ranibizumab and photodynamic therapy (PDT) with verteporfin (Visudyne), which until recently had been the standard of care for subfoveal CNV. Four hundred and twenty-three patients were randomized 1:1:1 to receive monthly intravitreal injections with ranibizumab 0.3 mg and sham PDT, ranibizumab 0.5 mg with sham PDT or monthly sham injections plus active verteporfin PDT. As in the MARINA trial, the primary endpoint in ANCHOR was the number of patients losing fewer than 15 letters of baseline visual acuity at 12 months; 94.3% of the patients receiving 0.3 mg ranibizumab and 96.4% of patients receiving 0.5 mg ranibizumab versus 64.3% in the verteporfin group achieved the primary endpoint. The percentages of patients experiencing an improvement over baseline visual acuity of at least 15 letters were 35.7% and 40.3% respectively in the ranibizumab-treated patients, versus only 5.6% in the verteporfin-treated patients. Mean visual acuity at month 12 increased by 8.5 letters in the 0.3-mg group and 11.3 letters in the 0.5-mg ranibizumab group. In contrast, mean visual acuity dropped by 9.5 letters in the verteporfin PDT group.

Measurement of choroidal neovascular lesions throughout the ANCHOR study revealed positive morphologic effects similar to those observed in the MARINA study. In general, average total lesion size remained relatively stable in the ranibizumab-treated patients over 1 year, while increasing significantly in the verteporfin-treated patients. Moreover, the average total area of leakage and the average total area of classic leakage both decreased significantly at 1 year in the ranibizumab-treated patients, while they increased in the verteporfin-treated group.

Serious adverse ocular events in ranibizumab-treated patients in the ANCHOR trial over 12 months included presumed endophthalmitis in 0.7% of patients and serious uveitis in 0.4% of patients. One case of retinal detachment was observed in the ranibizumab-treated patients (0.4%), as was 1 case of vitreous hemorrhage (0.4%). Lens damage as a result of intravitreal injection was not observed. Mild post-injection inflammation was the most common adverse event observed in the ANCHOR trial, occurring in 12% of patients. No statistically significant difference in serious system adverse events was observed between the ranibizumab and verteporfin arms of the study.

Several additional clinical trials of ranibizumab are ongoing at this time. The PIER study is a Phase IIIb, prospective, multicenter, randomized, double-masked, controlled study of 184 patients with predominantly classic or occult CNV randomized to receive ranibizumab or sham injections monthly for the first 3 months, followed by once every 3 months for a total of 24 months. The purpose of PIER is to help determine the optimal dosing schedule for ranibizumab. The 1-year results of the PIER study showed that 83% (0.3 mg) and 90% (0.5 mg) of ranibizumab-treated eyes lost less than 15 letters of visual acuity, compared with 49% of sham eyes. However, the percentage of eyes improving by 15 or more letters was only 12% (0.3 mg) and 13% (0.5 mg) in ranibizumab-treated eyes, compared with 10% of sham eyes (reported at the Retinal Physician Symposium, Bahamas, June 2006).

PRONTO is a 2-year, single site, open-label, uncontrolled study of 40 patients designed to evaluate the durability of response of ranibizumab and whether optical coherence tomography (OCT) can be used to guide treatment of neovascular AMD. As in the PIER study, patients receive monthly injections of ranibizumab for the first 3 months. Thereafter, the patient is assessed monthly by OCT, and every 3 months by fluorescein angiography. Patients are given additional ranibizumab injections only if central OCT thickness increases by ≥100 µm, if visual acuity declines by 5 or more letters associated with evidence of fluid on OCT, if there is new onset classic neovascularization, or if new macular hemorrhage is present. Preliminary visual acuity results through 1 year (Fung et al., *abstract*, Retina Society Meeting, Cape Town Oct. 2006) are thus far roughly comparable to visual acuity outcomes in the MARINA and ANCHOR trials. The PIER and PRONTO studies will help determine whether treatment with ranibizumab must be continued on a monthly basis, or whether less frequent dosing regimens can be utilized.

The FOCUS study [18] is a 2-year, phase I/II, multicenter, randomized, single-masked, controlled study of 162 patients with predominantly classic CNV. FOCUS is designed to compare the safety and efficacy of intravitreal ranibizumab (0.5 mg) combined with verteporfin PDT versus verteporfin PDT alone (combined with sham injection). Preliminary results at 12 months showed that 90.5% of patients treated with the combination of verteporfin PDT and ranibizumab lost fewer than 15 letters from baseline visual acuity, compared with 67.9% of control patients treated with verteporfin PDT alone. Adverse events in the ranibizumab-treated patients included intraocular inflammation in 11.4% and endophthalmitis in 1.9% (4.8% if presumed cases were included). Notably, ranibizumab-treated patients experiencing intraocular inflammation still had better visual acuity outcomes at 12 months than the control patients.

4.2.3 Monoclonal Antibodies: Bevacizumab (Avastin)

Bevacizumab (Avastin; Genentech) is a full-length humanized murine monoclonal antibody directed against human VEGF-A, and thus a closely-related drug to ranibizumab. It was approved by theFDA in 2004 for the intravenous treatment of metastatic colorectal cancer. Its potential for the treatment of CNV was first tested by Michels et al. [33] via intravenous infusion in a 12-week, open-label, uncontrolled study. Striking effects were observed on both visual acuity and the OCT and angiographic characteristics of the neovascular lesions. However, patients experienced a mean increase of 12 mmHg in systolic blood pressure, which was felt to be a deterrent to its common use.

This systemic side effect, combined with the promising visual and anatomic results from the intravenous infusion of bevacizumab, led investigators to consider the intravitreal injection of bevacizumab [42]. Since then, several retrospective, uncontrolled, open-label case series have been published regarding the use of intravitreal bevacizumab for the treatment of CNV secondary to AMD [3, 6, 40, 49]. As with ranibizumab, the effect of bevacizumab has been impressive.

Avery and colleagues [3] treated 79 patients with 1.25 mg of intravitreal bevacizumab monthly and reported the early results after 3 months' follow-up. Many of these patients had had prior failed treatment with verteporfin or pegaptanib. At 3 months, median Snellen visual acuity improved from 20/200 at baseline to 20/80. Mean central retinal thickness by OCT decreased by 67 µm at 3 months. No ocular or systemic adverse events were observed.

Spaide and colleagues [49] treated 266 patients with a monthly dose of 1.25 mg of intravitreal bevacizumab. By 3 months, Snellen visual acuity improved from a mean of 20/184 at baseline to 20/109, with 38.3% of patients experiencing some improvement in visual acuity. Mean central retinal thickness by OCT improved from 340 μm at baseline to 213 μm at 3 months. Again, no adverse ocular or systemic adverse events were observed.

In contrast to the intravenous administration of bevacizumab, intravitreal injection of bevacizumab did not result in the systemic side effect of hypertension in any of these studies. The systemic concentration of bevacizumab, when given intravenously, is obviously several times larger than the systemic concentrations seen after intravitreal injections, and no elevation in blood pressure has yet been reported in patients treated with intravitreal bevacizumab.

Animal and in vitro studies published thus far have failed to identify any specific toxicity associated with bevacizumab use. Luthra et al. [29] demonstrated that the viability of human RPE cells, rat neurosensory cells, and human microvascular endothelial cells in culture was normal after exposure to bevacizumab at concentrations of up to 1 mg/ml. Rabbit studies by Manzano et al. [31] found no changes in the ERG patterns of eyes injected with intravitreal bevacizumab at doses up to 5.0 mg. Mild vitreous inflammation was seen at the 5.0 mg dose, but not at lower doses. Bakri et al. [5] looked at the retinal histology of rabbit eyes injected with bevacizumab and again found no histologic changes compared with control eyes.

One important aspect in which ranibizumab and bevacizumab may differ is their pharmacokinetics. Because of its larger molecular weight, it is assumed that bevacizumab has a significantly longer half-life in the vitreous, and possibly systemically as well. A longer half-life may allow for less frequent injections to achieve the same biologic effect. Recent unpublished data, however, indicate that the half-lives of the two drugs may actually be quite similar. According to the package insert for Lucentis, the half-life of ranibizumab in the vitreous is approximately 3 days based on animal studies. Pharmacokinetic studies in rabbits reveal that the half-life of bevacizumab in the vitreous is only marginally longer at 4.3 days (Bakri et al., *abstract*, Retina Society Meeting, Cape Town, October 2006).

Although the limited data thus far suggest that bevacizumab is highly effective and safe for the treatment of CNV secondary to AMD, without a head-to-head prospective clinical trial, the relative efficacy and safety of bevacizumab compared with ranibizumab will remain unknown. Fortunately, the National Eye Institute has agreed to sponsor a trial comparing bevacizumab with ranibizumab in AMD patients with subfoveal CNV. This study, the CATT (Comparison of Treatment Trial) Study, will randomize patients into one of four treatment arms: monthly intravitreal injection of ranibizumab, monthly injection of bevacizumab, monthly injection of ranibizumab followed by treatment on an as-needed basis, and monthly injection of bevacizumab followed by as-needed treatment. Until the results of the CATT Study are available, bevacizumab is nonetheless an attractive treatment option due to its cost advantage over ranibizumab, especially for those patients without drug insurance coverage or with large drug co-payment requirements.

Summary for the Clinician

- Pegaptnanib is a VEGF-165 isoform-specific inhibitor.
- Pegaptanib is safe.
- Pegaptanib-treated patients still on average lose vision over time.
- Ranibizumab inhibits all VEGF isoforms.
- Ranibizumab is safe.
- Ranibizumab-treated patients on average gain vision over time.
- Ranibizumab is the current standard of care for most cases of CNV.
- Bevacizumab inhibits all VEGF isoforms.
- Intravitreal use of bevacizumab is off-label.
- Bevacizumab appears to have a similar safety and efficacy profile as ranibizumab, but this is yet to be confirmed by randomized clinical controlled trials.

4.3 Anti-VEGF Therapy: Practical Considerations

4.3.1 Intravitreal Injection Technique

It appears that the greatest risks associated with the use of current anti-VEGF therapies for the treatment of AMD (endophthalmitis, retinal detachment, lens trauma) come from the intravitreal injection itself. Therefore, proper injection technique and careful antiseptic practices are important.

Supplies that are recommended for prepping the eye include 5% povidine–iodine solution, povidine–iodine sticks, and a sterile lid speculum. At our center, we use sterile gloves, a sterile drape, and an empty sterile 1 cc tuberculin syringe to mark the sclera. Alternatively, one can use a caliper to mark the location for the injection procedure. The drug is drawn from the drug vial using a filtered needle attached to a tuberculin syringe. The needle is then changed to a sterile 30-gauge needle prior to the injection. Preinjection prophylactic antibiotic drops may also be used, although no benefit of antibiotic prophylaxis has been established.

The eye should first be anesthetized. In our hands, topical anesthesia appears to work just as well as subconjunctival injection of lidocaine, but either method can be used. For topical anesthesia, a cotton tip applicator is soaked with tetracaine and placed under the upper or lower eyelid in the conjunctival fornix, so that it rests against the superotemporal or inferotemporal bulbar conjunctiva at the site where the injection is planned. The patient should be instructed to look in the opposite direction and remain that way, so as not to scratch the cornea on the cotton tip applicator. After 3–5 min, the applicator can be removed and the eye prepped with 5% povidine–iodine solution placed directly on the eye, and povidine sticks used to clean the eyelids, lashes, and periocular skin. Gloves are then worn and the sterile lid speculum placed to hold the eyelids open. A sterile drape can be placed over the eye if desired, but is not necessary. The patient is then asked to fix their gaze in the direction opposite to where the injection is planned, so as to provide the best possible exposure. Providing the patient with an object to fixate upon, such as their own raised thumb, can improve stability of the eye during the injection.

A sterile 1-cc syringe is used as a ruler to mark the site of injection. The safest point of injection in phakic patients is 4 mm posterior to the limbus, and the round tip of the tuberculin 1-cc syringe happens to be exactly 4 mm in diameter. (A sterile caliper can also be used.) The syringe containing the drug is then used to inject the drug into the vitreous cavity through the pars plana with a 30-gauge needle (0.05 cc total volume in the case of ranibizumab or bevacizumab, 0.1 cc total volume in the case of pegaptanib). The needle is withdrawn and a dry cotton tip applicator is immediately applied over the injection site for a few seconds to help prevent prolapse and incarceration of vitreous in the wound, which can serve as a possible wick for the introduction of bacteria. Antibiotic drops are then placed in the eye and the lid speculum is removed. The eye pressure is monitored following the injection to confirm that it returns to normal. Finally, the patient is sent home with prophylactic antibiotic drops to be used for 3 days.

Most compliant patients do not need to be rechecked in the clinic until they are due for their next injection 4–6 weeks later, presuming you give them clear instructions on the signs and symptoms of infection or retinal detachment and are confident that they will call you immediately if they were to develop these symptoms. Povidine–iodine can be quite irritating to the corneal epithelium. It is therefore normal for patients to have some degree of irritation, burning, and tearing following their injection, in addition to varying amounts of subconjunctival hemorrhage. The wise physician will warn their patients of these possibilities at the time of injection in order to prevent the inevitable after-hours telephone call. However, any antiseptic-associated discomfort should resolve by the following day. Therefore, any pain or decreased vision reported by the patient on post-injection day 1 or later should be taken very seriously.

4.3.2 Safety Considerations

The observation that injection of intravitreal bevacizumab [4] or pegaptanib [1] for the treatment of proliferative diabetic retinopathy results in regression of neovascularization in the fellow eye provides compelling evidence that these molecules are indeed absorbed systemically to levels that are clinically relevant. Although no serious systemic concerns were raised by the MARINA, ANCHOR or VISION studies, it should be remembered that studies of this size are powered to detect only relatively large differences in rare events between the study groups. A modest increase in the risk of heart attack or stroke, for example, might not be detected by these studies. Given that serious systemic adverse events were noted in the clinical trials of intravenous bevacizumab for the treatment of metastatic colon cancer—perhaps most notably a 2-fold increase in the risk of serious thromboembolic events— these potent drugs should be used with caution, especially in patients with a history of stroke, myocardial infarction, angina or blood clot.

It should also be remembered that VEGF plays an important role in normal angiogenesis and vasculogenesis. Therefore, although usually not a consideration when treating a disease such as AMD, VEGF inhibitors should probably not be used in women who are pregnant or breastfeeding, and should be used only very cautiously in pre-pubescent children.

Because bevacizumab has been approved by the FDA only for the intravenous treatment of metastatic colon cancer, intravitreal injection of bevacizumab is an off-label use of the drug by an altered route of administration. This makes documentation of the informed consent process especially important when using bevacizumab. During informed consent, the physician should explain to patients that the safety and efficacy of bevacizumab has not been established with certainty, and that there may be unknown risks with its use. A bevacizumab-specific consent form is recommended, and can be found on the website of the Ophthalmic Mutual Insurance Company (OMIC—www.omic.com) [24].

4.3.3 Bevacizumab (Avastin) Preparation: Compounding Pharmacies

Bevacizumab comes in preservative-free 100-mg vials, containing 4 cc of a 25 mg/cc solution, intended for one-time use only for treatment of a single cancer patient. A single vial can theoretically be aliquoted out to provide up to 80 individual 0.05 cc intravitreal doses in 1-cc tuberculin syringes. While certainly economical, treating multiple macular degeneration patients with a single vial of bevacizumab does raise several important patient safety and professional liability issues. A federal standard for preadministration manipulation of compounded sterile preparations was established in January 2004, as codified by USP Chapter 797. Any physician who intends to use intravitreal bevacizumab should have the medication prepared only by a compounding pharmacy that complies fully with Chapter 797 [24]. The pharmacy should confirm the dose and sterility, provide proper storage instructions, and mark all aliquots with an expiration date. Although bevacizumab is a very stable drug with a shelf-life of many months, compounded aliquots will usually have an expiration date of only a few weeks due to sterility concerns. The use of bevacizumab past the expiration date specified by the compounding pharmacy is not recommended.

Summary for the Clinician

- The greatest risks of anti-VEGF therapy appear to arise from the intravitreal injection itself.
- Proper antiseptic and injection techniques are critical to minimize these risks.
- Anti-VEGF agents are potent drugs and should be used with all due caution and consideration
- Bevacizumab should be prepared by a qualified compounding pharmacy

4.4 Future Anti-VEGF Therapies

4.4.1 VEGF Trap

Pegaptanib, ranibizumab, and bevacizumab all act through inhibition of VEGF-A; they do not bind other members of the VEGF family. VEGF Trap (Regeneron, Tarrytown, NY, USA) is an experimental new drug designed to inhibit all members of the VEGF family: VEGF-A, -B, -C,

-D, and PlGF-1 and -2. VEGF Trap is a recombinant chimeric VEGF receptor fusion protein in which the binding domains of VEGF receptors 1 and 2 are combined with the Fc portion of immunoglobulin G to create a stable, soluble, high-affinity inhibitor. Not only does VEGF Trap bind all known members of the VEGF family, but it binds VEGF-A with higher affinity (kD <1 pmol/l) than any of the currently available anti-VEGF drugs [37]. Whether the broader spectrum and higher affinity of VEGF Trap equates to improved efficacy in the treatment of CNV secondary to AMD is yet to be determined.

VEGF Trap is currently undergoing phase I clinical trials. The CLEAR-AMD 1 Study is a randomized, multicenter, placebo-controlled, dose escalation study designed to assess the safety, tolerability, and bioactivity of VEGF Trap [37]. The study enrolled 25 patients who had CNV secondary to AMD, with lesions ≥12 disc areas in size, with ≥50% active leakage, and with ETDRS visual acuity of ≤20/40. Patients were randomized to receive either placebo, or one of three doses of VEGF Trap (0.3, 1.0, or 3.0 mg/kg) as a single intravenous dose, followed by a 4-week observation period, then three additional doses 2 weeks apart. Dose-limiting toxicity was observed for 2 out of 5 patients treated with the 3.0-mg/kg dose: 1 patient developed grade 4 hypertension and the other developed grade 2 proteinuria. Although reduced leakage on fluorescein angiography and reduced retinal thickening on OCT was observed in the patients treated with VEGF Trap, no corresponding reduction in choroidal neovascular lesion size or improvement in visual acuity was observed in these patients over the short 71-day study period. It was concluded that the maximum tolerated intravenous dose of VEGF Trap was 1.0 mg/kg.

The CLEAR-IT 1 Study is similarly designed to assess the safety, tolerability, and bioactivity of VEGF Trap through the intravitreal route of administration (Nguyen et al., *abstract*, Retina Society Meeting, Cape Town, October 2006). The study enrolled 21 patients using the same inclusion criteria as CLEAR-AMD 1, and randomized them to receive one of six doses of VEGF Trap as a single intravitreal injection: 0.05, 0.15, 0.5, 1.0, 2.0 or 4.0 mg. After 43 days of follow-up, no adverse ocular or systemic events were observed. Mean decrease in excess foveal thickness for all patients was 72%. The mean increase in ETDRS visual acuity was 4.75 letters and visual acuity remained stable or improved in 95% of patients. Notably, 3 out of 6 patients treated with the higher doses (2.0 or 4.0 mg) gained ≥3 lines of visual acuity by day 43.

Clearly, VEGF Trap shows promise as a novel treatment for CNV secondary to AMD.

4.4.2 Small Interfering RNAs

In 1998, Fire and Mello and colleagues [14] discovered that injection of gene-specific double-stranded RNA into cells results in the potent silencing of that gene's expression. They had stumbled upon one of the fundamental mechanisms by which the cell regulates gene expression and protects itself against viral infection: RNA interference. For their discovery, Fire and Mello were awarded the Nobel Prize in Physiology and Medicine in 2006.

The components of the RNA interference machinery have since been identified. Double-stranded RNA binds to a protein complex called Dicer, which cleaves it into multiple smaller fragments. A second protein complex called RISC then binds these RNA fragments and eliminates one of the strands. The remaining strand stays bound to RISC, and serves as a probe that recognizes the corresponding messenger RNA transcript in the cell. When the RISC complex finds a complementary messenger RNA transcript, the transcript is cleaved and degraded, thus silencing that gene's expression [39].

Small interfering RNAs (siRNAs) have quickly become important tools in genetic research. Their potential as therapeutic agents is being explored in many areas of medicine, and ophthalmology is no exception. Reich and Tolentino [39, 50] were the first to apply siRNA technology to the treatment of choroidal neovascularization, and their research has progressed to the phase II clinical trial stage, with a drug called bevasiranib/Cand5 (Acuity Pharmaceuticals, Philadelphia, PA, USA). Bevasiranib/Cand5 is an siRNA inhibitor of VEGF designed for intravitreal injection. A phase I, open-label, dose escalation study of 15 patients revealed no serious ocular or systemic adverse effects at doses up to 3.0 mg.

The CARE study (short for Cand5 Anti-VEGF RNAi Evaluation) is a phase II multicenter, randomized, double-masked, trial of bevasiranib/Cand5 in patients with CNV secondary to AMD (Brucker et al., Retina Society Meeting, Cape Town, October 2006; Thompson et al., AAO Meeting, Las Vegas, November 2006). One hundred and twenty-seven patients with predominantly classic, minimally classic, or retinal angiomatous proliferation lesions (occult with no classic lesions excluded) were randomized to receive one of three doses of the drug (0.2 mg, 1.5 mg, and 3.0 mg) at baseline and at 6 weeks. The primary endpoint was the mean change in ETDRS visual acuity from baseline at 12 weeks, which was -4 letters (0.2 mg), -7 letters (1.5 mg), and -6 letters (3.0 mg). The authors have theorized that these disappointing results stem from the fact that bevasiranib/Cand5 only blocks the production of new VEGF—VEGF already present at the time of injection is not inhibited. The investigators postulated that a baseline combination treatment with a VEGF protein blocker may be required to "mop up" the preexisting VEGF load. The half-life of VEGF is short and it does not explain why the results were not seen by the 12-week mark with siRNA treatment. The efficacy of the proposed treatment combination remains to be shown. The investigators envision the role of bevasiranib/Cand5 more as being a long-term "maintenance" drug. The CARE trial raised no safety concerns, with only 1 patient developing uveitis.

Other therapeutic targets for siRNAs are being investigated. siRNAs directed against the VEGFR-1 receptor have shown promise in a mouse model of CNV [47], and are currently in clinical development (Sirna-027; Sirna Therapeutics, Boulder, CO, USA).

4.4.3 Receptor Tyrosine Kinase Inhibitors

Non-RNA inhibitors of VEGF receptor tyrosine kinase activity have been identified, and their anti-angiogenic properties are being investigated for use in the treatment of systemic malignancy, as well as CNV. One advantage of this class of drugs over those discussed thus far in this chapter is the possibility of an oral route of administration, thereby avoiding the ocular complications associated with frequent intravitreal injections.

One promising compound is PTK787, which is a nonselective inhibitor of all known VEGF receptors [53]. PTK787 has been shown to inhibit retinal neovascularization in a hypoxic mouse model [30, 38]. Phase I/II clinical trials of PTK787 (Vatalanib; Novartis, East Hanover, NJ, USA) have been carried out in patients with both solid and hematologic malignancies. A multicenter phase I trial of PTK787/Vatalanib in patients with macular degeneration—the ADVANCE study—is currently enrolling patients. Patients with all CNV lesion types will receive photodynamic therapy with Visudyne at baseline, and will be randomized to receive concurrent treatment with either 500 mg or 1,000 mg of oral PTK787/Vatalanib, or placebo, once daily for 3 months (Joondeph, *abstract*, Retina Society Meeting, Cape Town, October 2006). ADVANCE is designed to assess the safety and efficacy of the drug.

AG-013958 (Pfizer, San Diego, CA, USA) is a selective VEGFR and PDGFR inhibitor that is currently in phase I/II testing. The route of administration being examined is subtenons injection. The preliminary results of 21 patients with subfoveal CNV indicated that adverse events were mild [21].

Summary for the Clinician

- VEGF Trap shows promise as a novel treatment for CNV.
- SiRNAs may become an important new class of drugs in the future.
- Early phase II results of an siRNA inhibitor of VEGF have been disappointing.
- Receptor tyrosine kinase inhibitors may allow for oral treatment of CNV in the future.

4.5 Conclusion

Anti-VEGF treatment has enabled a sizeable proportion of treated patients to attain significant visual improvement or to maintain vision. Future research will hopefully continue to build on these advances and make restoration of vision a reality for the majority of these patients.

References

1. Adamis AP, Altaweel M, Bressler NM, Cunningham ET Jr, Davis MD, Goldbaum M, Gonzales C, Guyer DR, Barrett K, Patel M; Macugen Diabetic Retinopathy Study Group (2006) Changes in retinal neovascularization after pegaptanib (Macugen) therapy in diabetic individuals. Ophthalmology 113:23–28
2. Aiello LP, Avery RL, Arrigg PG, Keyt BA, Jampel HD, Shah ST, Pasquale LR, Thieme H, Iwamoto MA, Park JE et al (1994) Vascular endothelial growth factor in ocular fluid of patients with diabetic retinopathy and other retinal disorders. N Engl J Med 331:1480–1487
3. Avery RL, Pieramici DJ, Rabena MD, Castellarin AA, Nasir MA, Giust MJ (2006) Intravitreal bevacizumab (Avastin) for neovascular age-related macular degeneration. Ophthalmology 113:363–372
4. Avery RL, Pearlman J, Pieramici DJ, Rabena MD, Castellarin AA, Nasir MA, Giust MJ, Wendel R, Patel A (2006) Intravitreal bevacizumab (Avastin) in the treatment of proliferative diabetic retinopathy. Ophthalmology 113:1695 (e1–15)
5. Bakri SJ, Cameron JD, McCannel CA, Pulido JS, Marler RJ (2006) Absence of histologic retinal toxicity of intravitreal bevacizumab in a rabbit model. Am J Ophthalmol 142:162–164
6. Bashshur ZF, Bazarbachi A, Schakal A, Haddad ZA, El Haibi CP, Noureddin BN (2006) Intravitreal bevacizumab for the management of choroidal neovascularization in age-related macular degeneration. Am J Ophthalmol 142(1):1–9
7. Brown DM, Kaiser PK, Michels M, Soubrane G, Heier JS, Kim RY, Sy JP, Schneider S; ANCHOR Study Group (2006) Ranibizumab versus verteporfin for neovascular age-related macular degeneration. N Engl J Med 355:1432–1444
8. Chakravarthy U, Adamis AP, Cunningham ET Jr, Goldbaum M, Guyer DR, Katz B, Patel M (2006) VEGF Inhibition Study in Ocular Neovascularization (V.I.S.I.O.N.) Clinical Trial Group Year 2 efficacy results of 2 randomized controlled clinical trials of pegaptanib for neovascular age-related macular degeneration. Ophthalmology 113:1508–1521
9. De Vries C, Escobedo JA, Ueno H, Houck K, Ferrara N, Williams LT (1992) The fms-like tyrosine kinase, a receptor for vascular endothelial growth factor. Science 255:989–991
10. Dumont DJ, Jussila L, Taipale J, Lymboussaki A, Mustonen T, Pajusola K, Breitman M, Alitalo K (1998) Cardiovascular failure in mouse embryos deficient in VEGF receptor-3. Science 282:946–949
11. Ehrmann RL, Knoth M (1968) Choriocarcinoma. Transfilter stimulation of vasoproliferation in the hamster cheek pouch. Studied by light and electron microscopy. J Natl Cancer Inst 41:1329–1341
12. Ferrara N (2004) Vascular endothelial growth factor: basic science and clinical progress. Endocr Rev 25:581–611
13. Ferrara N, Henzel WJ (1989) Pituitary follicular cells secrete a novel heparin-binding growth factor specific for vascular endothelial cells. Biochem Biophys Res Commun 161:851–858
14. Fire A, Xu S, Montgomery MK, Kostas SA, Driver SE, Mello CC (1998) Potent and specific genetic interference by double-stranded RNA in Caenorhabditis elegans. Nature 391:806–811
15. Fong GH, Zhang L, Bryce DM, Peng J (1999) Increased hemangioblast commitment, not vascular disorganization, is the primary defect in flt-1 knock-out mice. Development 126:3015–3025
16. Gragoudas ES, Adamis AP, Cunningham ET Jr, Feinsod M, Guyer DR (2004) VEGF Inhibition Study in Ocular Neovascularization Clinical Trial Group. Pegaptanib for neovascular age-related macular degeneration. N Engl J Med 351:2805–2816
17. Greenblatt M, Shubik P (1968) Tumor angiogenesis: transfilter diffusion studies in the hamster by the transplant chamber technique. J Natl Cancer Inst 41:111–124
18. Heier JS, Boyer DS, Ciulla TA, Ferrone PJ, Jumper JM, Gentile RC, Kotlovker D, Chung CY, Kim RY; FOCUS Study Group (2006) Ranibizumab com-

bined with verteporfin photodynamic therapy in neovascular age-related macular degeneration: year 1 results of the FOCUS Study. Arch Ophthalmol 124:1532–1542
19. Hicklin DJ, Ellis LM (2005) Role of the vascular endothelial growth factor in tumor growth and angiogenesis. J Clin Oncol 23:1011–1027
20. Kaipainen A, Korhonen J, Mustonen T, van Hinsbergh VW, Fang GH, Dumont D, Breitman M, Alitalo K (1995) Expression of the fms-like tyrosine kinase 4 gene becomes restricted to lymphatic endothelium during development. Proc Natl Acad Sci USA 92:3566–3570
21. Kaiser PK (2006) Antivascular endothelial growth factor agents and their development: therapeutic implications in ocular diseases. Am J Ophthalmol 142:660e1–e10
22. Keck PJ, Hauser SD, Krivi G, Sanzo K, Warren T, Feder J, Connolly DT (1989) Vascular permeability factor, an endothelial cell mitogen related to PDGF. Science 246:1309–1312
23. Keyt BA, Berleau LT, Nguyen HV, Chen H, Heinsohn H, Vandlen R, Ferrara N (1996) The carboxyl-terminal domain (111-165) of vascular endothelial growth factor is critical for its mitogenic potency. J Biol Chem 271:7788–7795
24. Klesert TR (2005) So you want to try intravitreal Avastin. Retina Times 14:18–21
25. Kvanta A, Algvere PV, Berglin L, Seregard S (1996) Subfoveal fibrovascular membranes in age-related macular degeneration express vascular endothelial growth factor. Invest Ophthalmol Vis Sci 37:1929–1934
26. Leung DW, Cachianes G, Kuang WJ, Goeddel DV, Ferrara N (1989) Vascular endothelial growth factor is a secreted angiogenic mitogen. Science 246:1306–1309
27. Levy AP, Levy NS, Wegner S, Goldberg MA (1995) Transcriptional regulation of the rat vascular endothelial growth factor gene by hypoxia. J Biol Chem 270:13333–13340
28. Liu Y, Cox SR, Morita T, Kourembanas S (1995) Hypoxia regulates vascular endothelial growth factor gene expression in endothelial cells. Identification of a 5' enhancer. Circ Res 77:638–643
29. Luthra S, Narayanan R, Marques LE, Chwa M, Kim DW, Dong J, Seigel GM, Neekhra A, Gramajo AL, Brown DJ, Kenney MC, Kuppermann BD (2006) Evaluation of in vitro effects of bevacizumab (Avastin) on retinal pigment epithelial, neurosensory retinal, and microvascular endothelial cells. Retina 26:512–518
30. Maier P, Unsoeld AS, Junker B, Martin G, Drevs J, Hansen LL, Agostini HT (2005) Intravitreal injection of specific receptor tyrosine kinase inhibitor PTK787/ZK222 584 improves ischemia-induced retinopathy in mice. Graefes Arch Clin Exp Ophthalmol 243:593–596
31. Manzano RP, Peyman GA, Khan P, Kivilcim M (2006) Testing intravitreal toxicity of bevacizumab (Avastin). Retina 26:257–261
32. Michaelson IC (1948) The mode of development of the vascular system of the retina with some observations on its significance for certain retinal disorders. Trans Ophthalmol Soc UK 68:137–180
33. Michels S, Rosenfeld JR, Puliafito CA, Marcus EN, Venkatraman AS (2005) Systemic bevacizumab (Avastin) therapy for neovascular age-related macular degeneration: twelve-week results of an uncontrolled open-label clinical study. Ophthalmology 112:1035–1047
34. Miller JW, Adamis AP, Shima DT, D'Amore PA, Moulton RS, O'Reilly MS, Folkman J, Dvorak HF, Brown LF, Berse B et al (1994) Vascular endothelial growth factor/vascular permeability factor is temporally and spatially correlated with ocular angiogenesis in a primate model. Am J Pathol 145:574–584
35. Mordenti J, Cuthbertson RA, Ferrara N, Thomsen K, Berleau L, Licko V, Allen PC, Valverde CR, Meng YG, Fei DT, Fourre KM, Ryan AM (1999) Comparisons of the intraocular tissue distribution, pharmacokinetics, and safety of 125I-labeled full-length and Fab antibodies in rhesus monkeys following intravitreal administration. Toxicol Pathol 27:536–544
36. Ng EW, Shima DT, Calias P, Cunningham ET Jr, Guyer DR, Adamis AP (2006) Pegaptanib, a targeted anti-VEGF aptamer for ocular vascular disease. Nat Rev Drug Discov 5:123–132
37. Nguyen QD, Shah SM, Hafiz G, Quinlan E, Sung J, Chu K, Cedarbaum JM, Campochiaro PA; CLEAR-AMD 1 Study Group (2006) A phase I trial of an IV-administered vascular endothelial growth factor trap for treatment in patients with choroidal neovascularization due to age-related macular degeneration. Ophthalmology 113:1522–1538

38. Ozaki H, Seo MS, Ozaki K, Yamada H, Yamada E, Okamoto N, Hofmann F, Wood JM, Campochiaro PA (2000) Blockade of vascular endothelial cell growth factor receptor signaling is sufficient to completely prevent retinal neovascularization. Am J Pathol 156:697–707
39. Reich SJ, Fosnot J, Kuroki A, Tang W, Yang X, Maguire AM, Bennett J, Tolentino MJ (2003) Small interfering RNA (siRNA) targeting VEGF effectively inhibits ocular neovascularization in a mouse model. Mol Vis 9:210–216
40. Rich RM, Rosenfeld PJ, Puliafito CA, Dubovy SR, Davis JL, Flynn HW Jr, Gonzalez S, Feuer WJ, Lin RC, Lalwani GA, Nguyen JK, Kumar G (2006) Short-term safety and efficacy of intravitreal bevacizumab (Avastin) for neovascular age-related macular degeneration. Retina 26:495–511
41. Robinson C, Stinger S (1991) The splice variants of vascular endothelial growth factor (VEGF) and their receptors. J Cell Sci 114:853–865
42. Rosenfeld PJ, Moshfeghi AA, Puliafito CA (2005) Optical coherence tomography findings after an intravitreal injection of bevacizumab (Avastin) for neovascular age-related macular degeneration. Ophthalmic Surg Lasers Imaging 36:331–335
43. Rosenfeld PJ, Brown DM, Heier JS, Boyer DS, Kaiser PK, Chung CY, Kim RY; MARINA Study Group (2006) Ranibizumab for neovascular age-related macular degeneration. N Engl J Med 355:1419–1431
44. Senger DR, Galli SJ, Dvorak AM, Perruzzi CA, Harvey VA, Dvorak HF (1983) Tumor cells secrete a vascular permeability factor that promotes accumulation of ascites fluid. Science 219:983–985
45. Shahar J, Avery RL, Heilweil G, Barak A, Zemel E, Lewis GP, Johnson PT, Fisher SK, Perlman I, Loewenstein A (2006) Electrophysiologic and retinal penetration studies following intravitreal injection of bevacizumab (Avastin). Retina 26:262–269
46. Shalaby F, Rossant J, Yamaguchi TP, Gertsenstein M, Wu XF, Breitman ML, Schuh AC (1995) Failure of blood-island formation and vasculogenesis in Flk-1-deficient mice. Nature 376:62–66
47. Shen J, Samul R, Silva RL, Akiyama H, Liu H, Saishin Y, Hackett SF, Zinnen S, Kossen K, Fosnaugh K, Vargeese C, Gomez A, Bouhana K, Aitchison R, Pavco P, Campochiaro PA (2006) Suppression of ocular neovascularization with siRNA targeting VEGF receptor 1. Gene Ther 13:225–234
48. Shweiki D, Itin A, Soffer D, Keshet E (1992) Vascular endothelial growth factor induced by hypoxia may mediate hypoxia-initiated angiogenesis. Nature 359:843–845
49. Spaide RF, Laud K, Fine HF, Klancnik JM Jr, Meyerle CB, Yannuzzi LA, Sorenson J, Slakter J, Fisher YL, Cooney MJ (2006) Intravitreal bevacizumab treatment of choroidal neovascularization secondary to age-related macular degeneration. Retina 26:383–390
50. Tolentino MJ, Brucker AJ, Fosnot J, Ying GS, Wu IH, Malik G, Wan S, Reich SJ (2004) Intravitreal injection of vascular endothelial growth factor small interfering RNA inhibits growth and leakage in a nonhuman primate, laser-induced model of choroidal neovascularization. Retina 24:132–138
51. Weis SM, Cheresh DA (2005) Pathophysiological consequences of VEGF-induced vascular permeability. Nature 437:497–504
52. Wells JA, Murthy R, Chibber R, Nunn A, Molinatti PA, Kohner EM, Gregor ZJ (1996) Levels of vascular endothelial growth factor are elevated in the vitreous of patients with subretinal neovascularisation. Br J Ophthalmol 80:363–366
53. Wood JM, Bold G, Buchdunger E, Cozens R, Ferrari S, Frei J, Hofmann F, Mestan J, Mett H, O'Reilly T, Persohn E, Rosel J, Schnell C, Stover D, Theuer A, Towbin H, Wenger F, Woods-Cook K, Menrad A, Siemeister G, Schirner M, Thierauch KH, Schneider MR, Drevs J, Martiny-Baron G, Totzke F (2000) PTK787/ZK 222584, a novel and potent inhibitor of vascular endothelial growth factor receptor tyrosine kinases, impairs vascular endothelial growth factor-induced responses and tumor growth after oral administration. Cancer Res 60:2178–2189

Chapter 5

Intravitreal Injections: Techniques and Sequelae

Heinrich Heimann

Core Messages

- Through the introduction of new treatment strategies for exudative age-related macular degeneration, the number of intravitreal injections has increased dramatically over the past few years. It is likely that this form of therapy will become the most common surgical intervention in ophthalmology within a short period of time.
- Although severe ocular adverse events associated with intraocular injections are rare, the rate can increase significantly if certain standards for intraocular interventions are not followed. Several guidelines on the technique for intravitreal injections have been published in recent years. Strict adherence to these guidelines is advisable.
- Endophthalmitis is the most feared complication of intravitreal injections. It is usually caused by bacterial contamination during or immediately after the injection and occurs in about 0.1% of injections and in about 1% of patients with repeated injections.
- Ocular hypertension and cataract development are not typically seen after anti-VEGF therapy.
- Based on the studies and data currently available, no major difference in the risk profile of the anti-VEGF drugs used at present can be seen.
- Triamcinolone is associated with a higher rate of secondary ocular hypertension (40%) and need for glaucoma surgery (1%) than anti-VEGF agents. It also has a higher rate of cataract progression in about 40% of patients within the first year of treatment.

5.1 Introduction

The introduction of new drugs for the treatment of age-related macular degeneration (AMD) has led to a significant change in ophthalmological practice. Until a few years ago, intravitreal injections were reserved for a small number of rare diseases (e.g., endophthalmitis, viral retinitis). Within a short period of time, the numbers of injections have increased and are now second only to cataract surgery as the most common treatment in most tertiary centers across Europe and the United States. It is likely that intravitreal injections with the anti-vascular endothelial growth factor (VEGF) type of action will soon become the most common intraocular procedure performed worldwide. With intravitreal injection we can obtain a high intraocular concentration of a drug, with minimal systemic exposure.

This tremendous and rapid change indicates a significant challenge for ophthalmological units; a tidal wave of intraocular injections, re-injections, and follow-up examinations has to be integrated into daily routine without compromising patients' safety. It is therefore mandatory to maintain essential safety standards for all injections whilst avoiding unnecessary and costly examinations and safety measures. In order to maximize the number of patients that can be treated, the workload associated with each patient has to be minimized within the treating unit; therefore, it is likely that more and more pre- and postoperative examinations will be shifted to places outside the centers where the injections are performed. In a relatively short period of time, ophthalmologists and optometrists who are currently not performing intraocular injections will be confronted with a larger number of patients following intravitreal injections. In this chapter, the techniques, complications, and guidelines for intravitreal injections are reviewed. Because of the recent shift in the application of intravitreal drugs, the chapter focuses on studies of anti-VEGF substances and triamcinolone.

5.2 Complications of Intravitreal Injections

With an appropriate technique, the intravitreal injection of a drug is a straightforward surgical procedure that carries a low rate of serious complications (Table 5.1). Yet, the first published multicenter study showed that the disregard

Table 5.1 Complications of intravitreal injections

Complication	Peri-operative	Early (>7 days)	Late (>7 days)	Incidence	Related to injected substance
Conjunctival hemorrhage	X	X		~20–40%	–
Conjunctival scarring			X		
Punctate keratitis	X	X		~30%	–
Pain	X	X		~30%	
Traumatic cataract	X	X	X	<1%	–
Cataract progression			X	First year: ~15% ~40% (triamcinolone)	X
Central retinal artery occlusion	X	X		<1%	–
Vitreous reflux	X	X		~20%	–
Vitreous hemorrhage	X	X	X	<1%	–
Vitreous floaters	X	X	X	~30%	X
Intraocular inflammation	X	X		~20%	X
Uveitis/pseudo-endophthalmitis		X		~1%	X
Endophthalmitis		X	X	~0.15% per injection ~1% per patient with multiple injections	X
Retinal detachment		X	X	<1%	–
Ocular hypertension	X	X	X	Triamcinolone ~40%	X

of basic standards for intraocular surgery can quickly increase the rate of complications to unacceptable levels. In the initial stages of the VISION trial, the rates of bacterial endophthalmitis were more than 4-fold higher than those after routine cataract surgery [8, 14]. Serious adverse events occurred in 19% of patients (169 out of 892), although serious adverse events were also noted in 15% of patients (45 out of 298) with sham treatment [8]. These figures underline that intravitreal injections should be treated as intraocular surgery and conducted according to the standards applied to all intraocular procedures, e.g., asepsis of the operating field and a sterile technique throughout the process. Even with the greatest care, complications associated with intravitreal injections will never be avoided completely; however, as demonstrated in the recent large prospective trials, in only very few cases will these complications lead to a long-term reduction in visual acuity or discontinuation of the treatment if dealt with in a timely and appropriate fashion [4, 8, 14, 29].

5.2.1 Methodology

In this chapter, the complications associated with intraocular injections are reviewed. A methodological review is flawed by several problems:

1. The most serious side effects of intravitreal injections (e.g., endophthalmitis, retinal detachment, glaucoma, cataract) are rare following anti-VEGF treatment and occur in less than 1% of injections and in about 1–2% of patients undergoing repeated injections. Only randomized prospective trials with large patient numbers are able to reflect the true rate of complications associated with the drug examined and the treatment protocol applied. Such trials have been published for pegaptanib and ranibizumab (Table 5.2) [4, 8, 14, 29].
2. For the two other currently most commonly used drugs, bevacizumab and triamcinolone, such studies do not exist and it is unlikely that this will be the case in the near future.
3. Other important, potentially sight-threatening complications of injections are intraocular inflammation, cataract development, and a rise in intraocular pressure (IOP). The examination methods, time points, and definitions for the detection of these complications vary from study to study.
4. Different protocols for the performance of intravitreal injections have been used. The differences in the injection technique (e.g., subconjunctival anesthesia, perioperative drug treatment, etc.) can have a significant influence on the complication rate.

5.2.2 Perioperative Complications

Complications following intravitreal injections can be divided according to their occurrence into perioperative, early postoperative, and late (Table 5.1). Furthermore, complications from the intraocular injection procedure itself have to be distinguished from possible biological side-effects of the injected substance.

5.2.2.1 Conjunctival Hemorrhage

Conjunctival hemorrhage is related to the trauma caused by manipulations during the injection, e.g., forceps or needle injuries. Obviously, when subconjunctival anesthesia is used, the need for two injections increases the risk of this complication. In one series, subconjunctival hemorrhages could be seen in 18% of patients with intravitreal injections and topical anesthesia versus 40% in patients with subconjunctival anesthesia [22]. Nevertheless, even with topical anesthesia, hemorrhage can be seen in up to 37% of patients [7].

In the vast majority of cases, conjunctival hemorrhages is more cosmetically disturbing than harmful. They clear spontaneously within 7–14 days and do not require any therapy. Very rarely, they can progress to cause significant anterior segment problems that require surgical intervention. The risk of significant conjunctival hemorrhage seems to be increased in patients with anticoagulant therapy, e.g., warfarin [15]. In contrast to their relative insignificance in the majority of cases, conjunctival hemorrhage is often perceived as a serious side-effect from the patients' point of view. Particularly in an outpatient setting without a scheduled short-term follow-up examination, patients have to be instructed about

Table 5.2 Ocular adverse events in studies of pegaptanib and ranibizumab

	Follow-up (months)	Number of patients	Number of injections	Endophthalmitis (*n*)	Per patient (%)	Per injection (%)
Pegaptanib						
VISION [14]						
0.3 mg		295				
1.0 mg		301				
3.0 mg		296				
First year	12	892	7,545	12	1.3	0.16
Second year		374	4,091	4	1.0	0.1
Ranibizumab						
MARINA [29]						
0.3 mg	24	238	NA	2	0.8	
0.5 mg	24	240	NA	3	1.2	
Total		478	10,443	5	1.0	0.05
ANCHOR [4]	12					
0.3 mg	12	137	1,507	0	0	0
0.5 mg	12	140	1,568	2	0.14	
Total		277	3,075	2	0.07	0.006
Control groups						
VISION (sham injection)	24	298				
ANCHOR (PDT)	12	140			0	
MARINA (sham injection)	24	238			0	

Inflammation (%)	Uveitis (%)	Cataract (%)	Cataract surgery (%)	Glaucoma (%)		Retinal detachment (%)
16		Split in different grades, highest grade 17%		>35 mmHg 9		
14		18		9		1
13		22		15		0.3
			<1			
						1.6
17	1.2	15	5.1	>30 mmHg 13.0	>40 mmHg 2.3	–
21	1.2	15	7.2	17.6	2.3	–
19	1.2		6.1			–
12		11	5.3	>30 mmHg 8.8	>40 mmHg 2.9	0.7
8		12.9	1.2	8.6	2.9	–
						0.3
16		26	18			
3		7.0	0	>30 mmHg 4.2	>40 mmHg 0.7	0.7
12	0	15.7		>30 mmHg 3.4	>40 mmHg 0	0.4

their appearance and natural course. Strategies to minimize their incidence include the use of topical versus subconjunctival anesthesia and the use of a cotton bud for conjunctival manipulation instead of forceps.

5.2.2.2 Conjunctival Scarring

Repeat injections, especially when combined with subconjunctival anesthesia, will lead to conjunctival scarring. Significant conjunctival scarring or ocular surface disorders as a result of multiple intravitreal injections have not been reported in larger studies to date. However, if repeated injections are necessary, it is recommended to record the position of the injection and to avoid repeated injection in the same location if possible.

5.2.2.3 Pain

Pain can be related to the anesthesia, the needle entry through the conjunctiva and sclera, and the rise in IOP associated with the injection. When subconjunctival anesthesia is used, patients experience pain associated with the subconjunctival injection, but less pain when the needle enters the posterior segment. In the VISION trial, 34% of patients (subconjunctival anesthesia and intravitreal injection) versus 28% of the controls (subconjunctival anesthesia and sham injection) experienced pain [8]. When topical anesthesia is used, the pain associated with the subconjunctival injection is avoided; however, the intravitreal injection is more painful [22]. Overall, the patients' expected levels of pain and discomfort are usually greater than those from the actual experience [30].

5.2.2.4 Punctate Keratitis and Corneal Edema

Punctate keratitis was detected in 32% of patients in the VISION trial versus 27% of controls [8]. It has not been noted as a complication in other trials. The most likely cause is a combination of the anesthesia of the ocular surface, a reduced blink reflex after corneal anesthesia, flushing of the corneal surface with antiseptic solution, the prolonged exposure of the cornea for the duration of the injection, and irregularities of the ocular surface after the injection. A combination of these factors and the intermittent rise in IOP can also cause corneal edema; this was noted in 9% of patients in the VISION trial [8]. However, to date there are no suggestions that the corneal surface or the corneal endothelium can be affected through a direct toxic effect of the injected substances. To avoid damage to the corneal epithelium, the exposure time following topical anesthesia should be minimized. Alternatively, ocular lubricants can be applied following the procedure.

5.2.2.5 Vitreous Reflux

The intravitreal injection of 0.1 ml of fluid is associated with a rise in IOP to around 45 mmHg [3]. During removal of the needle, vitreous, liquefied vitreous or fluid can exit the posterior segment through the needle path into the subconjunctival space or transconjunctivally to the ocular surface. This phenomenon can be observed in about 20% of injections [3]. Two problems can be associated with a vitreous prolapse:
1. A substantial amount of the injected drug can be misplaced.
2. A "vitreous wick" can serve as an entry site for bacteria from the ocular surface and may significantly increase the risk of postoperative endophthalmitis [5].

The rate of vitreous reflux is dependent on the needle, the injected volume, the consequential rise in IOP, and the injection technique used. Vitreous reflux can be avoided using sharp small-gauge needles (e.g., 27-, 30- or 31-gauge) and/or a short scleral tunnel for injection by pulling the conjunctiva over the injection site and using a slightly angled scleral path with the injection needle.

5.2.2.6 Traumatic Cataract

With the appropriate training of surgeons carrying out the injection and the injection technique, the rate of traumatic cataract should be minimal. Yet, sudden head movements of the patient or accidental moving of the needle tip toward the lens can never be fully avoided, and even intralenticular injections have been reported [19].

In the VISION trial, the rate of traumatic cataract was 0.07% (5 out of 892) [8]. The importance of the appropriate injection technique is underlined by the fact that, in this trial, 2 of the 5 lens injuries occurred on the same day in one center [8]. In the MARINA trial, lens damage was noted in 0.2% (1 out of 477) [29]. In the ANCHOR trial, no lens damage was noted during the first year in 277 patients with multiple injections [4].

5.2.2.7 Cataract Progression

Any intraocular manipulation is likely to be associated with an increase in cataract formation over time. The analysis of this complication is made difficult by several factors:
1. Different systems for grading and diverse definitions of "cataract progression" have been used in studies on intravitreal injections.
2. The systems for cataract grading currently used are still biased by subjective differences in the grading of lens opacities by different examiners.
3. The majority of published studies are retrospective in nature and a precise recording of cataract progression does not seem to be achievable with such study designs.
4. A difference in cataract progression may only be seen after several years of follow-up. To date, most studies cannot provide the necessary data because follow-ups are limited to 1 or 2 years.
5. A significant amount of cataract progression is likely to occur in the age group of patients with AMD unrelated to any intervention.

The latter is underlined by the rates of cataract progression that were noted in the control groups of prospective trials. These were 16% in the MARINA trial (sham injection), 7% in the ANCHOR trial (photodynamic therapy + sham injection), and 26% in the VISION trial (sham injection) [4, 8, 14, 29]. In comparison, similar or slightly higher rates of cataract progression could be noted in the treatment groups (MARINA 15%, ANCHOR 11–13%, and VISION 17–22%) [4, 8, 14, 29]. Very few patients underwent cataract surgery during the trial periods in these studies. Overall, there seems to be little or no cataractogenicity of repeated intraocular injections with anti-VEGF substances compared with their respective control groups within the first 2 years.

In contrast to the intravitreal application of anti-VEGF substances, intravitreal triamcinolone is associated with a higher rate of cataract development. By and large, cataract surgery has been performed in 20–45% of patients within the first year of the initial injection [21, 33]. The rate of cataract formation and consecutive surgery is time-dependent. In a prospective 2-year trial, cataract surgery was performed in 54% of patients (15 out of 28) with diabetic macular edema treated with intravitreal triamcinolone compared with 0% (0 out of 21) in the control group [12].

The cataractogenicity of local and systemic steroids has long been established; yet, the precise mechanisms are not clearly understood [20]. In the majority of cases, steroid use is associated with posterior subcapsular cataract formation. In addition, cortical cataracts and, to a lesser extent, nuclear cataract progression can also be seen following intravitreal triamcinolone injection [11, 33]. Interestingly, there seems to be a highly significant association of the second major complication of intravitreal triamcinolone, the rise in IOP, with the progression of subcapsular posterior and cortical cataracts [11]. A higher rate of cataract progression should therefore be expected in patients who are classified as steroid responders according to a rise in IOP following the injection.

5.2.2.8 Retinal Perforation

Entering the posterior segment with a sharp instrument carries the potential risk of retinal injury. This can occur when the entry site is too posterior (>5 mm), the needle is too long and advanced too far, the needle is pointed in the wrong direction or detached retina or choroid are in the way of the needle. No such retinal injuries have been reported in recent multicenter trials [4, 8, 14, 29]. Inspection of the retinal periphery before and after the injection should be included in the routine injection procedure. With appropriate training of surgeons, retinal injuries should be avoidable.

5.2.2.9 Vitreous Floaters

Vitreous floaters are commonly noticed by patients following intravitreal injections. In the VISION trial, they were perceived in 33% of patients in the treatment group versus 8% of patients with sham injections [14]. Due to the crystalline structure of the injected substance, floaters are more prevalent following triamcinolone injections. Floaters usually subside within the first week without the need for additional therapeutical measures.

5.2.2.10 Vitreous Hemorrhage

Vitreous hemorrhage is another potential complication of intravitreal injections. It can be caused by the injection itself during which the needle penetrates the choroids to reach the posterior chamber as well as by post-injection changes within the vitreous, leading to vitreous traction with preretinal hemorrhage. Its incidence, however, is relatively low; furthermore, the diseases most commonly treated with intravitreal injections, e.g., exudative AMD or diabetic retinopathy, are frequently associated with vitreous hemorrhage not related to surgical interventions.

In the VISION trial, the rate of vitreous hemorrhage was 0.21% (16 out of 7,545) [8]. However, only 9 of the 16 incidents were judged to be associated with the injection procedure. In the MARINA trial, the rates of vitreous hemorrhage were 0.4% (2 out of 477) in the treatment group versus 0.8% (2 out of 236) in the group with sham treatment [29]. Usually, no treatment is required for vitreous hemorrhage secondary to intravitreal injections. Pars plana vitrectomy can be considered in advanced cases or those without spontaneous regression.

5.2.2.11 Retinal Toxicity

Retinal toxicity is a potential complication of intravitreally applied drugs. Such toxicity, can lead to changes in the electroretinogram, may cause visible changes through alterations of the fundus pigmentation and can lead to gross photoreceptor and macular malfunction. Cases of retinal toxicity or presumed toxicity have been documented following intravitreal application of tissue plasminogen activator, methotrexate, amikacin and hyaluronidase [6, 17, 35].

So far, there have been no reports of presumed toxicity of anti-VEGF drugs, including bevacizumab, in vivo or in vitro with the currently used dose regimen [4, 8, 10, 29]. However, some concerns remain that constant VEGF suppression might increase the long-term risks of toxicities for retinal tissue [25].

The question of possible toxicity of triamcinolone has been raised in in vitro studies on rabbits and on cultured human retinal pigment epithelial (RPE) cells [32, 36]. This toxicity has been linked to the concentration of the drug, the preservative in commercial preparations or the direct contact of the triamcinolone crystals with the retina [21, 32, 36]. In clinical series, no evidence of triamcinolone toxicity has been reported so far [21].

5.2.2.12 Intraocular Inflammation

Anti-VEGF substances are humanized antibodies, or aptamers, that potentially can cause an intraocular immune reaction. Clinical studies have therefore specifically looked at intraocular inflammation following their intravitreal application. Intraocular inflammatory cells, however, can also be seen after any manipulation of the eye or the ocular adnexa, including intravitreal injections or sham injections.

A dose-related increase in intraocular inflammation has been documented for two drugs after intravitreal application, ranibizumab and hyaluronidase. Early phase I/II studies of ranibizumab were associated with a relatively high rate of low-grade to moderate intraocular inflammation in up to 78% of patients [16]. This might have been due to the lyophilized preparation of the antibody. In a further dose-escalating study, Rosenfeld et al. found a dose-dependent response; injections up to 500 μg of ranibizumab seem to be well tolerated, but higher doses were accompanied by more intraocular inflammation [28]. In the large prospective clinical trials of ranibizumab (up to 500 μg) and pegaptanib (up to 3 mg), the rates of (mostly low-grade) anterior and posterior chamber inflammation were significantly lower and were seen in up to 20% within the treatment groups. There was no correlation between the level of intraocular inflammation and the injected drug dose and a comparable rate and severity of events could be seen in the respective control groups [4, 8, 14, 29]. Typically, intraocular inflammations following ranibizumab and pegaptanib can be seen on day 1 after the injection and usually subside without treatment within 14 days. Anti-inflammatory treatment is not necessary in most cases. There does not seem to be an increased risk of more severe inflammation with repeated injections that would indicate an amplification of the immune response as a reaction to the injected proteins. In contrast, lower intraocular inflammation scores were seen following repeated injections in a dose-escalating study with more frequent and higher dosed injections compared with the currently recommended doses of ranibizumab [28].

Another drug that was documented to cause a biological reaction following intravitreal injection is bovine hyaluronidase. Increased intraocular inflammatory responses with a dose relationship could be seen. The rates of moderate or severe iritis in the study by Kupperman et al. were 0% (observation) and 8% (saline injection) in the control groups versus 20% (7.5 IU hyaluronidase), 37% (55 IU), and 40% (75 IU) [24] in the treatment groups.

Intraocular inflammatory reactions (with the exception of pseudo-endophthalmitis or endophthalmitis, see Sect. 5.2.2.13) do not seem to be a particular problem following intravitreal triamcinolone [21]. When injected into the anterior chamber and capsular bag following routine cataract surgery, there is a dose-related reduction of the anterior chamber inflammatory response [13]. In one series of 759 consecutive intravitreal injections, no significant anterior chamber reaction could be noted [23]. This is probably due to the immunosuppressive effect of the drug.

5.2.2.13 Uveitis and Pseudo-endophthalmitis

The vast majority of inflammatory reactions in the anterior and posterior chamber following intravitreal injections are of low grade and do not require any treatment. They are usually thought to be associated with the injection procedure. Occasionally, severe intraocular inflammatory reactions can be seen. In these rare cases it is important, although sometimes extremely difficult, to differentiate a sterile inflammatory process from an inflammatory reaction associated with infectious endophthalmitis. To complicate things further, the term "pseudo-endophthalmitis" has been introduced. This has almost exclusively been used for severe intraocular inflammations following intravitreal triamcinolone injections.

Low-grade inflammatory reactions following intravitreal injections are thought to be a reaction to the injection procedure, whereas severe, noninfectious reactions might be caused by the drug itself (or its solvent) [29]. To distinguish low-grade inflammation from clinically significant inflammatory reactions, the latter are often classified as uveitis. In a phase I/II study of ranibizumab, one case of a severe recurrent uveitis was noted [16]; the uveitis recurred after each injection of the drug, underlining the likelihood of a biological reaction to the injected antibody. In the larger prospective studies of ranibizumab, uveitis could be seen in 1 of the 277 cases in the ANCHOR trial and in 1.2% of cases (6 out of 478) in the MARINA trial. In the Bevacizumab Safety Survey, 10 cases of uveitis out of a total of 5,228 patients (0.19%) were reported [10]. No severe intraocular inflammations other than endophthalmitis were reported to occur following pegaptanib injection in the VISION trial [14].

Pseudo-endophthalmitis (synonyms: sterile, noninfectious or toxic endophthalmitis) is characterized by intraocular changes or a severe inflammatory reaction mimicking the clinical picture of infectious endophthalmitis. This reaction is almost exclusively seen following intravitreal injection of unaltered, commercially available triamcinolone. Three different paths can lead to its manifestation:

1. Immune reaction to the vehicle of the injected drug, leading to severe intraocular uveitis.
2. Collection of triamcinolone crystals in the anterior chamber, mimicking the picture of a hypopyon. This can particularly seen in eyes with previous vitrectomy and defects in the lens capsule or zonular fibers, or when part

of the injected triamcinolone is misdirected alongside the anterior vitreous surface.
3. The crushing of triamcinolone crystals in small-gauge cannulae (30- or 31-gauge), leading to an almost immediate and dense vitreous haze following the injection.

There is no unambiguous clinical sign to differentiate pseudo-endophthalmitis from infectious endophthalmitis. However, some clinical features are more commonly associated with pseudo-endophthalmitis:
1. Clinical signs develop within the first few hours of the injection. This does not exclude infectious endophthalmitis, but newly diagnosed intraocular inflammation days after the injection should is more indicative of infectious endophthalmitis and rather than pseudo-endophthalmitis.
2. Pain, periorbital swelling and photophobia are usually absent in pseudo-endophthalmitis. However, it should be kept in mind that pain is also absent in about 20% of infectious endophthalmitis.
3. Dense vitreous infiltrates and pseudo-hypopyon seen in pseudo-endophthalmitis are accompanied by a relatively low-grade anterior chamber reaction (e.g., very few anterior chamber cells above the crystals).
4. Anterior chamber taps or vitreous biopsies fail to isolate bacterial or fungal organisms.

Some authors advocate purification of commercially available triamcinolone before intravitreal injection in order to eliminate the vehicle and to lower the occurrence of toxic reactions. With this technique, only one case of pseudo-endophthalmitis could be seen after 759 injections in a series by Kreissig et al. [23]. In contrast, in a series of 922 injections without removal of the vehicle, 8 cases of pseudo-endophthalmitis were seen (0.87%) [26].

Pseudo-endophthalmitis usually subsides without any specific therapy over 7–14 days. In contrast, infectious endophthalmitis can progress extremely quickly without appropriate treatment with potentially devastating consequences. Weighing the potential risks of treating a case of pseudo-endophthalmitis with intraocular antibiotics against delaying treatment of infectious endophthalmitis, it seems justified to recommend treatment with intraocular antibiotics in uncertain cases.

5.2.2.14 Endophthalmitis

Infectious endophthalmitis is the most feared complication of intravitreal injections and has been reported after application of all currently used preparations. The prevention of postoperative endophthalmitis is one of the key issues influencing the organization and implementation of intravitreal injections on a larger scale. The first large multicenter studies of intravitreal anti-VEGF treatment revealed several problems that need to be considered when integrating this type of therapy into routine practice:
1. The endophthalmitis rates per patient following repeated intraocular injections are significantly higher than rates reported after routine cataract surgery. This underlines the importance of appropriate hygiene standards and techniques for intraocular injections.
2. The rate of endophthalmitis can be lowered by adherence to certain standards, e.g., sterile environment, and appropriate disinfection [8]. This, in return, has a major impact on the costs and the logistics of patient treatment.
3. With timely and appropriate treatment, devastating outcomes can be avoided and the majority of patients will go on and continue the therapy if more injections are needed [8].

Prevention and timely treatment are key issues to lower the rates of post-injection endophthalmitis and its potentially devastating outcomes. This concerns not only the injection itself, but also the pre-operative examination and postoperative care of the patient:
1. Patients with acute or chronic infections of the anterior segment and ocular adnexa, e.g., conjunctivitis or blepharitis, should first undergo treatment of the infectious disease before proceeding to the injection.
2. The preparation of the ocular surface should aim to minimize the bacterial contamination during the injection. Additional measures, e.g., sterile drapes and the use of a lid speculum, have been associated with a decrease in postoperative endophthalmitis in one study [8].

3. The preparation of drugs and any modification processes (e.g., separation from the solvent of commercially available triamcinolone) have to be performed under sterile conditions.
4. Patients at higher risk of endophthalmitis (e.g., those post-filtering surgery, with immunosuppression, with diabetes) have to be identified, informed about their increased risk and monitored more closely.
5. Patients have to be informed about possible signs and symptoms of endophthalmitis.
6. Patients should be provided with clear instructions and pathways of whom to contact and where to be examined if symptoms or signs of endophthalmitis develop.
7. Ophthalmologists performing intravitreal injections should be familiar with the current treatment recommendations for postoperative endophthalmitis and should be able to perform an injection of intravitreal antibiotics in cases of presumed infectious endophthalmitis. Any delay in initiation of treatment can lower the chances of a successful treatment outcome.
8. Patients with routine topical eye medications (e.g., glaucoma drops or artificial tears) should discard their old eye drop bottles and resume with new bottles due to the possibility of bacterial contamination of old opened bottles.

Currently, it is unclear whether or not scheduled follow-up visits can lower the rate of devastating outcomes in cases of infectious endophthalmitis, e.g., by detecting clinical signs of endophthalmitis before patients become symptomatic and seek medical attention. The necessity of follow-up visits, the extent of these examinations, their frequency and timing would depend on such information, and this would have a major impact on the costs and logistics of routine application of intravitreal drugs. No universally accepted guidelines have been established on this matter so far and recommendations regarding postoperative follow-up examinations differ significantly between studies and current guidelines (Table 5.1).

In the three major trials published on intravitreal anti-VEGF therapy, endophthalmitis rates were between 0.006% and 0.16% per injection and between 0.07% and 1.3% per patient [4, 8, 14, 29]. There were a total of 19 cases of presumed infectious endophthalmitis, with 11 out of 19 being culture-positive. The most commonly isolated organism was *Staphylococcus aureus*. In the Bevacizumab Safety Survey, 1 case of endophthalmitis in 5,228 patients with 7,113 injections has been reported [10]. However, these data come from a self-reporting survey with the potential of under-reporting serious adverse events.

Post-injection endophthalmitis has been a particular concern in conjunction with the intravitreal use of triamcinolone. In a review of 922 patients treated at different institutions with intravitreal triamcinolone, 8 patients with infectious endophthalmitis were identified, leading to an endophthalmitis rate of 0.87% [26]. In contrast, Kreissig et al. observed only 1 case of endophthalmitis following 759 injections (0.1%) in 645 eyes (0.1%) [23]. There are differences between infectious endophthalmitis following intravitreal injection of triamcinolone and that after anti-VEGF therapy or other intravitreally applied drugs:

1. There seems to be a higher risk of infectious endophthalmitis following triamcinolone injection. This is likely to be due to the immunosuppressive steroid effect of the drug. Also, more patients at higher risk of endophthalmitis are usually included in the populations treated with triamcinolone (e.g., those with diabetes).
2. Severe pain associated with the onset of endophthalmitis seems to be less common.
3. The clinical course is often prolonged, but more foudroyant, and the rate of eyes with total visual loss, phthisis or enucleation may be higher compared with other causes of infectious post-injection endophthalmitis.
4. The spectrum of cultured organism shows a greater variation of different bacterial species causing endophthalmitis.
5. The histology of enucleated globes demonstrates differences with regard to the morphology of the inflammatory infiltrations, possibly due to local variation in the triamcinolone concentration and its immunosuppressive effects.

The current first-line treatment for infectious endophthalmitis is intravitreal injection of antibiotics and/or pars plana vitrectomy in advanced cases. The choice of antibiotic depends on the suspected organism. Usually, a broad spectrum antibiotic is chosen because in most cases, therapy has to be initiated before culture results are available. Because the majority of cultured species are gram-positive bacteria, vancomycin (1 mg/0.1 ml) has been the most commonly used agent. Cephalosporins, e.g., ceftazidime (2.25 mg/0.1 ml), cover some gram-negative bacteria as well. Aminoglycosides, e.g., amikacin (0.4 mg/0.1 ml), have a broad gram-negative coverage, but have been associated with retinal toxicity [35].

Reported outcomes of endophthalmitis following intravitreal injections with pegaptanib have been surprisingly good compared with postoperative endophthalmitis of other etiology. In the VISION trial, only 1 out of 12 cases of endophthalmitis suffered a significant visual loss and 8 were within 10 letters of visual loss compared with baseline [8]. In contrast, 5 out of 8 cases with bacterial endophthalmitis following triamcinolone injection had a significant decrease in visual acuity, with 3 eyes losing light perception [26]. One of the reasons for the good outcomes of endophthalmitis in the VISION trial might be the intensified instructions and methodical follow-up examinations of patients participating in such well-conducted clinical trials. It underlines the importance of these aspects to routine intravitreal therapy in day-to-day practice.

Summary for the Clinician

- Infectious endophthalmitis following intravitreal injections typically occurs within the first week of injection.
- About two thirds of cases are culture-positive, e.g., *Staphylococcus aureus*.
- Clinical signs are periocular pain, swelling, redness, photophobia, decrease in visual acuity.
- There is a good outcome in the majority of cases when treated promptly.
- Treatment is with intravitreal injections of antibiotics, e.g., vancomycin (1 mg/0.1 ml) or ceftazidime (2.25 mg/0.1 ml).

5.2.2.15 Retinal Artery and Vein Occlusion

Central retinal artery occlusions can be observed in patients with an acute and extreme increase in IOP immediately after the injection. It is an unusual finding if a volume of 0.5 ml is injected. In the VISION trial, 4 cases out of 7,545 injections were reported [8]. All cases resolved after paracentesis without long-term complications. Checking the visual acuity should be performed immediately after the injection. Patients with central retinal artery occlusion usually have no light perception. Most current guidelines also recommend performing ophthalmoscopy to check perfusion of the retinal artery after the injection.

Retinal artery or vein occlusions outside the immediate postoperative course are even rarer. One case of a central retinal artery occlusion has been reported in the Bevacizumab Safety Survey [10]. Single cases of retinal arterial emboli and vein occlusion were reported by Heier et al. following ranibizumab injections [16]. No other retinal vascular occlusion has been described in the larger studies of anti-VEGF therapy. Few cases of retinal vascular occlusion have been reported following intravitreal injection of other drugs, mainly antiviral agents [17]. Based on the data currently available, there does not seem to be an increased risk of retinal vascular disease following intravitreal injections with the exception of acute central retinal artery occlusion during or immediately after the injection.

5.2.2.16 Retinal Detachment

Surgical manipulations in the posterior segment carry the risk of inducing retinal detachment or its precursors. This is also true for intravitreal injections, as they can lead to vitreous reflux that might result in increased vitreous traction. Furthermore, initiation of posterior vitreous detachment might also be caused through repeated surgical manipulations in the posterior segment with low-grade inflammations. The injection of gas, for example, induces posterior vitreous detachment in a high number of cases [27]; this is one of the major events preceding rhegmatogenous retinal detachment.

Several cases of retinal detachment have been seen after intravitreal anti-VEGF treatment. However, the detachment rates were lower than expected and no major differences from the control groups were seen. In the MARINA trial, no retinal detachment and 2 retinal breaks were found in 477 eyes with intravitreal Lucentis therapy versus 1 detachment and no breaks in 236 eyes of the control group [29]. In the ANCHOR trial, 1 detachment was seen in 277 treated eyes as well as in 143 eyes of the control group treated with photodynamic therapy [4]. In the VISION trial, 4 cases of rhegmatogenous retinal detachment were seen in the first year of follow-up of 892 patients, with an additional two detachments in 374 patients during the second year; no detachments were noted in the control group [8]. Three cases of retinal detachment were reported in 5,228 summarized in the Bevacizumab Safety Survey [10]. Jonas observed no cases of retinal detachment in 348 patients treated with intravitreal triamcinolone [21]. In summary, the risk of the development of a retinal detachment seems to be low with the drugs currently used for intravitreal injections.

In contrast to the results of the studies of anti-VEGF therapy and triamcinolone, a high rate of 9.5% of patients with post-injection retinal detachment (128 out of 1,344) was seen in the controls as well as in the treatment group in two trials on the intravitreal use of hyaluronidase for vitreous hemorrhage [24]. However, this is most likely due to the high incidence of retinal detachment in the study population (patients with vitreous hemorrhage), including the high number of tractional retinal detachments in this cohort.

Immediately following the injection of 0.1 ml, IOP reaches 46 mmHg on average if no vitreous reflux is noted. This will quickly return to the normal values within the first 30 min [3]. Between 3 and 24 h after injection, the IOP is comparable to baseline values [9].

The injected volume of ranibizumab is 0.05 ml, bevacizumab is usually approximately 0.05 ml, and the volume of pegaptanib is 0.09 ml of fluid. With this volume, IOP measurements are on average 4–5 mmHg higher at 30 min post-injection and 2–4 mmHg at 60 min compared with the baseline [28, 29]. IOPs above 30 mmHg were noted in up to 17% of patients after ranibizumab injection [29]. The rate of paracentesis for release of acutely elevated IOP in the VISION trial was low (3% in the first year and 4% in the second year) and seem to be possibly due to the preferred practice pattern in a participating center rather than a significantly elevated IOP [8]. In addition, pegaptanib is delivered through an incorporated needle that is quite large, allowing for the possibility of spontaneous reflux through the needle track. To avoid major increases in IOP during or immediately after the injection, care must be taken to remove excess fluid or air from the syringe and needle before injection and to ensure that no additional resistance, e.g., blocking of the needle or plunger, is present before entering the globe with the needle.

In addition to the purely volume-related increases in IOP, relatively early and clinically significant rises in IOP within the first week of the injection of intravitreal triamcinolone have been reported [31]. This could either be due to an early steroid-associated effect of IOP rise or a presumed blockade of the trabecular meshwork outflow by triamcinolone crystals.

5.2.2.17 Acute Rise in Intraocular Pressure

Intraocular injections will lead to a rise in the IOP in relation to the injected volume. During the injection, the rise in the IOP is related to the force applied to the plunger and the diameter of the needle. This is sometimes difficult to judge and one case of globe rupture has been reported following intraocular injection of triamcinolone [34].

5.2.2.18 Ocular Hypertension and Glaucoma

Sustained rises in IOP following intravitreal injections can either be due to a pharmacological effect of the injected agent or vehicle, structural changes within the globe following the injections, secondary effects of singular or repetitive intraocular inflammations after one or more injections, or an aging process independent of the treatment performed. The data currently available demonstrate that only drug-related effects seem to play a significant role and that a sustained rise in IOP is almost exclusively associated with triamcinolone injections.

Regarding anti-VEGF therapy, data of three major prospective randomized trials with a follow-up of up to 2 years are available [4, 8, 14, 29]. IOP rises have specifically been addressed in these studies. No significant differences in sustained rises in IOP were seen compared with control groups, and no pressure-lowering surgical interventions have been reported. In the Bevacizumab Safety Survey, no cases of ocular hypertension or secondary glaucoma were identified [10].

The induction of secondary ocular hypertension after intravitreal triamcinolone injection has been well documented. In summary, the following observations can be made [21]:
1. A sustained rise in IOP can be observed in about 40% of treated patients.
2. About 9% will have IOPs above 30 mmHg.
3. About 1% of patients will have insufficient lowering of IOP with medical treatment and will have to undergo glaucoma surgery.
4. Following a first injection, a comparable reaction and rise in IOP can be expected with repeated injections.
5. In most cases, increased IOP values can be detected about 1 week after the injection, with a peak incidence between 1 and 2 months.
6. The duration of the pressure increase seems to be dose-dependent (about 3–4 months with 4 mg and about 7–9 months with 20–25 mg).
7. Higher doses of injected triamcinolone do not cause greater elevation of IOP, but prolonged pressure elevation.
8. Pre-existing glaucoma or ocular hypertension does not seem to increase the risk of increased pressure.
9. Younger patients seem to have a higher rate of secondary ocular hypertension.
10. There does not seem to be any significant difference in the responses to various groups of glaucoma medications.

Summary for the Clinician

- Perioperative complications include conjunctival hemorrhage (20–40%), pain (30%), punctate keratitis (30%), vitreous reflux (20%), vitreous floaters (20%), traumatic cataract (<1%), a rise in IOP (average IOP 46 mmHg if 0.1 ml is injected), and central retinal artery occlusion (<1%).
- Postoperative complications include intraocular inflammation (20%), cataract progression (7–26% within first year), endophthalmitis (0.15% per injection, 1% in patients with multiple injections), and retinal detachment (<1%).
- Complications associated with intravitreal triamcinolone injections include a higher rate of cataract progression (20–45% within the first year), ocular hypertension (about 40% of all patients, about 1% requiring filtration surgery), "pseudo-endophthalmitis" (suspected immune reaction to vehicle or drug, <1%), and a possibly higher rate of infectious endophthalmitis (0.8% per injection).

5.3 Surgical Technique for Intravitreal Injection

Intravitreal injections are relatively straightforward intraocular procedures with a low rate of severe ocular side effects. However, based on treatment strategies that are currently are transferred into daily practice, the number of patients who will receive up to 12 intravitreal injections per year over the next few years is likely to increase exponentially—and with it the number of severe adverse ocular events. Because patient safety is a key issue in all surgical interventions, it is therefore necessary to incorporate this expected high number of future patients into the daily routine of operating theaters and outpatient clinics with acceptable safety standards.

Many recommendations regarding several aspects of the procedure are not evidence-based. Some parts can be transferred from studies and practice patterns of routine cataract surgery.

Other features have been conceived from recently conducted and published studies. In most cases, guidelines represent a consensus statement of authorities in the field.

5.3.1 Guidelines and Preferred Practice Survey

The synopsis of three major guidelines is displayed in Table 5.3. The consensus statement of mainly US-based retinal specialists was published in Retina in 2004 and is based on a review of more than 15,000 injections [1, 17]. The recommendations of the German Ophthalmological Society, the Retinological Society, and the Association of Ophthalmologists in Germany was published in 2005 [18]. The guidelines of the Royal College of Ophthalmologists became available on the internet in 2006 (http://www.rcophth.ac.uk/). The display of guidelines is accompanied by a survey of the preferred practice patterns for intravitreal triamcinolone injections of 562 ophthalmologists performing intravitreal injections in the UK in 2004 [2].

5.3.2 Preoperative Assessment and Preparation

5.3.2.1 Concomitant Eye Diseases

Bacterial infections of the anterior segment and ocular adnexa increase the risk of endophthalmitis and should be treated before performing an intravitreal injection. Patients with glaucomatous diseases should have adequately controlled IOP before injection. Although the risks and the amount of postoperative rises in IOP is higher for patients with glaucoma, it is not seen as a contraindication for intravitreal injections including triamcinolone. The value of a pre-injection provocation test with steroid eye drops is questionable and this is usually not performed.

5.3.2.2 Preoperative Assessment

A thorough preoperative assessment including funduscopy should be performed before any intravitreal injection to confirm the need for the injection and to rule out possible contraindications or to detect conditions that might complicate the injection, e.g., retinal detachment, vitreous hemorrhage or increased IOP. Measurement of the IOP immediately before the injection is recommended by the Royal College guidelines.

5.3.2.3 Preoperative Medication

The value of preoperative topical antibiotics to reduce the number of bacteria on the ocular surface is a point of debate. It has been optional in some of the major trials of anti-VEGF therapy and is sometimes advocated in patients with a presumed allergy to iodine. The disadvantage of the uncritical application of broad-spectrum antibiotics is the induction of resistance of bacteria to antibiotic treatment. There seems to be no advantage of topical antibiotics over disinfection with povidone-iodine. In the guidelines, the use of preoperative antibiotics is optional.

5.3.2.4 Location

In the USA the vast majority of injections are given in the outpatient clinic. The German guidelines recommend performing the injection in an operating theater according to the standards for day-case surgical interventions. The Royal College guidelines recommend alternatively a dedicated room in the outpatient department. The preferred practice pattern survey showed that the majority of injections in the UK were carried out in operating theaters.

5.3.2.5 Preparation of the Eye and Ocular Adnexa

The standard for preoperative disinfection of the ocular surface and eyelids is povidone-iodine 5% and 10% (skin). A forceful scrubbing of the lid margins is not recommended to avoid expression of bacteria from the lid glands. Pupillary dilatation is recommended by all guidelines in all routine cases except for those with contraindications. Although subconjunctival anesthesia has

Table 5.3 Current guidelines and preferred practice survey for intravitreal injections

Guidelines	German Ophthalmological Society	Consensus Statement Retina	Royal College of Ophthalmologists http://www.rcophth.ac.uk/	Preferred practice survey Royal College of Ophthalmologist Specialist register
Country, year	Germany, 2005 [18]	USA, 2004 [1]	United Kingdom, 2006	United Kingdom, 2006 [2]
Preparation				
Location	Operating theater	–	Operating theater or dedicated room in outpatients clinic	77% operating theater 19% outpatients
Removal of vehicle (triamcinolone)	Recommended	–	–	5.8%
Pretreatment antibiotics	Recommended in high-risk cases	Optional	Optional	
Mydriatics	Yes	Yes	Yes	78%
Topical anesthesia	Yes		Yes	
Subconjunctival anesthesia	Optional	Optional	Optional	
Conjunctival disinfection	10 ml povidone-iodine 5%	Povidone-iodine	5% povidone-iodine drops 3 min before injection	94% povidone iodine
Lid disinfection	Povidone-iodine 10%	Povidone-iodine No scrubbing of lid margins	Povidone-iodine 10%	
Hand disinfection	Yes	–	Yes	
Gloves	Yes	Yes	Yes	86%
Sterile drape	Yes	Optional	Yes	63%
Lid speculum	Yes	Yes	Yes	
Preoperative intraocular pressure measurement			Yes	

Table 5.3 *(continued)* Current guidelines and preferred practice survey for intravitreal injections

Guidelines				Preferred practice survey
Injection				
Cannula	27- or 30-gauge	27-gauge or smaller length 12.7 to 0.15.75 mm	27- to 30- gauge length 12.7 to 15.75 mm	54% 27-gauge 22% 30-gauge
Distance to limbus	3.5 mm	Pseudophakic 3.5 mm Phakic 4.0 mm	Pseudophakic 3.0 to 3.5 mm Phakic 3.5 to 4.0 mm	
Conjunctival shift	Yes	–	–	
Needle positioning	Advance 6–7 mm	Advance at least 6 mm	–	
Injection	Not too quickly	Moderately slow	Slowly and carefully	
Blockade sclerotomy	Yes	Yes	–	
Paracentesis	Optional, not routinely recommended	Optional, not routinely recommended	Optional, not routinely recommended	11% before (sometimes) 40% after (sometimes)
Antibiotic drops immediately after injection	–	–	Yes	
Postoperative care				
Visual acuity check	Yes	Yes	Yes	
Ophthalmoscopy	Yes	Yes	No	
Slit-lamp examination	No	No	Yes	
Intraocular pressure check	30–60 min	Monitor pressure after injection	Within 30 min	26% same day 23% next day
Topical antibiotics	Optional for 3 days	Optional	For 3 days	58%
Follow-up examination	First day post-injection	To be contacted by physician's office within 1 week	–	

been used in some of the major studies, standard practice is topical anesthesia with eye-drops with or without a pledget. Paracentesis before injection is not recommended unless higher volumes are injected (≥0.2 ml).

5.3.2.6 Preparation of the Surgeon

A hand-wash and disinfection according to routine standards for surgical interventions as well as wearing of surgical gloves are recommended as per universal precautions. However, surgical gowns or face masks are not worn in the majority of centers.

5.3.2.7 Preparation of the Drug

Most drugs for intravitreal injections are provided in syringe and needle packets ready for injection. When the injectable volume is drawn from larger vials (e.g., bevacizumab or triamcinolone), sterile conditions have to be ensured throughout the preparation of the drug. Removal of the solvent before triamcinolone injections has been associated with a lower rate of intraocular inflammation and is recommended by the German guidelines.

5.3.3 Injection

5.3.3.1 Syringe and Needle

Twenty-seven or 30-gauge needles measuring between 12.7 and 15.75 mm long are usually recommended. In every case, air within the syringe and needle should be removed before the injection. Testing that no major resistance is present (e.g., clogging of the needle with triamcinolone crystals or the rigid plunger of the syringe) before injection is also recommended. When injecting triamcinolone it is helpful to have a syringe with a Luer lock, so that the needle does not become detached from the syringe during injection.

5.3.3.2 Position of the Injection

The injection should be positioned between 3.0 and 4.0 mm posterior to the limbus, depending on the lens status. Usually, the first injection is performed temporally and inferiorly. In most cases of repeated injections, previous injection sites are avoided because of fibrotic reactions in this area. The exact position of an injection should be noted within the patient's notes. However, given the need for monthly injections for some medications it will be virtually impossible to avoid a site inferiorly that has not been injected before.

5.3.3.3 Entry Path

The German guidelines recommend pulling the conjunctiva over the entry site in order to achieve a step-like entry path and to lower the risk of vitreous reflux. Usually, a straight needle path, pointing at the center of the eyeball is recommended. With relatively large needles that sometimes are pre-installed from the manufacturer and cannot be exchanged, a slightly angled scleral entry path is needed in order to avoid vitreous reflux.

5.3.3.4 Advancement of Needle and Injection

The needle should be advanced 6–7 mm toward the center of the eyeball to avoid injection along the anterior vitreous surface. Checking the position of the needle tip with indirect ophthalmoscopy or with the operating microscope is not recommended because these manipulations may increase the risk of unintentional movements of the needle tip and iatrogenic trauma. The injection should be carried out in one slow but steady movement. Caution should be used if increased resistance is felt at the beginning or during the injection. The needle should be withdrawn in one movement with a cotton applicator covering the injection site and replacing the conjunctiva in order to avoid vitreous reflux and a vitreous wick.

5.3.4 Postoperative Assessment

5.3.4.1 Assessment Immediately Following the Injection

Immediately after the injection, the visual function (hand movements and light perception) should be checked. In addition, funduscopy should be performed to rule out central retinal artery occlusion, retinal detachment or vitreous hemorrhage. If central retinal artery occlusion is present and does not resolve spontaneously within the first few minutes, paracentesis should be performed. Paracentesis is not recommended routinely. The IOP should be checked within the first 60 min of injection. The Royal College guidelines also recommend a slit-lamp examination following the injection.

> **Summary for the Clinician**
>
> - Check vision and assess central retinal artery perfusion immediately post-injection.
> - Perform paracentesis only if the central retinal artery is occluded.
> - Carry out an IOP check within 30–60 min.
> - Administer topical antibiotics for 3 days.

5.3.4.2 Topical Therapy

The value of postoperative topical antibiotics is debatable and recommendations vary among the different guidelines. Again, the reduction in number of bacteria on the ocular surface has to be measured against the relatively low incidence of endophthalmitis when appropriate standards for the injection are used and the definite induction of resistance to antibiotics by routine application of broad-spectrum antibiotics. Recommendations concerning the type of drug to be used also vary.

> **Summary for the Clinician**
>
> - Exclude patients with suspected bacterial infections of the anterior segment (e.g. blepharitis, conjunctivitis).
> - Provide a designated treatment room or operating theater.
> - Use preoperative antisepsis with 10% povidone-iodine (lids) and 5% povidone-iodine (conjunctiva).
> - Carry out hand disinfection and wear gloves.
> - Use a sterile drape and lid speculum.
> - Use preoperative mydriatics.
> - Use topical anesthesia.
> - Use a 27- or 30-gauge cannula.
> - Ensure the injection site is 3.5–4.0 mm from the limbus, preferably in the temporal inferior quadrant.
> - Carry out conjunctival shift.
> - Ensure needle advancement of 6–7 mm.
> - Carry out moderately slow injection.

5.3.4.3 Follow-up Examinations

There is some variation regarding the necessity of follow-up examinations. In addition, regional variations in the availability of such examinations also play a role. The German guidelines advocate a full examination on the first day after the injection. Since most cases of endophthalmitis occur several days after injection, examination 1 day post-injection may miss a true infection. The US consensus statement recommends (telephone-based) contact between the patient and the treating institution. In any case, patients should be well informed about possible symptoms and signs of severe ocular events, e.g., pain, decrease in vision, inflammation and photophobia, and the means of contact and emergency treatment should such situations arise.

References

1. Aiello LP, Brucker AJ, Chang S et al (2004) Evolving guidelines for intravitreous injections. Retina 2004;24 [5 Suppl]:S3–19
2. Anijeet DR, Hanson RJ, Bhagey J et al (2006) National survey of the technique of intravitreal triamcinolone injection in the United Kingdom. Eye (in press)
3. Benz MS, Albini TA, Holz ER et al (2006) Short-term course of intraocular pressure after intravitreal injection of triamcinolone acetonide. Ophthalmology 2006;113(7):1174–1178
4. Brown DM, Kaiser PK, Michels M et al (2006) Ranibizumab versus verteporfin for neovascular age-related macular degeneration. N Engl J Med 355(14):1432–1444

5. Chen SD, Mohammed Q, Bowling B et al (2004) Vitreous wick syndrome—a potential cause of endophthalmitis after intravitreal injection of triamcinolone through the pars plana. Am J Ophthalmol 137(6):1159–1160; author reply 1160–1161
6. Chen SN, Yang TC, Ho CL et al (2003) Retinal toxicity of intravitreal tissue plasminogen activator: case report and literature review. Ophthalmology 110(4):704–708
7. Costa RA, Jorge R, Calucci D et al (2006) Intravitreal bevacizumab for choroidal neovascularization caused by AMD (IBeNA Study): results of a phase 1 dose-escalation study. Invest Ophthalmol Vis Sci 47(10):4569–4578
8. D'Amico DJ, Patel M, Adamis AP et al (2006) Pegaptanib sodium for neovascular age-related macular degeneration: two-year safety results of the two prospective, multicenter, controlled clinical trials. Ophthalmology 113(6): 992–1001.e6
9. Dwinger MC, Pieper-Bodeewes I, Eter N et al (2005) [Variations in intraocular pressure (IOP) and necessity for paracentesis following intravitreal triamcinolone injection]. Klin Monatsbl Augenheilkd 222(8):638–642
10. Fung AE, Rosenfeld PJ, Reichel E (2006) The International Intravitreal Bevacizumab Safety Survey: using the internet to assess drug safety worldwide. Br J Ophthalmol 90(11):1344–1349
11. Gillies MC, Kuzniarz M, Craig J et al (2005) Intravitreal triamcinolone-induced elevated intraocular pressure is associated with the development of posterior subcapsular cataract. Ophthalmology 112(1):139–143
12. Gillies MC, Sutter FK, Simpson JM et al (2006) Intravitreal triamcinolone for refractory diabetic macular edema: two-year results of a double-masked, placebo-controlled, randomized clinical trial. Ophthalmology 113(9):1533–1538
13. Gills JP, Gills P (2005) Effect of intracameral triamcinolone to control inflammation following cataract surgery. J Cataract Refract Surg 31(8):1670–1671
14. Gragoudas ES, Adamis AP, Cunningham ET Jr et al (2004) Pegaptanib for neovascular age-related macular degeneration. N Engl J Med 351(27):2805–2816
15. Gupta R, Negi A, Vernon SA (2005) Severe sub conjunctival haemorrhage following intravitreal triamcinolone for refractory diabetic oedema. Eye 19(5):590–591
16. Heier JS, Antoszyk AN, Pavan PR et al (2006) Ranibizumab for treatment of neovascular age-related macular degeneration: a phase I/II multicenter, controlled, multidose study. Ophthalmology 113(4):633–642.e4
17. Jager RD, Aiello LP, Patel SC et al (2004) Risks of intravitreous injection: a comprehensive review. Retina 24(5):676–698
18. Jaissle GB, Szurman P, Bartz-Schmidt KU (2005) [Recommendation for the implementation of intravitreal injections—statement of the German Retina Society, the German Society of Ophthalmology (DOG) and the German Professional Association of Ophthalmologists (BVA)]. Klin Monatsbl Augenheilkd 222(5):390–395
19. Jalil A, Chaudhry NL, Gandhi JS et al (2007) Inadvertent injection of triamcinolone into the crystalline lens. Eye 21(1):152–154
20. Jobling AI, Augusteyn RC (2002) What causes steroid cataracts? A review of steroid-induced posterior subcapsular cataracts. Clin Exp Optom 85(2):61–75
21. Jonas JB, Kreissig I, Degenring R (2005) Intravitreal triamcinolone acetonide for treatment of intraocular proliferative, exudative, and neovascular diseases. Prog Retin Eye Res 24(5):587–611
22. Kaderli B, Avci R (2006) Comparison of topical and subconjunctival anesthesia in intravitreal injection administrations. Eur J Ophthalmol 16(5):718–721
23. Kreissig I, Degenring RF, Jonas JB (2006) [Intravitreal triamcinolone acetonide. Complication of infectious and sterile endophthalmitis]. Ophthalmologe 103(1):30–34
24. Kuppermann BD, Thomas EL, de Smet MD et al (2005) Safety results of two phase III trials of an intravitreous injection of highly purified ovine hyaluronidase (Vitrase) for the management of vitreous hemorrhage. Am J Ophthalmol 140(4):585–597
25. Michels S (2006) Is intravitreal bevacizumab (Avastin) safe? Br J Ophthalmol 90(11):1333–1334

26. Moshfeghi DM, Kaiser PK, Scott IU et al (2003) Acute endophthalmitis following intravitreal triamcinolone acetonide injection. Am J Ophthalmol 136(5):791–796
27. Ochoa-Contreras D, Delsol-Coronado L, Buitrago ME et al (2000) Induced posterior vitreous detachment by intravitreal sulfur hexafluoride (SF6) injection in patients with nonproliferative diabetic retinopathy. Acta Ophthalmol Scand 78(6):687–688
28. Rosenfeld PJ, Schwartz SD, Blumenkranz MS et al (2005) Maximum tolerated dose of a humanized anti-vascular endothelial growth factor antibody fragment for treating neovascular age-related macular degeneration. Ophthalmology 112(6):1048–1053
29. Rosenfeld PJ, Brown DM, Heier JS et al (2006) Ranibizumab for neovascular age-related macular degeneration. N Engl J Med 355(14):1419–1431
30. Roth DB, Scott IU, Gulati N et al (2006) Patient perceptions of discomfort and changes in vision and functional status associated with intravitreal triamcinolone injection. Am J Ophthalmol 142(3):492–494
31. Singh IP, Ahmad SI, Yeh D et al (2004) Early rapid rise in intraocular pressure after intravitreal triamcinolone acetonide injection. Am J Ophthalmol 138(2):286–287
32. Szurman P, Kaczmarek R, Spitzer MS et al (2006) Differential toxic effect of dissolved triamcinolone and its crystalline deposits on cultured human retinal pigment epithelium (ARPE19) cells. Exp Eye Res 83(3):584–592
33. Thompson JT (2006) Cataract formation and other complications of intravitreal triamcinolone for macular edema. Am J Ophthalmol 141(4):629–637
34. Ung T, Williams CP, Canning CR (2006) Globe rupture as a complication of intravitreal injection of triamcinolone. Eye (in press)
35. Widmer S, Helbig H (2006) Presumed macular toxicity of intravitreal antibiotics. Klin Monatsbl Augenheilkd 223(5):456–458
36. Yu SY, Damico FM, Viola F et al (2006) Retinal toxicity of intravitreal triamcinolone acetonide: a morphological study. Retina 26(5):531–536

Chapter 6

Combination Therapies for Choroidal Neovascularization

Richard F. Spaide

Core Messages

- Choroidal neovascularization (CNV) is a tissue invasion of more than just blood vessels, there is also infiltration with inflammatory cells, myofibroblasts, fibrocytes, and glial cells.
- A two-component model of CNV is thought to be composed of a vascular component and an extravascular component. Macular damage is potentially possible through the actions of either component.
- The vascular component arises through the orchestrated interaction of a number of growth factors, the most important being vascular endothelial growth factor (VEGF). Platelet-derived growth factor is important for maintaining pericyte viability.
- The vascular component of CNV can be selectively targeted with antiangiogenic agents such as anti-VEGF and anti-PEDF (pigment epithelial-derived factor) drugs. Other growth factors are more difficult to selectively target at present because of the lack of suitable pharmacologic agents. The vascular component may be nonselectively targeted through the use of corticosteroids or photodynamic therapy (PDT).
- The extravascular component can be targeted in a nonselective manner with corticosteroids. Selective targeting of tumor necrosis factor (TNF) α is possible through anti-TNF biologics.
- Given the redundancy and complex interaction among biologic systems involved in the production of CNV, it is likely that a monotherapeutic approach will not be as successful as a combined use of multiple agents in improving patient outcomes.
- The combined use of PDT and intravitreal triamcinolone appears to be better than the use of PDT alone, although there is a much greater risk of side-effects.
- Combinatorial use of additional agents is currently being investigated. Because of the very promising results of anti-VEGF antibody and antibody fragment studies, these drugs form the cornerstone of most combination studies at present.

6.1 Introduction

Choroidal neovascularization (CNV) is a process occurring in age-related macular degeneration (AMD) leading to severe loss of visual function. The name of the disease is derived from its fluorescein angiographic appearance in which hyperfluorescence related to the abnormal accumulation of vessels can be seen. By histopathologic examination CNV looks more like granulation tissue, with the invasion not only of blood vessels, but also of inflammatory cells and mesenchymal cells (Fig. 6.1). The vascular foundation is not inappropriate, however, because several of the most important attributes of CNV are related to vessels, namely bleeding and leakage. Inhibition of blood vessels offers the possibility of not only decreasing the damage caused by bleeding and leakage, but also secondarily decreasing the invasion of other cell types that may induce damage through inflammation or scarring.

Angiogenesis is a process honed through millions of years of evolution to be a complex multistage process requiring orchestrated interactions among pro- and anti-angiogenic stimuli, cells, proteases, and rheologic factors. As in any important biological process there are feedback and control mechanisms with built-in redundancies to modulate the complex interaction among a variety of entities. Selective targeting offers the easiest, most direct route to trying to control pathologic processes, but redundancies in these processes often means a single agent will not completely reverse or inhibit any complex pathologic response. Combinatorial approaches to disease treatment offer several theoretical advantages over monotherapeutic targeting. Because of redundancies in biologic processes such as angiogenesis, targeting of more than one effector may be necessary. Combinatorial approaches also allow targeting of more than one component of a disease process at a time; angiogenesis, scarring, and inflammation may be targeted simultaneously. Combination approaches may increase the overall efficacy while decreasing the potential for side-effects. Each individual part of a combination therapy may contribute to overall efficacy, but because each drug may be used in relatively low doses and may have side-effect profiles that do not overlap, the cumulative side-effect incidence and severity profile may be reduced for any given level of efficacy compared with high-dose single agent use. With more therapeutic modalities being developed there are an ever-increasing number of treatment permutations possible. A rational concept for treating CNV through combination therapies involves addressing known pathophysiologic aspects of the disease with available and potential future tools that can be developed [82]. This chapter reviews angiogenesis, the pathobiology of CNV, the potential targets of therapy, and provides a conceptual framework for combination therapies.

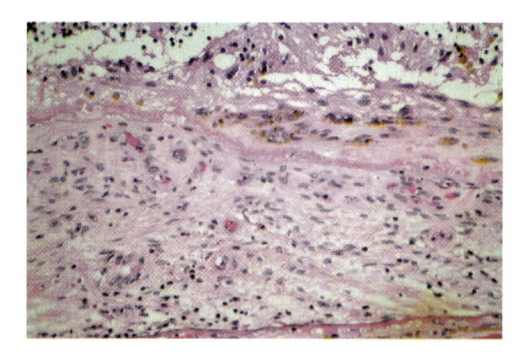

Fig. 6.1 Choroidal neovascularization secondary to age-related macular degeneration is a tissue invasion of a multitude of cells, many of which are inflammatory. The actual vascular component is a small minority of the lesion and grows in with, and to an extent because of, the extravascular component. (Photograph courtesy of Hans Grossniklaus, MD)

6.2 Angiogenesis

Angiogenic stimuli, particularly vascular endothelial growth factor-A (VEGF-A), activate vascular endothelial cells and lead to the formation of gaps between endothelial cells of the capillary wall [22, 74]. The capillary wall becomes more permeable allowing plasma proteins, such as fibrinogen, to extravasate leading to the formation of a provisional matrix to support the newly growing vessel. The endothelial cells form a bud and the advancing edge of the bud expresses integrins and matrix metalloproteinases to help the endothelial cells degrade the extracellular matrix [79]. The advancing cells move away from the pre-existing vessel toward the angiogenic stimulus. The endothelial cells in the vascular sprout proliferate, and additional cells, circulating endothelial progenitor cells, which are bone marrow-derived precursors that home to sites of angiogenesis, take up a vascular endothelial cell phenotype, and contribute to vessel formation [8, 53]. Lumen formation and anastomotic connection between neighboring sprouts lead to capillary loops. At this stage the cells form a thin-walled pericyte-poor vessel. Recruitment and differentiation of mural cell precursors occur and these cells in turn support the vascular endothelial cells through mechanisms that can include paracrine secretion of growth factors [1, 20, 39]. Blocking VEGF inhibits endothelial cell proliferation in the early stages of angiogenesis. Inflammatory cells are frequently seen in and around areas of angiogenesis in adults.

6.2.1 Development of CNV

In the development of CNV the process of angiogenesis appears to be somewhat more complicated. Gathering information about the angiogenic stimuli in CNV is difficult because of the lack of appropriate animal models. Information about VEGF levels and CNV in humans is surprisingly limited, and information about other cytokines is even sparser. The formation of blood vessels seems to occur only if the forces stimulating vessel growth outweighed those inhibiting vessel growth. Vascular growth, particularly in CNV, appears to be influenced by both stimulatory and inhibitory modulators. Increased levels of VEGF alone do not appear to be sufficient to cause CNV [69]. One cytokine that has the potential to inhibit angiogenesis is pigment epithelial-derived factor (PEDF). Decreased levels of PEDF appear to be permissive for the growth of vessels in CNV [11]. High levels of PEDF, though, paradoxically may increase the growth of CNV [5]. Inhibition of the receptor 1 for VEGF (VEGFR-1) decreases PEDF production and secretion [68]. VEGF downregulates PEDF expression and PEDF appears to compete with VEGF for binding to VEGFR-2 [91]. Curiously, many studies have shown an increase in both factors in ocular angiogenesis [21, 54, 58, 61, 66]. Other studies have shown a decrease in PEDF in ocular neovascularization [11, 40], with the exception of disciform scars [11]. The ratio between VEGF and PEDF is probably important in the development of CNV, but it is clear that the tissue effects are not simply proportional to the linear ratio between the two.

6.2.2 Cancer and Angiogenesis

Much of what we know about angiogenesis was gained from studying cancer. The treatment of cancer first relied on extrication, then on attempts to selectively inhibit or attack the cancer cells directly with radiation or drugs. Later realization that cancer was a tissue growth that often included supportive and nutritive components offered expanded treatment opportunities. Preventing or limiting tumor vasculature growth may limit the growth potential of the cancer as well. Cancer cells grow, and to grow they recruit new vessels to supply these metabolic demands. Inhibition of vascularization through monoclonal antibodies directed against VEGF was earlier shown to limit the growth of human tumor xenografts in animals [49]. Further advancement of this approach led to the development of bevacizumab (Avastin; Genentech, South San Francisco, CA, USA), a monoclonal antibody directed against VEGF [28].

An early clinical trial examining the effects of bevacizumab in breast cancer patients already under chemotherapy showed no prolongation of life [63]. However, patients with advanced colon cancer being treated with chemotherapy showed a statistically significant prolongation of life from a mean of 15.6 months to 20.3 months with the addition of bevacizumab [42]. The difference in the response between breast and colon cancer has been attributed, in part, to different angiogenic proteins produced by the tumors. In breast cancer multiple angiogenesis mediators are expressed including VEGF, fibroblast growth factor, placental growth factor, transforming growth factor β and the proportion of these mediators may shift with the stage of the cancer [60, 73]. Colon cancer, a more aggressive tumor, may rely predominantly on VEGF for angiogenesis. Because it appears that angiogenic pathways are more numerous and redundant as breast cancer progresses a later study of patients with previously untreated breast cancer was performed [36]. Those patients treated with a combination of bevacizumab and paclitaxel had an increase in response rate (28%) compared with paclitaxel alone (14%), but most patients did not respond. Early results of anti-VEGF treatment for cancer suggest that incremental improvement may be possible for some types of cancer at certain stages in development, and only when used in combination with chemotherapeutic agents.

Angiogenesis arises from multiple stimuli, and blocking only one molecule may not be enough to satisfactorily inhibit vascular development [73]. The combined targeting of angiogenesis is generating interest in cancer therapy. The response of vessels to antiangiogenic treatment is dependent on the maturity of the vessels. Withdrawal or the blocking of VEGF can cause regression of new vessels particularly if they do not have periendothelial support cells such as pericytes or smooth muscle cells [10, 23]. Blocking VEGF/VEGFR-2 signaling did not cause vascular regression in a C6 tumor angiogenesis model among vessels with pericytes, apparently because of Ang-1/Tie2 signaling between the pericytes and the endothelial cells [23]. Simultaneous targeting of pericytes by blocking the platelet-derived growth factor receptor and endothelial cells by blocking the VEGFR-2 receptor caused vascular regression in the newly developed tumor vessels [23]. This simultaneous blockade did not have an effect on the normal vessels of the host tissue, indicating that newly developed vessels have a plasticity not found in older, established vessels. VEGF inhibition in spontaneous RIP-Tag2 tumors and implanted Lewis lung carcinomas in mice caused regression of vascular endothelial cells and the vessels were less tortuous, more uniform in caliber, and had fewer branches and sprouts [55]. Histopathological examination showed empty sleeves of basement membrane, reduced numbers of pericytes and altered pericyte phenotype. Restoration of VEGF resulted in a rapid regrowth of the regressed vessels such that by 7 days the vessels were fully regrown, the regrowth occurred into the previously empty basement membrane tubes, and the pericyte phenotype returned to baseline [55]. These results suggest that the remnants of the vascular system left after VEGF inhibition act as scaffolding for the regrowth of vessels.

Summary for the Clinician

- Angiogenesis is a complex process with redundancies, as would be expected for a process central to development, growth, and survival.
- Growth of vessels requires actions of many effectors, including growth factors, integrins, and matrix metalloproteinases.
- The main mediator for angiogenesis is VEGF-A, which stimulates vascular leakage and vascular endothelial cell proliferation. Thin-walled tubes of vascular endothelial cells are formed. These initial steps of angiogenesis are very sensitive to VEGF withdrawal.
- After capillary tubes form, they become enveloped by pericytes, which offer structural support and also secrete growth factors to maintain the vessel. Withdrawal of VEGF at this stage is less successful in causing vascular regression.
- Inhibition of PDGF can cause pericyte regression, which when used with VEGF inhibition can cause vascular regression.

6.3 Normalization of Tumor Vasculature

Intense angiogenesis leads to the production of early vessels that are not graceful filigrees with the sequential hierarchy of arterioles, capillaries, and venules; instead, there is a plexus of loops, shunts, and saccular dilations. Leakage from these vessel walls is thought to increase tissue hydrostatic pressure, which may alter blood flow through the vascular network [16]. The heterogeneous blood flow distribution from shunts and hydrostatic pressure potentially results in regions where there is inadequate delivery of O_2 and metabolites in the tumor. Antiangiogenic treatment prunes the more immature, poorly formed vessels from the vascular complexes. This leaves vessels that adopt a more normal-appearing phenotype in a process called vascular normalization (Fig. 6.2) [44]. Normal vasculature has a hierarchical arrangement of arteries, arterioles, capillaries, and venules. The proangiogenic and antiangiogenic stimuli are in balance, maintaining a given degree of blood vessel density. With intense pro-angiogenic stimuli the vessels form loops, shunts, and gross dilations of vessels associated with leakage and increased tissue hydrostatic pressure. Antiangiogenic treatment, such as with VEGF withdrawal, leads to pruning of some of the most recent vessel growth, less tortuosity, and decreased leakage and tissue hydrostatic pressure. More profound levels of antiangiogenic treatment can lead to pronounced regression of the vessels, producing tissue ischemia. In this situation the perfusion is inadequate to maintain the associated tissue, resulting in regression of the cancer cells. In a similar manner CNV has the exuberant growth of vessels that appear to be pruned back to an extent, but not eliminated by current antiangiogenic treatments. This probably leads to normalization of the vessels within the CNV complex. More complete regression of the CNV vessels may be expected to cause regression or death of the extravascular component. Because of improved flow characteristics in the normalized vasculature after antiangiogenic treatment there may be a net improvement in the circulation within tumors [88]. In an editorial discussing the results of bevacizumab in the treatment of colon cancer the possibility was raised that the increased survival rates could have been due to the normalization of blood flow, which resulted in improved delivery of chemotherapeutic agents rather than more direct antiangiogenically induced tumor regression [62].

> **Summary for the Clinician**
>
> ■ Inhibition of intense pro-angiogenic stimuli causes a reduction in more abnormal-appearing vascular loops and shunts, and also decreases vascular leakage from areas of new vessel growth. This causes the vessels to adopt a more normal appearance.
> ■ Vascular normalization probably occurs with anti-VEGF treatment of CNV—the vessels may not be that evident by fluorescein angiography, but they are probably still there.

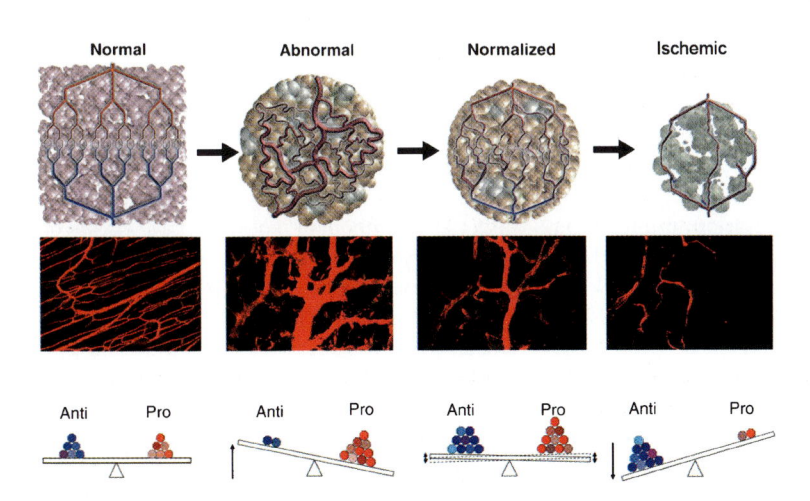

Fig. 6.2 Proposed role of vascular normalization within tumors in response to antiangiogenic treatment. (Figure modified from that in [44])

6.4 Two-Component Model of CNV

The constituents of cancer can be thought of as two principle components, tumor cells and vascular cells. Treatment of both components may have an improved effect compared with treatment with one component alone [2, 30]. It has been proposed that CNV can be considered a two-component system [82]. Histopathologic evaluation shows that CNV is really a tissue invasion of vascular cells and extravascular cells (Fig. 6.1) [32, 33]. The vascular component comprises endothelial cells, circulating endothelial progenitor cells, and pericytes. Invading extravascular cells include inflammatory cells such as macrophages, lymphocytes, granulocytes, foreign body giant cells, and also fibrocytes, myofibroblasts, retinal pigment epithelial (RPE) cells, and glial cells [26, 33, 48, 86]. Growth of vessels in pathologic conditions occurs because cells or tissues help recruit vessels to grow; the vessels do not stimulate themselves to grow. In CNV the amount of VEGF expressed is proportional to the number of inflammatory cells present and VEGF in CNV colocalizes with the inflammatory cells [33, 67]. VEGF in turn can induce expression of cellular adhesion molecules in vessels, and may participate in recruiting macrophages [19]. In CNV specimens the RPE cells expressed monocyte chemotactic protein (MCP), a cytokine involved in macrophage recruitment [33]. Depletion of monocyte cell lines inhibits the formation of CNV in experimental animal models [25]. Thus, self-reinforcing processes appear to be taking place in the initial steps of CNV. The outer retina has a physiologic hypoxia that may be a further stimulus for invading cells to produce angiogenic stimuli [4, 81]. Over time, CNV produces vascular invasion, proliferation, matrix formation with or without hemorrhage, remodeling of the tissue, and eventual vascular regression in involutional lesions [81]. This observed pattern strongly suggests a wound healing response instead of the growth of vessels in response to ischemia alone, where the invading vessels would recapitulate the organization of the choriocapillaris [32, 46, 81]. Both the vascular and extravascular components have the potential for inducing tissue damage independently and in concert.

Summary for the Clinician

- Choroidal neovascularization is actually a tissue comprising two principle components: a vascular component and an extravascular component.
- The vessels in CNV do not cause themselves to grow. The vessels grow in response to and with the help of cells surrounding the invading vessels. Histopathologic examination shows that the vessels constitute a minority of the volume of the invading tissue.
- Extravascular inflammatory cells are an important source of VEGF in CNV. Depletion of monocyte cell lines inhibits the formation of CNV in animal models.

6.5 Two-Component Model and Therapy

The goal of therapy for CNV would be to target the vascular component, the extravascular component or both. Inhibiting the vascular component directly addresses the vessels, but does not directly affect the extravascular component. With the reduction in blood supply there may be a corresponding reduction inn the extravascular component through ischemia and decreased delivery to the CNV complex. It is possible that with time compensatory or involutional changes may occur within the neovascular complex such as the enveloping of the new vessels by RPE cells or through eventual withdrawal or apoptosis of the extravascular cells. Existing therapies may target one component, but often have effects on the other component as well. Therapies principally directed against the vascular component include PDT and pharmacological approaches blocking VEGF (pegaptanib, bevacizumab, and ranibizumab). Initial data from studies examining anti-VEGF therapies have shown that there is continued growth with pegaptanib [31] or no growth, but no shrinkage, of the lesion size with ranibizumab [14, 75]. This suggests that there might be preservation and possibly normalization of the more mature portions of the neovascularization, possibly related to incomplete inhibition of angiogenic mediators [72]. Inhibition of VEGF may also decrease the inflammatory effects of induced cellular adhesion molecule expression and inflammatory cell recruitment to the lesion.

The strategy of inhibiting the extravascular component would include targeting the action of the extravascular cells or important cytokines (such as with immunomodulators [57]). In cancer treatment targeting cancer cells is difficult because of the narrow therapeutic window of chemotherapeutic agents, their poor selectivity for cancer cells compared with normal cells in the body, and because of the genetic instability of cancer cells [30]. In CNV, on the other hand, the invading cells are fairly consistent in their constituency from patient to patient and are genetically stable [82]. The problem of selectivity remains, however. This problem can be circumvented in some circumstances by local administration of the drug to the eye through intravitreal injection. This concentrates the drug in the eye and can suppress local undesired processes without having a significant systemic effect. For example, intravitreal injection of triamcinolone directly targets inflammatory processes in the eye that may be occurring as part of the growth of new vessels, without influencing the systemic inflammatory response. Inhibiting the extravascular component may indirectly have an effect on the vascular component through the secondary reduction in angiogenic cytokines or by reducing the tissue load needing vascular support. There are no published reports of pure inhibitors of the extravascular component of CNV at present, although corticosteroids inhibit many aspects of the extravascular component. Some therapies potentially inhibit both components and include thermal laser, radiation [41], and the combination of PDT and intravitreal triamcinolone [83].

Similar to cancer therapy, combination approaches are being considered for the treatment of CNV. Attacking both the vascular and extravascular components intuitively seems like a good approach. This brings about the need to look at additional agents that could attack or inhibit the extravascular component. Alternate approaches could include targeting one component twice if the attack is by different mechanisms, an approach being used in cancer trials [30]. For CNV the use of PDT combined with either pegaptanib or ranibizumab illustrates this idea. PDT damages both the neovascularization and normal choroidal vessels through the generation of singlet oxygen and free radicals. PDT causes both an increase in VEGF and a decrease in PEDF [77]. However, VEGF is a survival factor for vascular endothelial cells and has anti-apoptotic effects. Blocking VEGF may limit the ability of damaged resident choroidal vessels to sustain the oxidative damage induced by PDT. As a survival factor, the VEGF-165 isoform is the most potent and predominant type secreted after a variety of injuries including irradiation [12, 13, 35, 47, 70]. While PDT and anti-VEGF combinations may act together to stop neovascularization, blocking the injury-induced VEGF response may also lead to more collateral damage than either treatment method would have caused alone.

6.5.1 Are There Cytokines to Block Other Than VEGF?

Vascular endothelial growth factor generated great interest because it is one of the most important and powerful agents stimulating blood vessels to grow. There are a number of other potential factors to block besides VEGF in the treatment of CNV. The actual means of blocking each of these potential cytokines may not be readily available, but several factors can be inhibited with commercially available medications. PDGF is an intriguing cytokine to block because it plays a number of potential roles in producing a CNV lesion. PDGF is a family of homo- and heterodimeric proteins originally isolated from platelets. Subsequently, a number of cells have been found to produce PDGF [1]. The varying forms of PDGF exert their cellular effects through tyrosine kinase receptors. Ligand binding to the platelet-derived growth factor receptor (PDGFR) causes receptor dimerization, autophosphorylation, and leads to intracellular signaling. PDGF helps recruit pericytes and can enhance angiogenesis, in part by stimulating the expression of additional VEGF [34, 39, 52]. PDGF enhances recruitment of fibroblasts and has been shown to stimulate the production of collage, proteoglycans, and fibronectin [3, 15, 38, 45, 90]. PDGF also plays a role in recruiting inflammatory cells [51, 87]. PDGF has been related to increased tissue interstitial hydrostatic pressure [87], an important consideration in tumors [71] as well as in macular degeneration.

Tumor necrosis factor alpha (TNFα) is an acute phase reactant. It is a glycoprotein cleaved by macrophages and activated T lymphocytes from a longer peptide in response to a number of stimuli. TNF is involved in a variety of inflammatory pathways and participates in tissue damage from inflammation [43]. TNF can also cause hemorrhage and necrosis of tumor vasculature [17]. TNF is an important mediator of septic shock and vasoplegia, can regulate cell survival matrix metalloproteinase expression, stimulate production of other angiogenic factors and chemokines, and stimulate fibroblast growth and function [59, 89]. TNF is found in excised CNV specimens in the regions of macrophage infiltration [67]. In laser-induced choroidal neovascularization TNF expression is increased and blocking TNF with antibodies reduces the size of the resultant CNV [78]. Infliximab, an antibody that binds TNF, was anecdotally seen to cause regression in 3 patients with CNV [57].

6.6 Combination Therapies

The combination of more than one therapy against the tissue invasion of CNV has the potential to be efficacious if the treatments attack each of the two components or if each treatment attacks one component by more than one mechanism. A combinatorial approach allows attack against more than one aspect of CNV, with the potential for greater efficacy. The combination of agents targeting the process of CNV may lead to improved visual acuity, decreased treatment frequency or decreased severity of side-effects. In the treatment of cancer, the use of multiple agents in lower doses can lead to decreased side-effects with increased efficacy compared with single agents. In the treatment of CNV, combination therapies have often been associated with increased side-effects.

6.6.1 Anti-VEGF Biologics and Photodynamic Therapy

Anti-VEGF agents and PDT in combination both attack the vascular component by somewhat different mechanisms, but do not directly affect the extravascular component. Multiple logistic regression of the treatment effect of patients being treated with pegaptanib, many of whom also received PDT, found that PDT did not cause a significant treatment effect after taking account of pegaptanib. Although not specifically stated, this implies that the combination of the two treatments was not better than pegaptanib alone [22].

Combined use of PDT with ranibizumab resulted in improved acuity compared with PDT alone in the phase II FOCUS study [37]. A lyophilized version of ranibizumab used in the FOCUS study was associated with a high incidence of intraocular inflammation. Several patients treated with PDT and ranibizumab had decreased acuity associated with intraocular inflammation. The reason for the visual acuity loss in these patients was not known, but a protocol change was made to separate PDT and ranibizumab by 1 week. A later formulation of ranibizumab, used in phase III trials, was associated with a greatly reduced incidence of intraocular inflammation. We do not know if the combination of PDT with intraocular ranibizumab is better than ranibizumab alone. Early reports suggest that using PDT plus bevacizumab results in visual acuity improvement with a relatively low frequency of subsequent bevacizumab injections. PROTECT is an open-label multicenter phase II study involving 32 patients who were given verteporfin PDT at baseline and at months 3, 6, and 9 if leakage was present on fluorescein angiography. Patients were given four monthly injections of ranibizumab. One patient experienced an acute vision decrease and 3 had intraocular inflammation by 9 months' follow-up. The mean visual acuity change was an improvement of 2.4 letters by 9 months (Information from Frank Holz, MD, written communication 10 December 2006).

Photodynamic therapy has the unfortunate tendency to cause acute severe vision decrease, particularly in patients with occult CNV. The incidence of acute treatment-related visual acuity loss from PDT in patients who had had previous anti-VEGF treatment is not known, but it will probably be a finite number. The small proportion of patients having moderate visual acuity loss with anti-VEGF monotherapy is 5% or less at 1 year, making any PDT-induced loss of vision seem more troublesome. Using a reduced fluence of the laser during PDT may help reduce the likelihood of acute severe vision decrease in patients who had had previous anti-VEGF treatment.

6.6.2 Anecortave Acetate and Photodynamic Therapy

Anecortave acetate and PDT with verteporfin was not significantly different from PDT alone in a phase II study (Alcon, unpublished). Both treatments are directed against the vascular component and not the extravascular component.

6.6.3 Intravitreal Triamcinolone and Photodynamic Therapy

Patients treated with combined PDT and intravitreal triamcinolone seem to have a better visual acuity result with a lower treatment rate than with PDT alone. In one study of 26 patients [83], half of whom had had previous PDT, but with continued loss of vision, and half of whom had had no previous treatment were given PDT followed by an injection of 4 mg of triamcinolone. At the end of 1 year's follow-up these patients required slightly more than 1.2 treatments. The previously treated group had a visual acuity improvement of +0.44 lines, which was not significantly different from baseline. The previously untreated patients had an improvement of 2.5 lines, which was statistically significant. The principle short-term side-effect was increased intraocular pressure, which occurred in 10 of the 26 patients. A randomized trial of 61 patients with predominantly subfoveal CNV treated with PDT versus PDT and triamcinolone found that after a 12-month follow-up those treated with the combination had better acuity, smaller lesion sizes, and required fewer treatments than those who had had PDT alone [6]. Two nonrandomized comparative trials found that patients treated with the combination of PDT and triamcinolone did better in terms of visual acuity and treatment frequency than patients treated with PDT alone [18, 76]. Patient series uniformly showed a reduced treatment frequency for combined PDT and triamcinolone compared with that expected from PDT alone, with most studies showing improvement [9, 29, 56, 64] or stabilization of acuity [27, 50]. One study showed a significant decrease in visual acuity of patients treated with combined PDT and triamcinolone [24]. There are no data at present to suggest that there is a significant difference in outcomes if the triamcinolone is given before, at the same time as, or after the PDT.

The addition of triamcinolone to PDTR appeared to improve the outcome of patients compared with PDT alone. While PDT causes an increase in VEGF and a decrease in PEDF [85], treatment of RPE cell cultures with triamcinolone prevents both the increase in VEGF and the decrease in PEDF from PDT [65]. The main side-effects of intravitreal triamcinolone are cataract formation and increased intraocular pressure [80]. Of patients receiving intravitreal triamcinolone 40% will require topical medications and 1% will need a filtering operation to control their pressure. One of the more worrisome side-effects of PDT is acute severe vision decrease, which can occur in up to 4.5% of patients [7]. The advent of effective anti-VEGF agents in the forms of bevacizumab [84] or ranibizumab [14, 75] has changed the landscape of CNV treatment. Increased intraocular pressure, cataract, and acute severe vision decrease do not occur with intravitreal anti-VEGF agents. Therefore, there are not many compelling reasons to start patients on combined triamcinolone and PDT. (There are even fewer reasons to start patients on PDT alone.)

6.6.4 Triamcinolone and Anti-VEGF Therapy

Although both target the vascular component through partially overlapping mechanisms, the antivascular attacks do differ somewhat. In addition, corticosteroids address a variety of elements in the extravascular component that anti-VEGF agents do not. Current anti-VEGF agents have to be given relatively frequently, every 4 or 6 weeks, while intravitreal triamcinolone persists in the vitreous cavity for several months. It may be possible to decrease the treatment frequency with concurrent intravitreal triamcinolone. However, intravitreal triamcinolone carries an excessive incidence of side-effects. Subtenon injection of triamcinolone has a much lower incidence and severity of side-effects, but the efficacy of subtenon triamcinolone has not been established in the treatment of CNV.

6.6.5 Triamcinolone and Anecortave Acetate

Since both medications attack the vascular component through potentially the same mechanism a combination of the two potentially would be a corticosteroid-sparing strategy. However, corticosteroids address the inflammatory aspects of CNV while anecortave acetate does not. The nature of the interactions between anecortave acetate and triamcinolone are not known and it is possible that there may be competitive binding of the anecortave to sites compared with triamcinolone, potentially leading to less pronounced effects of the triamcinolone.

Summary for the Clinician

- Similar to cancer therapy, combinations of treatments, principally involving drugs, are being fashioned to target more than one aspect of CNV.
- Targeting of the vascular component can be done though nonspecific methods such as PDT or through specific targeting such as with anti-VEGF agents.
- Vascular endothelial growth factor is a survival factor for vascular endothelial cells. Nonselective destructive therapies may induce collateral damage to normal choroidal vessels.
- The extravascular component is a more heterogeneous population of cells and as such is not likely to have a single target for attack. Nonspecific drugs such as corticosteroids may target a number of different pieces of the extravascular component.
- Tumor necrosis factor is involved in tissue damage in other diseases, is present in CNV specimens, and blocking TNF anecdotally has shown early favorable results in CNV.
- Targeting multiple factors such as TNF and PDGF in addition to VEGF may address more aspects of the known pathophysiology of CNV than targeting VEGF alone

- Photodynamic therapy and intravitreal triamcinolone appear to have a better visual acuity response with fewer treatments needed compared with PDT alone.
- The high proportion of patients who have side-effects with combined PDT and triamcinolone along with the comparatively low rate of side-effects with anti-VEGF drugs means that combined PDT and intravitreal triamcinolone should not be used as first-line therapy in most patients.
- Anti-VEGF biologics have been successful at treating CNV and will probably be an important constituent of any combination therapy.
- The addition of PDT to the use of anti-VEGF therapy will probably not improve the visual acuity outcomes, but may reduce the treatment frequency.
- Photodynamic therapy has its own side-effect profile, including acute severe vision decrease. It may be possible to reduce the incidence of acute severe vision decrease in post anti-VEGF patients by using markedly reduced laser fluence.

6.7 Conclusion

Treatments for CNV are improving, with the latest results of the ranibizumab studies showing one-quarter to one-third of patients with a significant improvement in visual acuity. However, the mean visual acuity of patients recruited into CNV treatment studies has usually been between 20/80 and 20/100. So improvement in a minority of patients still leaves most with poor acuity. The principle goal of combination therapy would be to improve the proportion of patients experiencing improved acuity. A secondary goal would be to decrease the number of treatments needed to achieve improved acuity.

Acknowledgement

The author has no financial interests.

References

1. Abramsson A, Lindblom P, Betsholtz C (2003) Endothelial and nonendothelial sources of PDGF-B regulate pericyte recruitment and influence vascular pattern formation in tumors. J Clin Invest 112:1142–1151
2. Abdollahi A, Lipson KE, Sckell A et al (2003) Combined therapy with direct and indirect angiogenesis inhibition results in enhanced antiangiogenic and antitumor effects. Cancer Res 63(24):8890–8898
3. Abdollahi A, Li M, Ping G, Plathow C et al (2005) Inhibition of platelet-derived growth factor signaling attenuates pulmonary fibrosis. J Exp Med 201:925–935
4. Ahmed J, Braun RD, Dunn R, Linsenmeier RA (1993) Oxygen distribution in the macaque retina. Invest Ophthalmol Vis Sci 34:516–521
5. Apte RS, Barreiro RA, Duh E et al (2004) Stimulation of neovascularization by the anti-angiogenic factor PEDF. Invest Ophthalmol Vis Sci 45:4491–4497
6. Arias L, Garcia-Arumi J, Ramon JM et al (2006) Photodynamic therapy with intravitreal triamcinolone in predominantly classic choroidal neovascularization one-year results of a randomized study. Ophthalmology 84(6):743–748
7. Arnold JJ, Blinder KJ, Bressler NM et al (2004) Acute severe visual acuity decrease after photodynamic therapy with verteporfin: case reports from randomized clinical trials-TAP and VIP report no. 3. Am J Ophthalmol 137:683–696
8. Asahara T, Masuda H, Takahashi T et al (1999) Bone marrow origin of endothelial progenitor cells responsible for postnatal vasculogenesis in physiological and pathological neovascularization. Circ Res 85:221–228
9. Augustin AJ, Schmidt-Erfurth U (2006) Verteporfin and intravitreal triamcinolone acetonide combination therapy for occult choroidal neovascularization in age-related macular degeneration. Am J Ophthalmol 141:638–645
10. Bergers G, Song S, Meyer-Morse N, Bergsland E, Hanahan D (2003) Benefits of targeting both pericytes and endothelial cells in the tumor vasculature with kinase inhibitors. J Clin Invest 111:1287–1295
11. Bhutto IA, McLeod DS, Hasegawa T et al (2006) Pigment epithelium-derived factor (PEDF) and vascular endothelial growth factor (VEGF) in aged human choroid and eyes with age-related macular degeneration. Exp Eye Res 82:99–110
12. Boussat S, Eddahibi S, Coste A et al (2000) Expression and regulation of vascular endothelial growth factor in human pulmonary epithelial cells. Am J Physiol Lung Cell Mol Physiol 279: L371–L378
13. Brieger J, Schroeder P, Gosepath J, Mann WJ (2005) VEGF-subtype specific protection of SCC and HUVECs from radiation induced cell death. Int J Mol Med 15(1):145–151
14. Brown DM, Kaiser PK, Michels M et al (2006) Ranibizumab versus verteporfin for neovascular age-related macular degeneration. N Engl J Med 355:1432–1444
15. Canalis E (1981) Effect of platelet-derived growth factor on DNA and protein synthesis in cultured rat calvaria. Metabolism 30:970–975
16. Carmeliet P, Jain RK (2000) Angiogenesis in cancer and other diseases. Nature 407:249–257
17. Carswell EA, Old LJ, Kassel RL et al (1975) An endotoxin-induced serum factor that causes necrosis of tumors. Proc Natl Acad Sci USA 72:3666–3670
18. Chan WM, Lai TY, Wong AL et al (2006) Combined photodynamic therapy and intravitreal triamcinolone injection for the treatment of sub-

foveal choroidal neovascularisation in age related macular degeneration: a comparative study. Br J Ophthalmol 90:337–341
19. Cursiefen C, Chen L, Borges LP et al (2004) VEGF-A stimulates lymphangiogenesis and hemangiogenesis in inflammatory neovascularization via macrophage recruitment. J Clin Invest 113:1040–1050
20. Darland DC, Massingham LJ, Smith SR et al (2003) Pericyte production of cell-associated VEGF is differentiation-dependent and is associated with endothelial survival. Dev Biol 264:275–288
21. Duh EJ, Yang HS, Haller JA et al (2004) Vitreous levels of pigment epithelium-derived factor and vascular endothelial growth factor: implications for ocular angiogenesis. Am J Ophthalmol 137:668–674
22. Dvorak HF, Brown LF, Detmar M, Dvorak AM (1995) Vascular permeability factor/vascular endothelial growth factor, microvascular hyperpermeability, and angiogenesis. Am J Pathol 146:1029–1039
23. Erber R, Thurnher A, Katsen AD et al (2004) Combined inhibition of VEGF and PDGF signaling enforces tumor vessel regression by interfering with pericyte-mediated endothelial cell survival mechanisms. FASEB J 18:338–340
24. Ergun E, Maar N, Ansari-Shahrezaei S et al (2006) Photodynamic therapy with verteporfin and intravitreal triamcinolone acetonide in the treatment of neovascular age-related macular degeneration. Am J Ophthalmol 142:10–16
25. Espinosa-Heidmann DG, Suner IJ, Hernandez EP et al (2003) Macrophage depletion diminishes lesion size and severity in experimental choroidal neovascularization. Invest Ophthalmol Vis Sci 44:3586–3592
26. Espinosa-Heidmann DG, Reinoso MA, Pina Y et al (2005) Quantitative enumeration of vascular smooth muscle cells and endothelial cells derived from bone marrow precursors in experimental choroidal neovascularization. Exp Eye Res 80:369–378
27. Fackler TK, Reddy S, Bearelly S et al (2006) Retrospective review of eyes with neovascular age-related macular degeneration treated with photodynamic therapy with verteporfin and intravitreal triamcinolone. Ann Acad Med Singapore 35:701–705
28. Ferrara N, Hillan KJ, Novotny W (2005) Bevacizumab (Avastin), a humanized anti-VEGF monoclonal antibody for cancer therapy. Biochem Biophys Res Commun 333:328–335
29. Freund KB, Klais CM, Eandi CM et al (2006) Sequenced combined intravitreal triamcinolone and indocyanine green angiography-guided photodynamic therapy for retinal angiomatous proliferation. Arch Ophthalmol 124:487–492
30. Gasparini G, Longo R, Fanelli M, Teicher BA (2005) Combination of antiangiogenic therapy with other anticancer therapies: results, challenges, and open questions. J Clin Oncol 23:1295–1311
31. Gragoudas ES, Adamis AP, Cunningham ET Jr et al (2004) Pegaptanib for neovascular age-related macular degeneration. N Engl J Med 351:2805–2816
32. Grossniklaus HE, Green WR (2004) Choroidal neovascularization. Am J Ophthalmol 137:496–503
33. Grossniklaus HE, Ling JX, Wallace TM et al (2002) Macrophage and retinal pigment epithelium expression of angiogenic cytokines in choroidal neovascularization. Mol Vis 8:119–126
34. Guo P, Hu B, Gu W et al (2003) Platelet-derived growth factor-B enhances glioma angiogenesis by stimulating vascular endothelial growth factor expression in tumor endothelia and by promoting pericyte recruitment. Am J Pathol 162:1083–1093
35. Gupta VK, Jaskowiak NT, Beckett MA et al (2002) Vascular endothelial growth factor enhances endothelial cell survival and tumor radioresistance. Cancer J 8:47–54
36. Hampton T (2005) Monoclonal antibody therapies shine in breast cancer clinical trials. JAMA 293:2985–2989
37. Heier JS, Boyer DS, Ciulla TA et al (2006) Ranibizumab combined with verteporfin photodynamic therapy in neovascular age-related macular degeneration: year 1 results of the FOCUS Study. Arch Ophthalmol 124:1532–1542
38. Heldin CH, Westermark B (1999) Mechanism of action and in vivo role of platelet-derived growth factor. Physiol Rev 79:1283–1316
39. Hirschi KK, Rohovsky SA, Beck LH, Smith SR, D'Amore PA (1999) Endothelial cells modulate the proliferation of mural cell precursors via platelet-derived growth factor-BB and heterotypic cell contact. Circ Res 84:298–305

40. Holekamp NM, Bouck N, Volpert O (2002) Pigment epithelium-derived factor is deficient in the vitreous of patients with choroidal neovascularization due to age-related macular degeneration. Am J Ophthalmol 134:220–227
41. Hori K, Saito S, Tamai M (2004) Effect of irradiation on neovascularization in rat skinfold chambers: implications for clinical trials of low-dose radiotherapy for wet-type age-related macular degeneration. Int J Radiat Oncol Biol Phys 60:1564–1571
42. Hurwitz H, Fehrenbacher L, Novotny W et al (2004) Bevacizumab plus irinotecan, fluorouracil, and leucovorin for metastatic colorectal cancer. N Engl J Med 350:2335–2342
43. Husby G, Williams RC Jr (1988) Synovial localization of tumor necrosis factor in patients with rheumatoid arthritis. J Autoimmun 1:363–371
44. Jain RK (2005) Normalization of tumor vasculature: an emerging concept in antiangiogenic therapy. Science 307:58–62
45. Kamiyama K, Iguchi I, Wang X, Imanishi J (1998) Effects of PDGF on the migration of rabbit corneal fibroblasts and epithelial cells. Cornea 17:315–325
46. Kent D, Sheridan C (2003) Choroidal neovascularization: a wound healing perspective. Mol Vis 9:747–755
47. Kermani P, Leclerc G, Martel R, Fareh J (2001) Effect of ionizing radiation on thymidine uptake, differentiation, and VEGFR2 receptor expression in endothelial cells: the role of VEGF(165). Int J Radiat Oncol Biol Phys 50(1):213–220
48. Killingsworth MC (1995) Angiogenesis in early choroidal neovascularization secondary to age-related macular degeneration. Graefes Arch Clin Exp Ophthalmol 233:313–323
49. Kim KJ, Li B, Winer J et al (1993) Inhibition of vascular endothelial growth factor-induced angiogenesis suppresses tumour growth in vivo. Nature 362:841–844
50. Krebs I, Binder S, Stolba U (2006) A new treatment regimen in combined intravitreal injection of triamcinolone acetonide and photodynamic therapy. Graefes Arch Clin Exp Ophthalmol 244:863–867
51. Krettek A, Ostergren-Lunden G, Fager G et al (2001) Expression of PDGF receptors and ligand-induced migration of partially differentiated human monocyte-derived macrophages. Influence of IFN-gamma and TGF-beta. Atherosclerosis 156:267–275
52. Lindblom P, Gerhardt H, Liebner S et al (2003) Endothelial PDGF-B retention is required for proper investment of pericytes in the microvessel wall. Genes Dev 17:1835–1840
53. Lyden D, Hattori K, Dias S et al (2001) Impaired recruitment of bone-marrow-derived endothelial and hematopoietic precursor cells blocks tumor angiogenesis and growth. Nat Med. 2001(11):1194–1201
54. McColm JR, Geisen P, Hartnett ME. VEGF isoforms and their expression after a single episode of hypoxia or repeated fluctuations between hyperoxia and hypoxia: relevance to clinical ROP. Mol Vis 10:512–520
55. Mancuso MR, Davis R, Norberg SM et al (2006) Rapid vascular regrowth in tumors after reversal of VEGF inhibition. J Clin Invest 116:2610–2621
56. Mantel I, Ambresin A, Zografos L (2006) Retinal angiomatous proliferation treated with a combination of intravitreal triamcinolone acetonide and photodynamic therapy with verteporfin. Eur J Ophthalmol 16:705–710
57. Markomichelakis NN, Theodossiadis PG, Sfikakis PP (2005) Regression of neovascular age-related macular degeneration following infliximab therapy. Am J Ophthalmol 139:537–540
58. Martin G, Schlunck G, Hansen LL, Agostini HT (2004) Differential expression of angioregulatory factors in normal and CNV-derived human retinal pigment epithelium. Graefes Arch Clin Exp Ophthalmol 242:321–326
59. Maruotti N, Cantatore FP, Crivellato E et al (2006) Angiogenesis in rheumatoid arthritis. Histol Histopathol 21:557–566
60. Marx J (2003) Angiogenesis. A boost for tumor starvation. Science 301:452–454
61. Matsuoka M, Ogata N, Otsuji T et al (2004) Expression of pigment epithelium derived factor and vascular endothelial growth factor in choroidal neovascular membranes and polypoidal choroidal vasculopathy. Br J Ophthalmol 88:809–815
62. Mayer RJ (2004) Two steps forward in the treatment of colorectal cancer. N Engl J Med 350:2406–2408
63. Miller KD, Chap LI, Holmes FA et al (2005) Randomized phase III trial of capecitabine compared with bevacizumab plus capecitabine in patients with previously treated metastatic breast cancer. J Clin Oncol 23:792–799

64. Nicolo M, Ghiglione D, Lai S et al (2006) Occult with no classic choroidal neovascularization secondary to age-related macular degeneration treated by intravitreal triamcinolone and photodynamic therapy with verteporfin. Retina 26:58–64
65. Obata R, Inoue Y, Iriyama A et al (2007) Triamcinolone acetonide suppresses early proangiogenic response in RPE cells after photodynamic therapy in vitro. Br J Ophthalmol 91(1):100–104
66. Ogata N, Wada M, Otsuji T et al (2002) Expression of pigment epithelium-derived factor in normal adult rat eye and experimental choroidal neovascularization. Invest Ophthalmol Vis Sci 43:1168–1175
67. Oh H, Takagi H, Takagi C et al (1999) The potential angiogenic role of macrophages in the formation of choroidal neovascular membranes. Invest Ophthalmol Vis Sci 40:1891–1898
68. Ohno-Matsui K, Yoshida T, Uetama T et al (2003) Vascular endothelial growth factor up-regulates pigment epithelium-derived factor expression via VEGFR-1 in human retinal pigment epithelial cells. Biochem Biophys Res Commun 303:962–967
69. Oshima Y, Oshima S, Nambu H et al (2004) Increased expression of VEGF in retinal pigmented epithelial cells is not sufficient to cause choroidal neovascularization. J Cell Physiol 201:393–400
70. Ostendorf T, Kunter U, Eitner F et al (1999) VEGF(165) mediates glomerular endothelial repair. J Clin Invest 104:913–923
71. Pietras K, Rubin K, Sjoblom T et al (2002) Inhibition of PDGF receptor signaling in tumor stroma enhances antitumor effect of chemotherapy. Cancer Res 62:5476–5484
72. Rakic JM, Lambert V, Devy L et al (2003) Placental growth factor, a member of the VEGF family, contributes to the development of choroidal neovascularization. Invest Ophthalmol Vis Sci 44:3186–3193
73. Relf M, LeJeune S, Scott PA et al (1997) Expression of the angiogenic factors vascular endothelial cell growth factor, acidic and basic fibroblast growth factor, tumor growth factor beta-1, platelet-derived endothelial cell growth factor, placenta growth factor, and pleiotrophin in human primary breast cancer and its relation to angiogenesis. Cancer Res 57:963–969
74. Roberts WG, Palade GE (1995) Increased microvascular permeability and endothelial fenestration induced by vascular endothelial growth factor. J Cell Sci 108:2369–2379
75. Rosenfeld PJ, Brown DM, Heier JS et al (2006) Ranibizumab for neovascular age-related macular degeneration. N Engl J Med 355:1419–1431
76. Ruiz-Moreno JM, Montero JA et al (2006) Photodynamic therapy and high-dose intravitreal triamcinolone to treat exudative age-related macular degeneration: 1-year outcome. Retina 26:602–612
77. Schmidt-Erfurth U, Schlotzer-Schrehard U, Cursiefen C et al (2003) Influence of photodynamic therapy on expression of vascular endothelial growth factor (VEGF), VEGF receptor 3, and pigment epithelium-derived factor. Invest Ophthalmol Vis Sci 44:4473–4480
78. Shi X, Semkova I, Muther PS et al (2006) Inhibition of TNF-alpha reduces laser-induced choroidal neovascularization. Exp Eye Res 83:1325–1334
79. Silletti S, Kessler T, Goldberg J et al (2001) Disruption of matrix metalloproteinase 2 binding to integrin alpha vbeta 3 by an organic molecule inhibits angiogenesis and tumor growth in vivo. Proc Natl Acad Sci USA 98:119–124
80. Smithen LM, Spaide RF (2004) Photodynamic therapy and intravitreal triamcinolone for a subretinal neovascularization in bilateral idiopathic juxtafoveal telangiectasis. Am J Ophthalmol 138:884–885
81. Spaide RF (2005) Etiology of late-age-related macular disease. In: Holz F, Spaide RF (eds) Medical retina. Springer, New York
82. Spaide RF (2006) Rationale for combination therapies for choroidal neovascularization. Am J Ophthalmol 141:149–156
83. Spaide RF, Sorenson J, Maranan L (2005) Photodynamic therapy with verteporfin combined with intravitreal injection of triamcinolone acetonide for choroidal neovascularization. Ophthalmology 112:301–304
84. Spaide RF, Laud K, Fine HF et al (2006) Intravitreal bevacizumab treatment of choroidal neovascularization secondary to age-related macular degeneration. Retina 26:383–390
85. Tatar O, Adam A, Shinoda K et al (2006) Expression of VEGF and PEDF in choroidal neovascular membranes following verteporfin photodynamic therapy. Am J Ophthalmol 142:95–104

86. Tsutsumi-Miyahara C, Sonoda KH, Egashira K et al (2004) The relative contributions of each subset of ocular infiltrated cells in experimental choroidal neovascularisation. Br J Ophthalmol 88:1217–1222
87. Uutela M, Wirzenius M, Paavonen K et al (2004) PDGF-D induces macrophage recruitment, increased interstitial pressure, and blood vessel maturation during angiogenesis. Blood 104:3198–3204
88. Winkler F, Kozin SV, Tong RT et al (2004) Kinetics of vascular normalization by VEGFR2 blockade governs brain tumor response to radiation: role of oxygenation, angiopoietin-1, and matrix metalloproteinases. Cancer Cell 6:553–563
89. Yan L, Anderson GM, DeWitte M, Nakada MT (2006) Therapeutic potential of cytokine and chemokine antagonists in cancer therapy. Eur J Cancer 42:793–802
90. Yoshiji H, Kuriyama S, Noguchi R et al (2006) Amelioration of liver fibrogenesis by dual inhibition of PDGF and TGF-beta with a combination of imatinib mesylate and ACE inhibitor in rats. Int J Mol Med 17:899–904
91. Zhang SX, Wang JJ, Gao G et al (2006) Pigment epithelium-derived factor downregulates vascular endothelial growth factor (VEGF) expression and inhibits VEGF-VEGF receptor 2 binding in diabetic retinopathy. J Mol Endocrinol 37:1–12

Chapter 7

Nutritional Supplementation in Age-related Macular Degeneration

Hanna R. Coleman, Emily Y. Chew

Core Messages

- Oxidative stress may play an important role in the pathogenesis of age-related macular degeneration (AMD) as smoking is a major risk factor.
- The Age-Related Eye Disease Study (AREDS) showed that antioxidant vitamins C (500 mg), E (400 IU), beta-carotene (15 mg), zinc oxide (80 mg), and copper (as cupric oxide 2 mg) reduced the risk of developing advanced AMD (neovascular or geographic atrophy involving the center of the fovea) by 25% compared with placebo at 5 years' follow-up.
- The AREDS formulation also reduced the risk of moderate visual loss by 19% compared with placebo at 5 years' follow-up.
- There was no increased risk of mortality in the AREDS study in those participants assigned to the antioxidant vitamins and/or zinc.
- Observational data suggest that higher dietary intakes of lutein and omega-3 long-chain polyunsaturated fatty acids were associated with decreased risk of AMD.
- Lutein, zeaxanthin, omega-3 long-chain polyunsaturated fatty acids are currently investigated for their potential role in the treatment of AMD in a randomized, controlled clinical trial, AREDS2.

7.1 Introduction

Age-related macular degeneration (AMD) is the leading cause of visual loss in the US among patients over 65 years of age [14]. The disease is projected to increase at an alarming rate due to the increasing longevity of our elderly population [52]. The treatment of AMD has progressed over the years from the use of laser photocoagulation to photodynamic therapy, surgical procedures and anti-VEGF medications, but there is still no effective cure and visual impairment continues to be high [25, 26, 50, 54].

7.2 Risk Factors

A variety of risk factors have been identified for both early- and late-stage AMD [15, 20, 21, 27, 40, 42, 43, 44, 51, 53], the most consistent of which are age and smoking. Other factors that influence the risk of disease include gender, iris color, heredity, cardiovascular health, nutrient status, body mass index, and lifetime exposure to sunlight. Prevention of modifiable risk factors is a promising approach to reducing the burden of this condition [37, 45, 48].

Because smoking is known to deplete the body's antioxidative potential [1], components of cigarette smoke are oxidants, and diet and nutrition have been associated with advanced AMD, oxidative stress is thought to play a significant role in its pathogenesis. Oxidative processes occur in most biological functions, and multiple pathways have evolved to maintain the balance between the necessary free radicals that serve as regulatory molecules and the unchecked highly reactive molecules that initiate devastating cytotoxic reactions [30]. The retina is particularly susceptible to oxidative stress due to its high oxygen use and its chronic exposure to intense light. Furthermore, photoreceptor outer segments are especially vulnerable to oxidative damage because of their high polyunsaturated fatty acid content [17, 19]. The possibility that the anti oxidant balance can be positively altered by diet or vitamin supplementation has created much interest.

7.3 Age-Related Eye Disease Study

The Age-Related Eye Disease Study (AREDS) conducted by the National Eye Institute showed that the use of high doses of a combination of anti-oxidants (vitamin C, vitamin E, and beta-carotene) and zinc reduced the risk of development of advanced AMD by about 25% in participants with moderate AMD (AREDS category 3) or advanced AMD in one eye (AREDS category 4). The overall risk of moderate vision loss (>15 letters on the ETDRS chart) was reduced by 19% at 5 years [2]. In the study, the rate of participants with early AMD (AREDS categories 1 and 2) developing advanced AMD was exceedingly low, 1.3% in 5 years. Because of these small numbers, no beneficial effects of the combination treatment were seen. For this reason, the AREDS supplements are only recommended for persons with moderate to severe AMD (AREDS categories 3 or 4).

7.4 Lutein/Zeaxanthin

Continuing evidence is accumulating regarding the role of oxidative stress in the pathogenesis of AMD and the mechanisms involved [6, 11, 35, 55]. Of particular interest is the presence of macular pigment, which is composed primarily of the carotenoids lutein and zeaxanthin, two naturally occuring plant pigments [24, 46, 47]. The concentration of macular pigment is greatest at the inner retinal layers of the fovea and the small amounts that are present in the peripheral retina are found in rod outer segments [9, 49]. Studies suggest that an inverse relation exists between the risk of AMD and the amounts of lutein and zeaxanthin in the retina [7, 8, 10]. A high intake of green leafy vegetables containing lutein and zeaxanthin was associated with a reduction in the risk of neovascular AMD [32]. It has been postulated that the carotenoids may protect the retina from oxidative stress via two mechanisms: by absorbing the blue light that may be associated with photochemical damage, and by quenching reactive oxygen species [16, 22, 29, 36, 38].

At the beginning of the AREDS trial, lutein and zeaxanthin were not commercially available and beta-carotene, although not present in the retina, was used for its anti-oxidative potential. During the trial, supplementation of beta-carotene was shown to increase the risk of lung cancer and its associated mortality in smokers [5, 34]. Beta-carotene also increased the yellowing of the skin, but this was of no consequence healthwise. An amendment was made to the AREDS protocol to offer all smokers in the study the chance to stop the medication and consider randomization to placebo or zinc only. The current AREDS formulation with beta-carotene is thus not recommended for smokers and AREDS II will study the effect that eliminating beta-carotene from the original vitamin formulation has on the development and progression of AMD.

7.5 Zinc

Zinc was tested in the original formulation at high doses of 80 mg because of the beneficial results of treatment reported by a single-center, randomized, controlled clinical trial with a small sample size and short duration of follow-up [33]. Copper was added to offset the commonly seen side effect of copper-deficient anemia. The outcome measurement of a few letters gained in the zinc-treated group was considered to be of questionable clinical significance. Zinc treatment was also shown to be associated with decreased mortality in the AREDS (RR=0.73; 95% CI 0.60–0.89) [3]. The significance of this finding is not known as this is a selected population of volunteers in a randomized trial of vitamins and minerals. In AREDS, the use of zinc increased hospitalizations due to genitourinary problems. The most common problem was prostate enlargement in men. Other studies have reported that zinc may cause a decrease in HDL ("good") cholesterol or an increase in LDL ("bad") cholesterol. Nutritional experts continue to raise concerns about the widespread, common, and chronic use of such a large dose. AREDS II will study the effects of reducing the dose of zinc from the original AREDS formulation on the development and progression of AMD.

acid. In people reporting the highest levels of omega-3 long-chain polyunsaturated fatty acids (LCPUFA) intake there is a decreased likelihood of having neovascular AMD relative to people reporting the lowest levels of intake. These results and those from other observational analytic investigations [39] suggest that modifying diet to include more foods rich in ω-3 LCPUFAs could result in a reduction in the risk of having neovascular AMD [4, 13, 18].

7.6 Vitamin E

Vitamin E is commonly used at doses of 400 IU; however, a recent meta-analysis of vitamin E concluded that doses of vitamin E of 400 IU or higher were associated with an increased risk of mortality [31]. The analysis performed for this conclusion used prevalence data rather then incidence data from 19 studies and the cut-off point for exposure was arbitrarily set to 400 IU or higher. A follow-up analysis of studies using 400–440 IU of vitamin E in more than 15,000 participants showed that there was no strong basis for inferring increased mortality among participants exposed to these levels of vitamin E. The pooled risk ratio for these three studies was 0.998 with a risk difference of -1.8 per 10,000 persons in the direction of benefit. Based on these data, it would appear to be safe to take the 400-IU dose of vitamin E found in the AREDS formulation [12].

Summary for the Clinician

- Consider administering the AREDS formulation for patients with bilateral large drusen or advanced AMD in one eye.
- The AREDS formulation is contraindicated in cigarette smokers because the beta-carotene has been shown to increase the risk of lung cancer in smokers.
- Observational data from AREDS and other studies suggest that high levels of consumption of lutein/zeaxanthin-containing vegetables (i.e., spinach, kale, collard greens, etc.) and fish are associated with a lowered risk of advanced AMD.

7.7 Dietary Fat Intake

In the Beaver Dam Study, patients with the highest intake of saturated fat and cholesterol were at an 80% increased risk of early AMD. Similar results were found for advanced AMD, but were not statistically significant [28]. Saturated, monounsaturated, polyunsaturated, and transunsaturated fats increased the likelihood of progression for the highest fat intake quartile relative compared with the lowest fat intake quartile. Increased intake of fish reduced risk of AMD, particularly with consumption of two or more servings per week [41]. Dietary omega-3 fatty intake was inversely associated with AMD primarily among participants with low levels (below median) of linoleic acid intake, an omega-6 fatty

7.8 Age-Related Eye Disease Study 2

Based on all of the available nutritional evidence, the National Eye Institute developed the AREDS2 study, which started enrolling in the fall of 2006. Its primary objective is to determine whether oral supplementation with macular xanthophylls (lutein at 10 mg/day + zeaxanthin at 2 mg/day) and/or omega-3 long-chain polyunsaturated fatty acids (LCPUFAs, docosahexaenoic acid [DHA] 350 mg and eicosapentaenoic acid (EPA) 650 mg for a total of 1 g/day) will decrease the risk of progression to advanced AMD, compared with placebo. AREDS2 will also study the effects of these nutritional supplements on moderate vision loss and on the development of cataracts. This objective will be accomplished by collecting and assessing the data of approximately 4,000 participants aged 50–85 years, who at the time of enrollment, have sufficiently clear lenses for quality fundus photographs and have either bilateral large drusen or large drusen in one eye and advanced AMD (neovascular AMD or central geographic atrophy) in the fellow eye. Of the primary randomization agents, one-quarter of the patients will be assigned placebo, another quarter lutein/zeaxanthin, one-quarter omega-3 LCPUFAs, and the final quarter a combination of the two.

Because the study population in AREDS2 is at least moderately at risk of AMD, all participants will be offered the original AREDS formulation. Because of this opportunity, a second randomization was designed to evaluate the possibility of deleting beta-carotene and decreasing the current dose of zinc. The secondary randomization agents (AREDS-Type Supplement) formulations are divided into the four inclusion groups listed in Table 7.1.

Participants who are smokers are also then included in AREDS2 and they would be randomly assigned to either formulation 2 or formulation 3 in the AREDS supplements in the secondary randomization. It is also recognized that some participants may consider it difficult not to take the original AREDS formulation, the proven formulation for persons with moderate AMD, and they would be allowed to do so. It is also possible that some participants may not be able to tolerate the AREDS formulation and they would also be allowed to withdraw from this secondary randomization.

The savings gained from preventive therapy are enormous. It is estimated that about 55 million people in the USA may be at risk of macular degeneration. Of these, 8 million are at high risk, and are thus likely to benefit from the current combination of zinc and anti-oxidant therapy. If all 8 million people at a high risk of AMD took the supplement therapy, more than 300,000 of them could be saved from advanced AMD in the next 5 years.

Summary for the Clinician

- AREDS2 will test the roles of oral supplementation with lutein/zeaxanthin and/or omega-3 long chain polyunsaturated fatty acids in the treatment of AMD.
- AREDS2 will also evaluate the effects of eliminating beta-carotene and lowering the dose of zinc on the development of advanced AMD.

7.9 Conclusion

The economic benefit associated with the prevention of progression to advanced AMD in even a small proportion of cases is significant and will result in major cost savings to individuals and society at large [23]. The evidence that diet and nutrition play crucial roles in the pathogenesis of early AMD and its progression to AMD is now compelling; further studies are crucial in order to find the key micronutrient ingredients that will fully change our treatment and prevention of AMD in the future.

Table 7.1 The four formulations of the original Age-Related Eye Disease Study (AREDS) formulation that will be tested in the secondary randomization of the AREDS2

	1	2	3	4
Vitamin C	500 mg	500 mg	500 mg	500 mg
Vitamin E	400 IU	400 IU	400 IU	400 IU
Beta-carotene	15 mg	0 mg	0 mg	15 mg
Zinc oxide	80 mg	80 mg	25 mg	25 mg
Cupric oxide	2 mg	2 mg	2 mg	2 mg

References

1. Age-Related Eye Disease Study Research Group (2000) Risk factors associated with age-related macular degeneration. A case-control study in the Age-Related Eye Disease Study: Age-Related Eye Disease Study report number 3. Ophthalmology 107:2224–2232
2. Age-Related Eye Disease Study Group (2001) A randomized, placebo-controlled, clinical trial of high-dose supplementation with vitamins C and E, beta-carotene, and zinc for age-related macular degeneration and vision loss. AREDS Report No. 8. Arch Ophthalmol 119:1417–1436
3. Age-Related Eye Disease Study Group (2004) Associations of mortality with ocular disorders and an intervention of high-dose antioxidants and zinc in the Age-Related Eye Disease Study. AREDS Report No. 13. Arch Ophthalmol 122:716–726
4. Age-Related Eye Disease Study Research Group (2004) The relationship of dietary lipid intake and age-related macular degeneration: a case-control study in the Age-Related Eye Disease Study. AREDS Report No. 20. Arch Ophthalmol 122:716–726
5. Alpha-Tocopherol, Beta-Carotene Cancer Prevention Study Group (1994) The effect of vitamin E and beta-carotene on the incidence of lung cancer and other cancers in male smokers. N Engl J Med 330(15):1029–1035
6. Beatty S, Koh HH, Henson D, Bolton M (2000) The role of oxidative stress in the pathogenesis of age-related macular degeneration. Surv Ophthalmol 45:115–134
7. Beatty S, Murray IJ, Henson DB, Carden D, Koh H, Boulton ME (2001) Macular pigment and risk for age-related macular degeneration in subjects from a Northern European population. Invest Ophthalmol Vis Sci 42:439–446
8. Bernstein PS, Zhao DY, Wintch SW, Ermakov IV, McClane RW, Gellermann W (2002) Resonance Raman measurement of macular carotenoids in normal subjects and in age-related macular degeneration patients. Ophthalmology 109:1780–1787
9. Bone RA, Landrum JT, Friedes LM, Gomez CM, Kilburn MD, Menendez E, Vidal I, Wang W (1997) Distribution of lutein and zeaxanthin stereoisomers in the human retina. Exp Eye Res 64:211–218
10. Bone RA, Landrum JT, Mayne ST, Gomez CM, Tibor SE, Twaroska EE (2001) Macular pigment in donor eyes with and without AMD: a case-control study. Invest Ophthalmol Vis Sci 42:235–240
11. Cai J, Nelson KC, Wu M, Sternberg P Jr, Jones DP (2000) Oxidative damage and protection of the RPE. Prog Retinal Eye Res 19:205–221
12. Chew EY, Clemons T (2005) Vitamin E and the Age-Related Eye Disease Study supplementation for age-related macular degeneration. Arch Ophthalmol 123(3):395–396
13. Cho E, Hung S, Willett WC et al (2001) Prospective study of dietary fat and the risk of age-related macular degeneration. Am J Clin Nutr 73(2):209–218
14. Congdon N, O'Colmain B, Klaver CC, Klein R, Munoz B, Friedman DS, Kempen J, Taylor HR, Mitchell P; Eye Diseases Prevalence Research Group (2004) Causes and prevalence of visual impairment among adults in the United States. Arch Ophthalmol 122:477–485
15. Eye Disease Case Control Study Group (1992) Risk factors for neovascular age-related macular degeneration. Arch Ophthalmol 110:1701–1710
16. Eye Disease Case Control Study Group (1993) Antioxidant status and neovascular age-related macular degeneration. Arch Ophthalmol 111:104–109
17. Handleman GJ, Dratz E (1986) The role of antioxidants in the retina and retinal pigment epithelium and the nature of pro-oxidant induced damage. Adv Free Radic Biol Med 2:1–89
18. Herberger RA, Mares-Perlman JA, Klein R, Klein BE, Millen AE, Palta M (2001) Relationship of dietary fat to age-related maculopathy in the Third National Health and Nutrition Examination Survey. Arch Ophthalmol 119:1833–1838
19. Hogg R, Chakravarthy U (2004) Mini-review: AMD and micronutrient antioxidants. Curr Eye Res 29:387–401
20. Hyman L, Schachat AP, He Q, Leske MC (2000) Hypertension, cardiovascular disease, and age-related macular degeneration. Age-Related Macular Degeneration Risk Factors Study Group. Arch Ophthalmol 118:351–358
21. Klein R, Klein BE, Tomany SC, Cruickshanks KJ (2003) The association of cardiovascular disease with the long-term incidence of age-related maculopathy: the Beaver Dam Eye Study. Ophthalmology 110:1273–1280

22. Krinsky NI (2001) Carotenoids as antioxidants. Nutrition 17:815–817
23. Lanchoney DM, Maguire MG, Fine SL (1998) A model of the incidence and consequences of choroidal neovascularization secondary to age-related macular degeneration: comparative effects of current treatment and potential prophylaxis on visual outcomes in high risk patients. Arch Ophthalmol 116:1045–1052
24. Landrum JT, Bone RA (2001) Lutein, zeaxanthin, and the macular pigment. Arch Biochem Biophys 385:28–40
25. Macular Photocoagulation Study Group (1982) Argon laser photocoagulation for senile macular degeneration. Arch Ophthalmol 100:912–918
26. Macular Photocoagulation Study Group (1986) Argon laser photocoagulation for neovascular maculopathy. Three-year results from randomized clinical trials. Arch Ophthalmol 104:694–701
27. Macular Photocoagulation Study Group (1997) Risk factors for choroidal neovascularization in the second eye of patients with juxta foveal or subfoveal choroidal neovascularization secondary to age related macular degeneration. Arch Ophthalmol 115:741–747
28. Mares-Perlman JA, Brady WE, Klein R (1995) Dietary fat and age-related maculopathy. Arch Ophthalmol 113:743–748
29. Mares-Perlman JA, Fisher AI, Klein R, Palta M, Block G, Millen AE, Wright JD (2001) Lutein and zeaxanthin in the diet and serum and their relation to age-related maculopathy in the third national health and nutrition examination survey. Am J Epidemiol 153(5):424–432
30. Mayne ST (2003) Antioxidant nutrients and chronic disease: Use of biomarkers of exposure and oxidative stress status in epidemiologic research. J Nutr 133:933S–940S
31. Miller ER III, Pastor-Barriuso R, Dalal D, Riemersma RA, Appel LJ, Guallar E (2004) Meta-analysis: high-dosage vitamin E supplementation may increase all-cause mortality. Ann Intern Med 142(1):37–46
32. Moeller SM, Parekh N, Tinker L et al (2006) Associations between intermediate age-related macular degeneration and lutein and zeaxanthin in the carotenoids in Age-Related Eye Disease Study (CAREDS): ancillary study of the Women's Health Initiative. Arch Ophthalmol 124:1151–1162
33. Newsome DA, Swartz M, Leone NC, Elston RC, Miller E (1988) Oral zinc in macular degeneration. Arch Ophthalmol 106(2):192–198
34. Omenn GS, Goodman GE, Thornquist MD et al (1996) Effects of a combination of beta-carotene and vitamin A on lung cancer and cardiovascular disease. N Engl J Med 334:1150–1155
35. Roberts JE (2001) Ocular phototoxicity. J Photochem Photobiol 64:136–143
36. Schalch W, Dayhaw-Barker P, Barker FM (1999) The carotenoids of the human retina. In: Taylor A (ed) Nutritional and environmental influences of the eye. CRC Press, Boca Raton, pp 215–249
37. Seddon JM (2001) Epidemiology of age-related macular degeneration. In: Ryan SJ (ed) Medical retina, vol 2, 3rd edn. Mosby, St. Louis, pp 1039–1050
38. Seddon JM, Ajani UA, Sperduto RD et al (1994) Dietary carotenoids, vitamins A, C, E and advanced age-related macular degeneration. JAMA 272:1413–1420
39. Seddon JM, Rosner B, Sperduto RD et al (2001) Dietary fat and risk for advanced age-related macular degeneration. Arch Ophthalmol 119(8):1191–1199
40. Seddon JM, Cote J, Davis N, Rosner B (2003) Progression of age-related macular degeneration: association with body mass index, waist circumference, and waist-hip ratio. Arch Ophthalmol 121:785–792
41. Seddon JM, George S, Rosner B (2006) Cigarette smoking, fish consumption, omega-3 fatty acid intake, and associations with age-related macular degeneration: the US Twin Age-Related Macular Degeneration. Arch Ophthalmol 124:995–1001
42. Silvestri G, Johnston PB, Hughes AE (1994) Is genetic predisposition an important risk factor in age-related macular degeneration. Eye 8:564–568
43. Smith W, Mitchell P, Leeder SR (1996) Smoking and age-related maculopathy. Arch Ophthalmol 114:1518–1523
44. Smith W, Mitchell P, Leeder SR, Wang JJ (1998) Plasma fibrinogen levels, other cardiovascular risk factors and age-related maculopathy. The Blue Mountains Eye Study. Arch Ophthalmol 116:583–589
45. Smith W, Mitchell P, Leeder SR (2000) Dietary fat and fish intake and age-related maculopathy. Arch Ophthalmol 118(3):401–404

46. Snodderly DM, Brown PK, Delori FC, Auran JD (1984) The macular pigment. I. Absorbance spectra, localization and discrimination from other yellow pigments in the primate retinas. Invest Ophthalmol Vis Sci 25:660–673
47. Snodderly DM, Handelman GL, Adler AJ (2000) Distribution of individual macular pigment carotenoids in the central retina of macaque and squirrel monkeys. Invest Ophthalmol Vis Sci 45:115–134
48. Snow KK, Seddon JM (1999) Do age-related macular degeneration and cardiovascular disease share common antecedents? Ophthalmic Epidemiol 6(2):125–143
49. Sommerburg OG, Siems WG, Hurst JS, Lewis JW, Kliger DS, van Kuijk FJ (1999) Lutein and zeaxanthin are associated with photoreceptors in the human retina. Curr Eye Res 19:491–495
50. TAP Study Group (1999) Photodynamic therapy of subfoveal choroidal neovascularization in age-related macular degeneration with verteporfin: one-year results of 2 randomized clinical trials—TAP report. Treatment of age-related macular degeneration with photodynamic therapy(TAP) Study Group. Arch Ophthalmol 117:1329–1345
51. Taylor HR, West S, Munoz B, Rosenthal FS, Bressler SB, Bressler NM (1992) The long term effects of visible light on the eye. Arch Ophthalmol 110:99–104
52. Thylefors B (1998) A global initiative for the elimination of avoidable blindness. Am J Ophthalmol 125:90–93
53. Tomany SC, Klein R, Klein BE (2003) Beaver dam eye study. The relationship between iris color, hair color, and skin sun sensitivity and the 10-year incidence of age-related maculopathy: the Beaver Dam Eye Study. Ophthalmology 110:1526–1533
54. Verteporfin therapy of subfoveal choroidal neovascularization in age-related macular degeneration: two-year results of a randomized clinical trial including lesions with occult with no classic choroidal neovascularization—verteporfin in photodynamic therapy report 2. Am J Ophthalmol 131:541–160
55. Winkler BS, Boulton ME, Gottsch JD, Sternberg P (1999) Oxidative damage and age-related macular degeneration. Mol Vis 5:32

Chapter 8

New Perspectives in Geographic Atrophy Associated with AMD

Steffen Schmitz-Valckenberg, Monika Fleckenstein, Hendrik P.N. Scholl, Frank G. Holz

Core Messages

- The advanced atrophic form of age-related macular degeneration (AMD) is called "geographic" because the areas of atrophy tend to form well-demarcated borders of atrophy of the neurosensory retina, retinal pigment epithelium (RPE), and choroid that do not seem to be related to specific anatomic structures.
- Fundus autofluorescence (FAF) imaging allows for accurate delineation of atrophic patches. Thus, precise quantification of the area(s) of atrophy is possible, which is useful for clinical monitoring in the context of natural history or interventional studies addressing progression over time.
- Two large prospective studies of patients with geographic atrophy have shown a mean atrophy enlargement of 1.74 mm^2/year and 2.79 mm^2/year respectively. There is a wide range of atrophy progression among patients, which cannot be readily explained by baseline atrophy.
- Distinct phenotypic patterns of abnormal FAF in the junctional zone of atrophy are associated with significant differences in atrophy progression rates over time, and appear to have the strongest predictive value compared with other factors, including smoking, age, and baseline atrophy.

- No specific genetic or systemic risk factors have been identified for geographic atrophy (GA) vs. other AMD phenotypes including choroidal neovascularization (CNV).
- Measurement of visual acuity does not correlate well with the total GA size in earlier stages of the disease and may therefore not reflect the actual visual function of the patient, including stability of fixation, ability to read, and recognizing faces. Foveal sparing of atrophy may result in good central visual acuity, but not useful daily visual function because the residual island surrounded by atrophy is too small.
- Areas of increased FAF in the junctional zone of atrophy are correlated with decreased retinal sensitivity, which may reflect the pathophysiological role of increased lipofuscin accumulation.
- Fundus autofluorescence imaging has enhanced our understanding of the disease process and may be important for monitoring patients with GA over time and for future therapeutic interventions.

8.1 Introduction

8.1.1 Basics

Geographic atrophy of the retinal pigment epithelium is the advanced form of atrophic "dry" AMD. Geographic atrophy appears as sharply demarcated areas with depigmentation and enhanced visualization of deep choroidal vessels (Figs. 8.1, 8.2). It is called "geographic" because these areas do not seem related to specific anatomic structures [18]. The term geographic atrophy (GA) of the retinal epithelial pigment (RPE) is somewhat misleading as not only the RPE cells

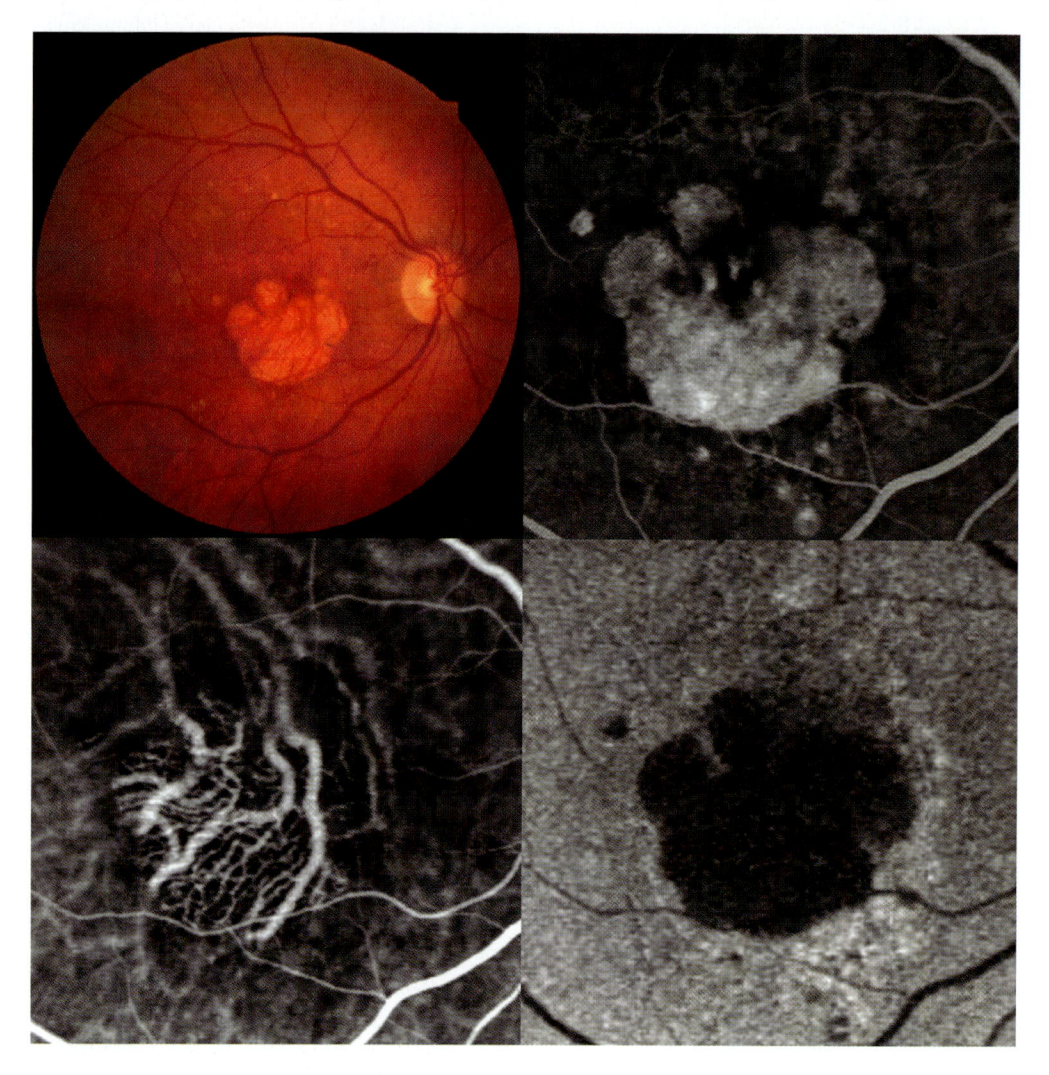

Fig. 8.1 Fundus photograph (*top left*), fluorescein angiography image (*top right*), indocyanine green (ICG) angiograph image (*bottom left*), and fundus autofluorescence (FAF) images (*bottom right*) of the right eye of a 57-year-old female patient with geographic atrophy (GA) of the retinal pigment epithelium (RPE) due to age-related macular degeneration (AMD). RPE atrophy shows well-demarcated borders that do not seem to be related to specific anatomic structures. There is one large central area of atrophy surrounded by several small atrophy satellites. Fluorescein angiography shows hyperfluorescence corresponding to atrophy because of transmission defect and staining. Larger choroidal vessels over the central atrophy can be seen in the fundus photograph and in the ICG angiography image. FAF intensity is markedly decreased over the atrophy because of the lack of RPE and lipofuscin (LF) accumulation

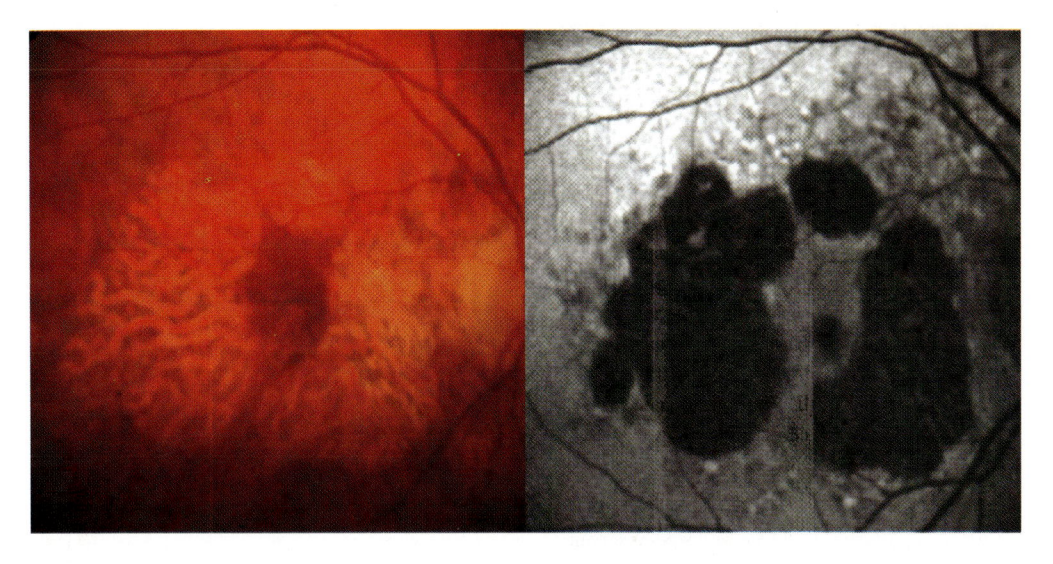

Fig. 8.2 Fundus photograph (*left*) and FAF image (*right*) of the right eye of a 78-year-old female patient showing multifocal RPE atrophy. The fovea is not involved, but areas of atrophy sandwich the residual foveal island resulting in the inability to read large letters or recognize faces, despite good central visual acuity

are atrophic, but also the layers anterior and posterior to the RPE cells, i.e., the choriocapillaris and the neurosensory retina [20]. However, the term GA has been established in the literature and should be used instead of "areolar choroidal atrophy," which is used for similar-appearing monogenetic retinal diseases with manifestations earlier in life [32, 42].

While choroidal neovascularization represents the most common form of advanced AMD, approximately 20% of AMD patients with advanced disease suffer from severe visual loss due to foveal involvement in GA of the RPE [17, 28, 29, 35, 55].

Patients with primary GA tend to be older than those with neovascular forms of AMD at the time of initial presentation. It has been speculated that GA occurs in eyes in which a neovascular angiogenic event has not developed.

8.1.2 Development and Spread of Atrophy

Geographic atrophy can occur primarily or subsequent to other forms of AMD. Development of atrophy in AMD is seen in the presence of macular changes at the level of the RPE and Bruch's membrane, such as pigmentary alterations and drusen [18, 20, 25, 42, 43]. Regression of confluent large, soft drusen leads to atrophy if these areas enlarge and coalesce. Calcified deposits seem to correlate with the occurrence of atrophy and to be pathogenetic for GA in comparison to other late-stage manifestations of AMD [2]. In some cases, GA develops following the collapse and flattening of RPE detachments [7].

Geographic atrophy may vary considerably in appearance. Atrophy may manifest as one single atrophic patch or multifocally with multiple areas of atrophy (Figs. 8.1, 8.2). In the early course of the disease, atrophy is typically limited to the perifoveal region [18, 20, 32]. Over time, the atrophy enlarges, several atrophic areas may coalesce, and new atrophic areas may occur (Fig. 8.3). This may result in a transient horseshoe configuration of atrophy. At more advanced stages, atrophic areas may form a ring or sandwich the atrophy-spared fovea in the center (Fig. 8.2). The fovea is usually not involved until late in the course of the disease. Besides a primary extrafoveal occurrence, the atrophy may also initially start in the foveal area. This manifestation is more rarely seen and can be typically observed, for example, after the collapse of an RPE detachment.

There is a high degree of symmetry between fellow eyes in total size of atrophy and atrophy configuration (Fig. 8.4) [4, 55]. Of note, peri-

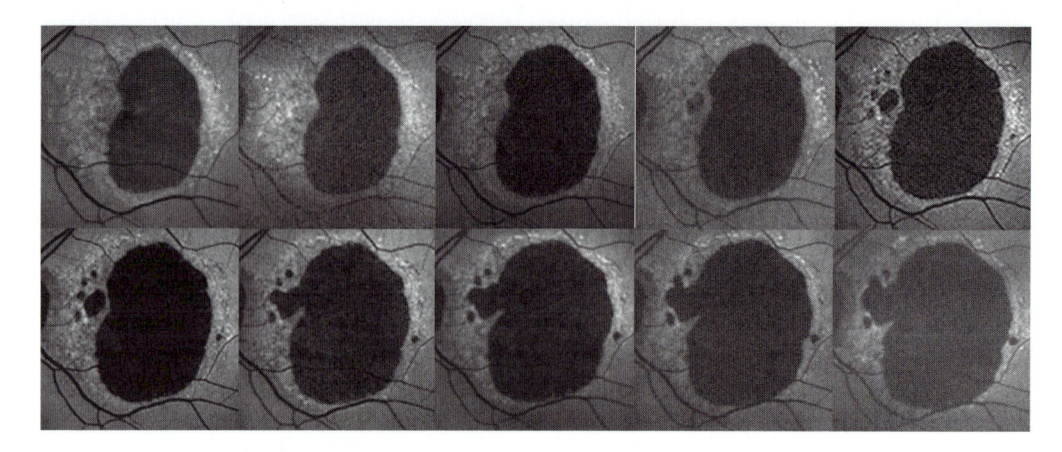

Fig. 8.3 Atrophy progression over a time period of more than 5 years. Over time, single new atrophic areas occur and coalesce with existing atrophy. Interestingly, existing atrophy enlarges or new atrophy occurs exactly where previously increased FAF had been observed

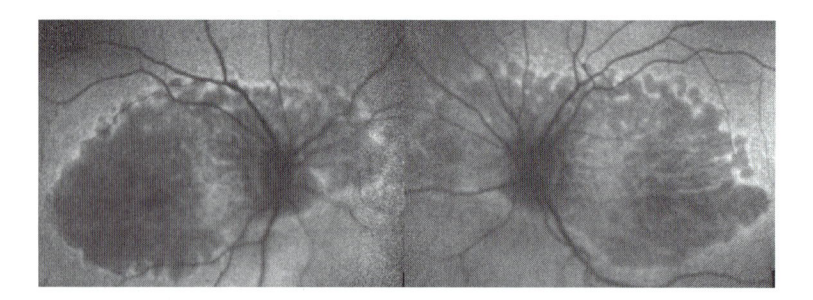

Fig. 8.4 Composite FAF images of both eyes of a 96-year-old patient with very advanced GA extending to the macula. The huge continuous area of atrophy includes large retinal areas within the temporal arcades, but also the optic disc and retinal areas nasally to the optic disc. Note the symmetric configuration of atrophy between the two eyes.

papillary atrophy is observed very commonly in eyes with GA and its prevalence in GA is higher compared with age-matched control eyes. Very advanced stages may show huge continuous atrophies including large retinal areas within the temporal arcades, the optic disc, and retinal areas nasally to the optic disc (Fig. 8.4).

8.2 Fundus Autofluorescence Imaging in Geographic Atrophy

The pathophysiologic mechanisms underlying the atrophic process in GA have been poorly understood to date. In human postmitotic RPE cells lipofuscin (LF) accumulates with age and in various retinal diseases such as Best's disease, Stargardt's disease or GA due to AMD [8]. It is thought to be mainly derived from the chemically modified residues of incompletely digested photoreceptor outer segment discs. Experimental findings suggest that certain molecular compounds of LF, such as A2-E, possess toxic properties and may interfere with normal cell function [50].

The accumulation of LF in postmitotic human RPE cells and its harmful effects on normal cell function has been largely studied in vitro with fluorescence microscopic techniques [8]. Delori and coworkers have shown that fundus autofluorescence (FAF) in vivo is mainly derived from RPE LF [13]. With the advent of confocal scanning laser ophthalmoscopy (cSLO) it has been possible to document FAF and its spatial distribution and intensity over large retinal areas in the living human eye [41, 52]. FAF imaging gives additional information above and beyond conventional imaging tools such as fundus photography, fluorescein angiography or optical coherence tomography.

As mentioned above, GA is characterized by areas of retinal atrophy. Due to the atrophy of RPE cells and therefore the lack of LF (dominant fluorophore for fundus autofluorescence) FAF imaging using the cSLO in patients with GA shows markedly decreased FAF intensity over atrophic patches (Fig. 8.1). Areas of atrophy can be accurately delineated, quantified with image analysis software, and atrophy progression rates can be calculated [11, 46]. Therefore, FAF imaging as an easy, feasible, noninvasive method is a useful tool to review GA patients over time.

Furthermore, it has been shown that areas with increased FAF intensities and therefore excessive RPE LF load surrounding atrophy in the so-called junctional zone of atrophy can be identified [41, 52]. Areas of increased FAF have been shown to precede the development of new areas of GA or the enlargement of preexisting atrophic patches (Fig. 8.3) [26]. In a cross-sectional analysis, the *FAM* (Fundus *A*utofluorescence in age-related *M*acular degeneration) Study Group has introduced a classification system for distinct patterns of abnormal elevated FAF in the junctional zone of GA [5]. This morphological classification was based on information that was solely detectable by FAF imaging.

Summary for the Clinician

- The scanning laser ophthalmoscope allows for imaging of RPE lipofuscin distribution in the living eye.
- Areas of atrophy are characterized by a low FAF signal due to lack of RPE LF.
- Areas of increased FAF and distinct patterns of FAF abnormalities can be identified in areas adjacent to the patches.

8.3 Quantification of Atrophy Progression

Progressive enlargement of GA over time has been assessed in several studies. The first quantitative data on the spread of atrophy were published by Schatz and McDonald in 1989 [44]. They showed in fundus photographs of 50 eyes an average growth rate of 139 µm/year in the horizontal direction. Sunness et al. described in 1999 in fundus photographs of 81 eyes a mean enlargement of 2.2 disc areas (DA; median 1.8) in a 2-year follow-up, which would be 2.79 mm^2/year (median 2.29 mm^2/year) assuming 2.54 mm^2 for 1 DA [55]. Furthermore, they classified the eyes into five different groups according to the total size of atrophy at baseline and stated that the enlargement of atrophy increased with increasing baseline atrophy for up to 5 DA of baseline atrophy, leveled off for the 5–10 DA group, and slightly decreased for the >10 DA group. In patients with GA in both eyes, no significant difference in atrophy enlargement between eyes was seen. The detection and quantification of atrophy was based on fundus photographs and involved several magnification steps. Both studies identified a great difference and range of atrophy enlargement within their cohorts, which could be explained neither by baseline atrophy nor by any other factor tested. For example, atrophy progression ranged in the latter study from 0 to 13.8 mm^2/per year.

Recently, the FAM Study group has published their data on atrophy progression over time [27, 48]. This longitudinal, multicenter, natural history study of patients with GA secondary to AMD was initiated to study FAF changes and their impact on the disease process using FAF imaging. FAF imaging permits atrophic areas to be easily detected, outlined, and quantified. By measuring the total size of atrophy at each visit, atrophy progression over time can be determined and differences between patients can be evaluated (Fig. 8.3). Atrophic areas can be identified and quantified using customized semi-automated image analysis software [11, 46]. The mean atrophy progression rate in the FAM Study with 1.74 mm^2/year (median 1.52 mm^2/year) is slightly smaller than the data from Sunness and coworkers (median 2.29 mm^2/year). Furthermore, it was confirmed that the slowest atrophy progression was found to be in the eyes with a total baseline atrophy of <1 DA, but no statistical significant difference in atrophy enlargement was shown for the other DA groups. Interestingly, variable rates of GA progression were dependent on the specific phenotype of abnormal FAF pattern at baseline (see Sect. 8.4.3).

> **Summary for the Clinician**
>
> - Atrophy enlargement varies between 0 and nearly 14 mm²/year with a mean rate of progression between 1.74 mm²/year and 2.79 mm²/year.
> - Very small areas show a slower spread of atrophy, but variations in atrophy enlargement cannot be totally explained by baseline atrophy.

8.4 Risk Factors

As the dry advanced form of AMD, GA represents a multifactorial complex disease involving genetic, other endogenous and exogenous risk factors. Population-based studies have examined the prevalence and epidemiologic risk factors of GA in comparison to CNV [17, 28, 29 35, 51]. More recently, genetic as well as natural history studies have given more insight into the potential risk factors of GA, and their results are promising to better elucidate the pathogenesis of GA and to develop future treatments for this disease.

8.4.1 Genetic Factors

Epidemiological studies in particular have suggested a substantial genetic compound of AMD [12, 24, 28, 45]. It is well known that age and a positive family history are two important risk factors for the prevalence of AMD in general. However, the FAM study failed to show a significant correlation between rate of atrophy progression and family history as well as age >80 years for patients who had been diagnosed with GA due to AMD previously [27]. Ethnicity seems to play a role in the prevalence of GA. There appears to be a lower occurrence in African-Americans and a lower prevalence of GA in Hispanic compared with white Americans [17, 36]. No clear gender difference in prevalence has been found.

In 2005, three independent groups reported at the same time an association between AMD and a complement factor H (CFH) variant [14, 23, 30]. CFH plays an important role in the regulation of the complement system, which is known to be a part of the immune system. Furthermore, the plasma level of CFH is influenced by age and smoking, and CFH is found in strong concentrations in the RPE/choroid complex of donor eyes [15, 22]. Other polymorphisms have been also identified in the context of AMD, namely in the genes coding for factor B (BF) and LOC387715 [19, 39]. Looking specifically at GA, no significant difference in the genetic polymorphism between the occurrence of GA and CNV has been found so far. While there are known genetic alterations for several hereditary retinal diseases (e.g., Stargardt's disease), which can resemble GA due to AMD, no specific genetic defect has yet been detected to cause advanced atrophic AMD [33, 34, 60].

8.4.2 Systemic Risk Factors

Extensive studies have been performed to examine possible relationships between AMD and systemic factors, such as hypertension, smoking, alcohol intake and cholesterol level. Despite a significant risk of smoking in developing AMD, their findings are not consistent [51]. Even more importantly, only a few studies have distinguished different stages and manifestations of AMD and have separately analyzed the occurrence of GA due to AMD. For example, the Blue Mountain Eye Study has shown that in women current or past smoking was a significant risk factor for the presence of GA; in men this did not reach statistical significance. The two large prospective natural history studies on GA patients have demonstrated that neither hypertension and hyperlipidemia nor body mass index >30 kg/m² are risk factors for a more rapid atrophy progression [27, 55]. No significant correlation between actual or previous history of smoking could be shown; however, there was a weak trend in smokers toward more rapid enlargement of atrophy.

There has been extensive speculation with regard to the role of light exposure in the pathogenesis of GA [61]. Ultraviolet or visible light can induce generation of reactive oxygen species in the retina, which may cause lipid peroxidation of photoreceptor outer segment membranes potentially contributing to LF accumulation in the RPE and, eventually, to the development of AMD. These assumptions have been partly confirmed in cell cultures and animal experiments [21, 50, 53]. However, until now, clinical and epidemiological studies have not been able to provide sound support of the view that cumulative sunlight exposure is associated with AMD [10, 58, 59]. However, it is difficult to accurately determine the amount of light exposure during the life span of a person who is 55 years and older and, therefore, at an age at which they are likely to develop AMD. For example, the ARED study was unable to show that a high-dose intake of vitamin and mineral supplements statistically significantly decreases the risk of the development of GA in the fellow eye of participants with unilateral advanced AMD or in participants without GA in any eye at baseline. Therefore, this large placebo-controlled, randomized study was unable to provide strong data in support of the hypothesis that reactive oxygen species might be involved in the GA disease process, which could be potentially scavenged by antioxidant vitamins [1].

The ophthalmologist is often confronted with the question whether or not cataract surgery should be performed in eyes with GA. There has been speculation regarding a possible association between cataract and AMD. Both are the most frequent causes of visual impairment in the elderly and their prevalence is strongly age-related [28]. Furthermore, both share common potential risk factors including smoking and sunlight exposure [58]. Cataract extraction, i.e., the exchange of an opaque, yellow and, therefore, blue-light filtering natural lens for a clear artificial lens, would consequently expose the macula to relatively more blue light than preoperatively [3]. Anecdotal reports and nonrandomized case series have suggested that cataract surgery in AMD patients may have an adverse effect regarding the progression of AMD and the development of CNV [37, 38]. The findings of prospective epidemiological and larger retrospective clinical studies have been inconsistent and inconclusive to date [16]. However, these studies analyzed AMD patients in general or differentiated only between early and late AMD manifestations. The study by Sunness and coworkers analyzing only GA patients mentions no significant differences in visual loss and atrophy enlargement between phakic and pseudophakic patients over time [55]. However, as long as speculation regarding an increased risk of CNV development and of adverse effects on disease progression is widely present and no systemic analysis of lens status and atrophy progression specifically for GA patients has been performed, the clinician will have difficulty in properly advising his GA patients. Even GA patients may be prevented from undergoing from cataract surgery, although they could potentially benefit from lens exchange, particularly affecting their difficulties in situations of dim illumination.

8.4.3 Ocular Risk Factors

As mentioned above, ocular risk factors for the development of GA encompass certain drusen characteristics, pigment alterations or RPE detachments. However, what factors influence the rate of atrophy enlargement once GA has commenced? There is evidence to suggest that number, distribution, and regression of drusen, as well as incipient atrophy, may play a role [43]. However, these characteristics are difficult to record and to quantify with conventional methods including fundus photograph and fluorescein angiography. FAF imaging, as a new modality, is superior for the evaluation and identification of additional disease markers. As already mentioned, it has been shown that areas with increased FAF intensities in the junctional zone of atrophy, and therefore, excessive RPE LF load, precede the development of new areas of GA or the enlargement of preexisting atrophic patches (Fig. 8.3) [26]. Additional analyses confirmed that FAF findings are suitable for identifying novel prognostic factors and for monitoring patients over time. The FAM Study has shown that eyes with larger areas of increased FAF outside atrophy were associated with higher rates of GA progression over time compared with eyes with smaller areas of increased FAF outside the atrophy at baseline [48]. These findings suggest that these areas are positively correlated with the degree of spread of GA over time (Fig. 8.5). A large area of increased FAF surrounding atrophy obviously represents a high-risk factor for the rate of GA progression and, therefore, for additional visual loss with enlargement of the absolute scotoma associated with GA. This is functionally relevant for the patient in terms of need for low-vision aids, ability to read, and quality of life.

A more recent analysis of the FAM Study of 195 eyes in 129 patients showed that variable rates of progression of GA are dependent on the specific phenotype of an abnormal FAF pattern at baseline (Figs. 8.6, 8.7) [27]. Atrophy enlargement was the slowest in eyes with no abnormal FAF pattern (median 0.38 mm^2/year), followed by eyes with the focal FAF pattern (median 0.81 mm^2/year), then by eyes with the diffuse FAF pattern (median 1.77 mm^2/year), and by eyes with the banded FAF pattern (1.81 mm^2/year; Figs. 8.8, 8.9). The difference in atrophy progression between the groups with no abnormal and focal FAF patterns and the groups with the diffuse and banded FAF patterns was statistically significant ($p<0.0001$). Overall,

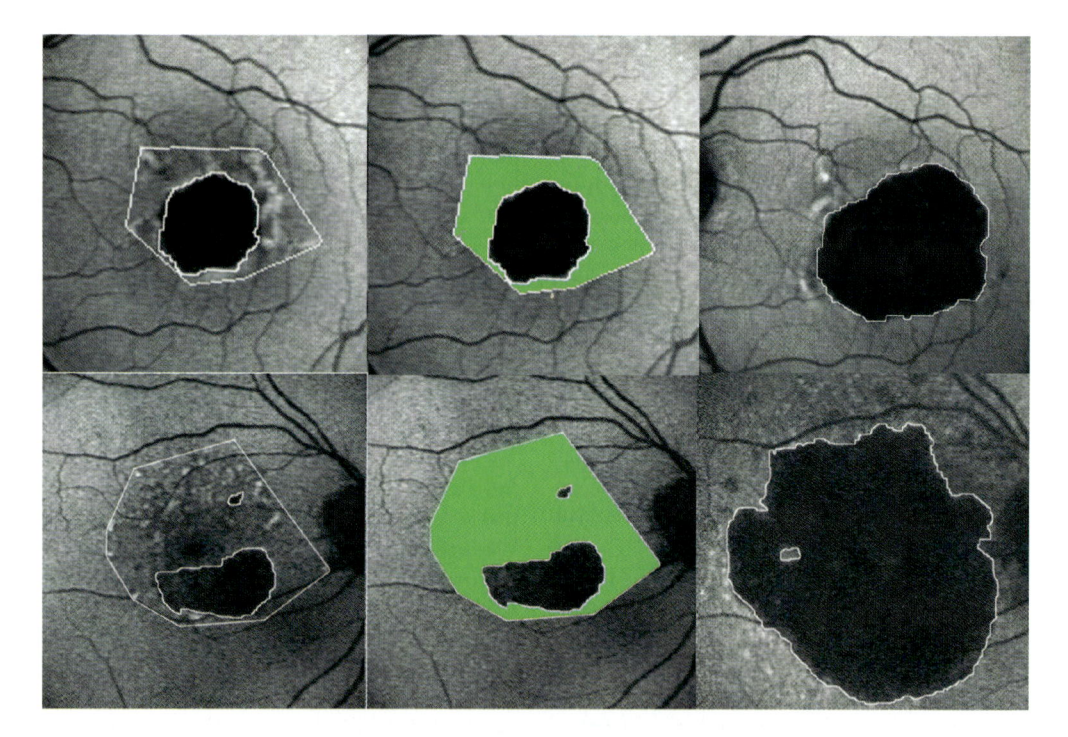

Fig. 8.5 Two examples of the influence of the extent of increased FAF around atrophy and atrophy progression. For the baseline images, areas of atrophy and the convex hull of increased FAF around atrophy are outlined (*left*). The *middle* image illustrated the extent of increased FAF at baseline as the difference between the convex hull and the total baseline atrophy (*green area*), which is nearly double the size in the lower (12.8 mm^2) compared with the upper example (6.5 mm^2). Looking at the *right* images, the lower patient had an atrophy progression rate of 3.10 mm^2/year over a time period of 5.6 years, while the upper patient experienced atrophy enlargement of 0.76 mm^2/year after 6.3 years

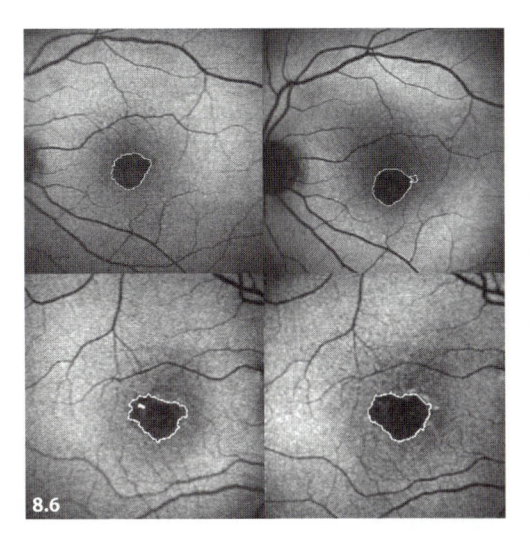

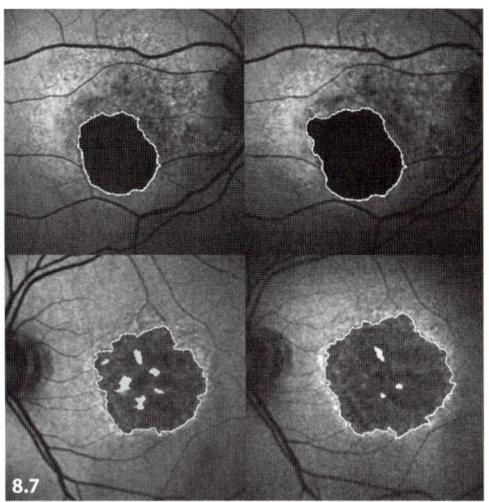

Figs. 8.6, 8.7 Relationship between specific FAF phenotypes and atrophy progression in patients with GA due to AMD showing the baseline FAF image *(left)* and follow-up FAF image *(right)* for each eye respectively. The examples with no abnormal FAF abnormalities (Fig. 8.6, *top*, atrophy progression 0.02 mm^2/year, follow-up 12 months) and with only small areas of focally increased autofluorescence at the margin of the atrophic patch (Fig. 8.6, *bottom*, 0.36 mm^2/year, follow-up 15 months) have less rapid atrophy enlargement compared with the examples with a diffuse fine granular FAF pattern (Fig. 8.7, *top*, 1.71 mm^2/year, follow-up 12 months) and with the banded type (Fig. 8.7, *bottom*, 2.52 mm^2/year, follow-up 18 months) of increased FAF surrounding the GA

phenotypic features of FAF abnormalities had a much stronger impact on atrophy progression than any other risk factor that has been addressed in previous studies on progression of GA due to AMD. These findings underscore the importance of abnormal FAF intensities around atrophy and the pathophysiological role of increased RPE LF accumulation in patients with GA due to AMD. Phenotypic differences may not be only responsible for the great range of atrophy enlargement within different patients (see above), but they may also reflect heterogeneity at the cellular and molecular level of the disease process. As there is a high degree of intraindividual symmetry, genetic determinants rather than nonspecific ageing changes may be involved in the disease process [4]. The findings on the role of polymorphisms in genes coding for CFH, BF, and LOC387715 are in accordance with the assumption that genetic factors may play a major role in the pathophysiology of AMD [14, 19, 23, 30, 39].

Natural history data and identification of high-risk characteristics will also help to test novel interventions in future clinical trials to slow down the spread of atrophy in order to preserve vision in patients with atrophic AMD.

Summary for the Clinician

- Smoking as well as genetic variations in the genes coding for the complement system and in LOC387715 are risk factors for AMD in general, but are not specific to particular phenotypes including GA.
- No statistically significant difference between atrophy progression and lens status (cataract versus pseudophakia) has been demonstrated so far.
- The extent of the area of increased FAF surrounding atrophy identified by SLO imaging is correlated with the rate of atrophy progression over time and reflects the pathophysiological role of RPE LF.

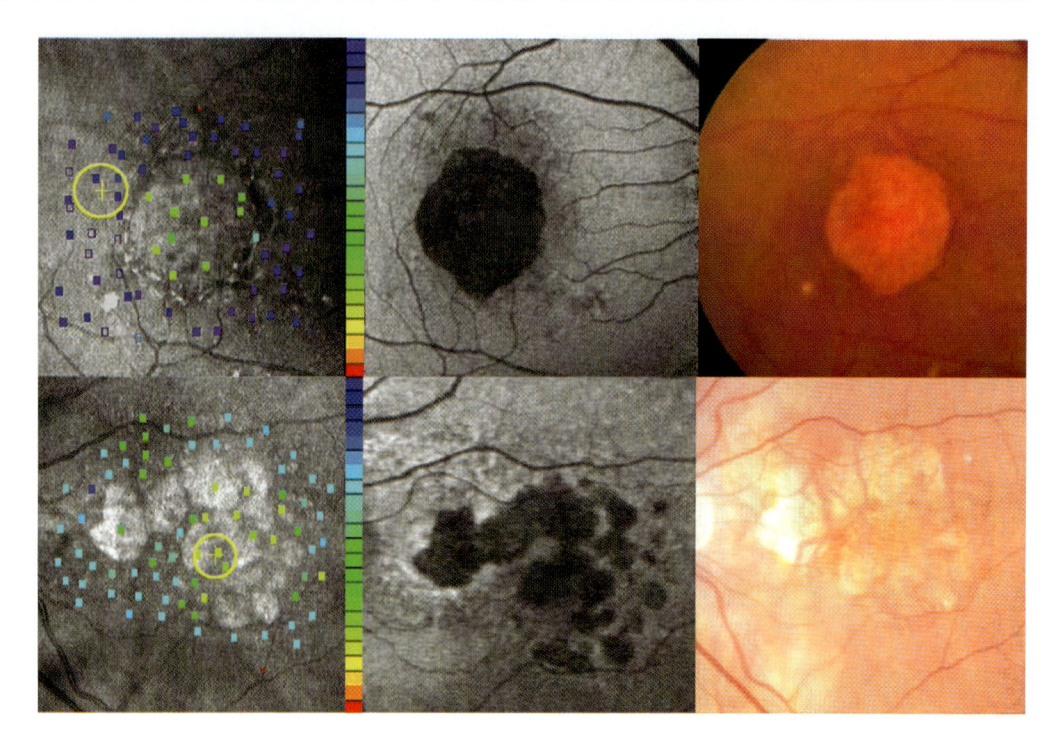

Fig. 8.8 Fundus photograph (*right*), FAF image (*left*) and results of fundus perimetry (FP) with Goldmann III size test points (*right*) for a GA eye with no increased FAF (*top*) and a GA eye with a diffuse trickling FAF signal in the junctional zone of atrophy (*bottom*). The *colored rectangles* on the FP image show the loss of local retinal sensitivity in comparison to age-adjusted normal values (scale on the right eye in 1-dB steps). The *yellow cross* surrounded by a *yellow circle* represents the center of fixation. The *upper* FP image has more blue rectangles, while the *lower* has more pale blue to green rectangles, indicating a stronger decrease in retinal function for the *lower* patient compared with age-correlated normal values

Summary for the Clinician

- Distinct phenotypic patterns of FAF abnormalities in the junctional zone of atrophy show significant differences in atrophy progression rates over time and are of predictive value, while others including smoking, age, and baseline atrophy have no or little influence. Atrophy enlargement is more rapid in eyes with the diffuse or banded pattern compared with eyes with the focal or nonexistent abnormal pattern.
- The high degree of intraindividual symmetry concerning FAF morphology and atrophy progression between fellow eyes suggests that genetic determinants rather than nonspecific ageing changes may be involved in the disease process.

8.5 Development of CNV in Eyes with GA

Age-related macular degeneration is a multifactorial disease and is known to occur in various manifestations. The FAF findings presented above suggest that even further phenotypes could be differentiated in GA patients. It is clinically well known that GA atrophy may manifest as a bilateral disease or unilaterally, involving only one eye [18, 20]. The fellow eye may be affected by any other AMD manifestation and stage, including CNV or disciform scar. Eyes showing typical early features of GA that develop CNV over time have also been described [56]. One other important aspect is the histological finding that eyes that were clinically diagnosed as having pure GA showed small, inactive CNV post-mortem, which indicates that CNV is more frequent than the clinical impression would suggest [20, 43].

When CNV develops in previously diagnosed GA patients, it may show an evanescent appearance and it is often difficult to outline its borders and to differentiate hyperfluorescence caused by CNV or by transmission defects of atrophic areas [55]. Here, careful examination for other characteristics of CNV such as hemorrhage is mandatory. In addition, optical coherence tomography investigation may be helpful.

The percentage of unilateral and bilateral GA patients, as well as the prevalence and the risk of development of CNV out of GA over time, is very inconsistent in different studies [27, 31, 44, 56]. Reported rates of CNV development for GA patients range between 1.5% and 49%. This makes it difficult to compare available data because it is well known that unilateral GA patients with CNV or disciform scars in the fellow eye are at particularly high risk. The best data so far are those obtained by Sunness and coworkers, who showed for patients with GA in one eye and CNV in the fellow eye a cumulative rate of CNV development of 18% at 2 years and 34% at 4 years, while the cumulative incidence for bilateral GA patients was 2% at 2 years and 11% at 4 years respectively [56].

Summary for the Clinician

- Choroidal neovascularization can develop before and after the occurrence of GA is seen in the same eye.
- Extensive atrophy protects against the development of CNV.
- No clear data on the conversion rates from GA to CNV and vice-versa are available.

8.6 Visual Function in GA Patients

Lacking not only the RPE, but also the neurosensory retina including the photoreceptors, atrophic areas constitute an absolute scotoma for the patient. Furthermore, patients have decreased vision in dim illumination and decreased contrast sensitivity [55]. Measurement of visual acuity does not correlated well with the total GA size in earlier stages of the disease and may therefore not reflect the actual visual function of the patient, including stability of fixation and the ability to read and to recognize faces. Using advanced technology, more accurate testing of patients' visual abilities can be achieved.

8.6.1 Measurement of Visual Acuity

Visual acuity measurement in the clinical setting will hardly reflect the actual visual function of the patient in the early course of the disease when the fovea is not involved. For example, a donut-like configuration of atrophy could result in a good central visual acuity because of sparing of the fovea (Fig. 8.2) [32]. However, the patient may be able to read single letters on the chart, but not larger words or recognize faces because the residual island of normal functioning foveal retina is too small. Therefore, visual acuity testing in the earlier courses of the disease may not give information about the actual abilities to cope with visual daily tasks and thus potentially underestimates the patient's visual function. Moreover, these findings explain the weak correlation between visual acuity and total size of atrophy when the fovea is not involved. This has also been statistically confirmed in prospective natural history studies [27, 55].

When the fovea is involved, a dramatic loss in visual acuity, including reading vision, is noted. Schatz and MacDonald showed for eyes with baseline visual acuity of 20/50 or better an 8% annual rate of deteriorating to 20/100 or worse [44]. For eyes with baseline visual acuity of 20/50 or better, the prospective natural history study of Sunness and coworkers showed a rate for a 3-line loss after 2 years of 41% and after 4 years of 70%; the proportion of eyes with visual acuity of 20/200 or less was 14% after 2 years and 27% after 4 years [55].

After foveal involvement, while atrophy continues to grow and to involve the whole macular area, subsequent further loss of visual acuity at a lower rate is observed. At 2 years, eyes with GA and visual acuity of 20/200 or worse at baseline had a 3-line loss rate of 15%; none of the eyes lost 6 or more lines. At this stage, a statistically significant correlation between visual acuity and total size of atrophy has been shown [54]. One other important role in visual function is now played by the stability of fixation. At this stage, the eccentric fixation pattern may be unstable at the beginning and gradually improve over time. In patients with bilateral GA and central scotoma, improvement of fixation and visual acuity in the worse-seeing eye has been observed in relation to deterioration in visual acuity of the better fellow eye [6, 57].

8.6.2 Contrast Sensitivity

A chief complaint of patients with GA is reading and performing other visual tasks in dim light. The worsening in visual acuity is greater in GA patients compared with patients with drusen and/or pigment alterations on the ETDRS acuity chart when a neutral density filter is placed over the eye [57]. Furthermore, dark adaptation is delayed for both rod and cone systems and GA patients have reduced contrast sensitivity even in the presence of good visual acuity [9]. These findings in visual function may be explained by retinal changes other than atrophy, e.g., increased LF accumulation at the level of the RPE and the onset of localized dysfunction of retinal areas [47, 49].

8.6.3 Reading Speed

Although requiring more time, the testing of reading speed particularly helps to assess the visual function in GA patients and is an important aspect of quality of life. Typical early complaints of patients are difficulties in reading, which continue to gradually deteriorate over time. As mentioned above, patients with foveal sparing may have good visual acuity, but an inability to read words or text in the early course of the disease because of extensive atrophy and therefore functional scotoma in the perifoveal region. Later, with foveal involvement, reading speed is dependent on the total size of atrophy and the location of the eccentric preferred retinal locus for fixation [54]. Fixation with the scotoma to the right and fixation with the scotoma superior have been shown to be the most frequent fixation patterns in an US population and to be advantageous for the reading rate compared with fixation with the scotoma to the left. While reading may be become more and more difficult with progression of atrophy, it is important that patients are equipped with appropriate magnifiers and are instructed to use high luminance while reading. Considering that location and stability of eccentric fixation can be potentially trained, patients should be encouraged to use these devices and to benefit from low vision interventions.

8.6.4 Fundus Perimetry

Using the SLO, fundus perimetry (FP) allows for exact correlation between fundus changes and functional impairment [40]. Since areas of GA can be identified using the infrared light source of the SLO, it is possible to determine and compare retinal threshold sensitivities in and around areas of GA. This is particularly interesting for retinal areas surrounding atrophy, in the so-called junctional zone. Here, the disease is presumably active [26]. As mentioned above, FAF imaging—a technology that is based on the SLO—allows different patterns of areas with increased FAF intensities to be identified in the junctional zone of atrophy in GA patients and thus areas with increased LF accumulation [5, 41, 52]. Combining both FP and FAF imaging, one study of 39 eyes in 39 patients showed an overall difference in reduction of retinal sensitivity in comparison to age-matched normal values between eyes with normal FAF in the junctional zone of atrophy and eyes with different degrees of increased FAF patterns [47]. The overall average reduction was greater when areas with increased FAF were detected in the eyes (44.9% versus 26.2% of the tested light stimuli) and was statistically significant using a multiple regression model, which takes the size of the total GA area and group affiliation as covariates (Fig. 8.8). The comparison of areas with increased FAF and areas with normal FAF within eyes that have areas of increased FAF also resulted in a higher percentage of locations with sensitivity loss than areas with increased FAF. These findings are in accordance with the data of Scholl et al. who found that in AMD eyes in general the scotopic sensitivity loss exceeds the photopic sensitivity loss in areas with increased FAF, using fine matrix mapping [49].

Even if these two studies demonstrated a functional correlate of decreased retinal sensitivity and areas with increased FAF and therefore the relevance of excessive LF accumulations in RPE cells in the context of developing AMD, no clear pattern of different degrees of elevated FAF and reduction of retinal sensitivity was found. Within eyes, different degrees of impaired retinal sensitivity were observed on retinal loci that showed similar FAF signals, while a similar decrease in retinal sensitivity was seen on retinal loci that had different FAF signals. This may indicate a more complex relationship among LF accumulation in the RPE, detected levels of FAF, and measured reduction of retinal dysfunction. Various explanations could be considered:

1. Increased FAF and LF accumulation represent an epiphenomenon and not a causative factor, i.e., excessive LF accumulation may be an expression of RPE cell dysfunction rather than being a cause of it.
2. A reproducible quantitative measurement of the FAF signal (gray levels) over localized retinal areas is not possible with the temporarily available instruments. This is largely because media opacities—with lens opacities being the most important factor—are associated with different degrees of absorption of light in the wavelength range used for excitation and emission in FAF imaging. Additional reasons are inconstant laser power of the SLO, different positions of patients at different examinations, and eye movements. Therefore, localized retinal areas are qualitatively distinguished with a normal background from areas with increased FAF, but a precise quantitative comparison of the FAF signal and the function measured by FP can not be performed.
3. The time course may play a role. To date, the time frame from detectable increased FAF signal, impaired photoreceptor function to developing atrophy along with an absolute scotoma has not been investigated. A possible relationship over time between increased FAF, visual function and atrophy of the RPE is illustrated in a theoretical model in Fig. 8.9. The gray values of the FAF image only show the FAF signals at the time of the examination. While it can be assumed that any area of increased FAF observed at a certain time had been before an area with normal background signal, it may not be possible to say whether an area with elevated FAF is in the process

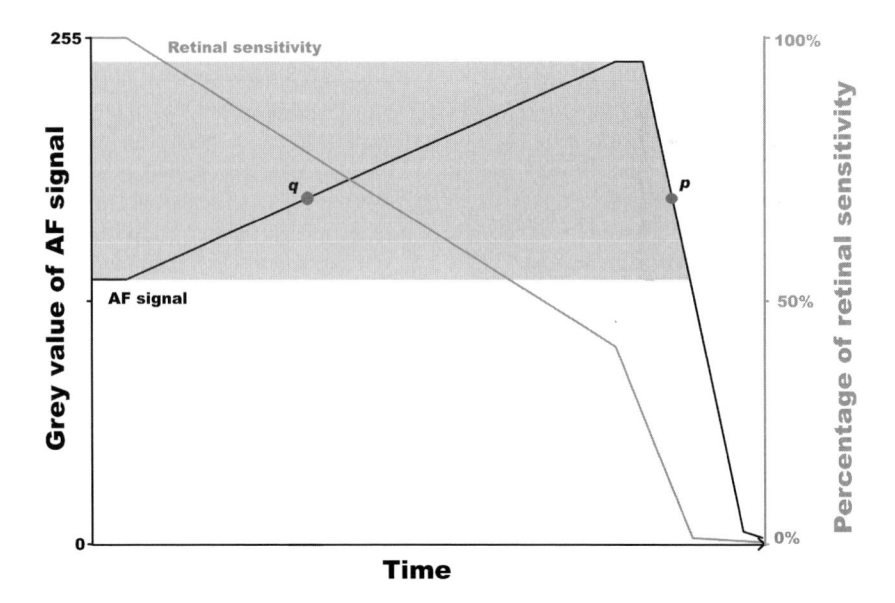

Fig. 8.9 Theoretical model for the relationship between FAF signal and retinal sensitivity over time in the junctional zone of GA. The *left vertical axis* shows the gray value of the detected FAF signal (0 = black, 255 = white), while the retinal function is illustrated by the right vertical axis (0% = no function, 100% = normal function). It may not be possible to determine whether an area with increased FAF is in the process of increasing accumulation of LF (point p) or is in the state of transferring from maximum LF accumulation to development of atrophy (point q). But this would be of great importance because retinal function would be assumed to be very different between the two points

of increasing accumulation of LF (point p) or whether it is in the state of turning from maximal accumulation of LF to development of atrophy (point q), i.e., if the gray value of the area is represented at the ascending or at the descending part of the FAF signal graph. Therefore, it is impossible to define the stage of the disease process of a localized area with increased FAF on a single FAF image without having previous or follow-up images. The time course of changes in FAF signals and the relationship between different degrees of increased FAF patterns and retinal sensitivity over time might be clarified in a longitudinal study with patients with GA using fundus FAF and FP with regular review.

Summary for the Clinician

- Measurement of visual acuity does not correlate well with the total GA size in earlier stages of the disease and may therefore not reflect the actual visual function of the patient, including stability of fixation, ability to read, and to recognize faces. Foveal sparing of atrophy may result in good visual acuity, but not useful daily visual function because the residual island surrounding the atrophy is too small.
- Typical visual complaints in patients with GA include difficulties in reading and decreased contrast sensitivity. Reading speed is dependent on the stability of fixation, which may change over time.
- Areas of increased FAF in the junctional zone of atrophy are correlated with decreased retinal sensitivity, which may reflect the pathophysiological role of increased LF accumulation and its harmful effects on normal cell function
- Changes in FAF intensity can so far only be graded in a qualitative fashion. The quantification of FAF signals would be very helpful to better interpret FAF findings.

References

1. Age-Related Eye Disease Study (AREDS) Research Group (2001) A randomized, placebo-controlled, clinical trial of high dose supplementation with vitamins C, E, beta carotene, and zinc for age-related macular degeneration and visual loss. Arch Ophthalmol 119:1417–1436
2. Age-Related Eye Disease Study (AREDS) Research Group (2005) A simplified severity scale for age-related macular degeneration. Arch Ophthalmol 123:1570–1574
3. Algvere PV, Marshall J, Seregard S (2006) Age-related maculopathy and the impact of blue-light hazard. Acta Ophthalmol Scand 84:4–15
4. Bellmann C, Jorzik J, Spital G, Unnebrink K, Pauleikhoff D, Holz FG (2002) Symmetry of bilateral lesions in geographic atrophy in patients with age-related macular degeneration. Arch Ophthalmol 120:579–584
5. Bindewald A, Schmitz-Valckenberg S, Jorzik JJ et al (2005) For the FAM Study Group. Classification of abnormal fundus autofluorescence patterns in the junctional zone of geographic atrophy in patients with AMD. Br J Ophthalmol 89:874–878
6. Bissell AJ, Yalcinbayir O, Akduman L (2005) Bilateral geographic atrophy: spontaneous visual improvement after loss of vision in the fellow eye. Acta Ophthalmol Scand 83:514–515
7. Blair CJ (1975) Geographic atrophy of the retinal pigment epithelium. Arch Ophthalmol 93:19–25
8. Boulton M, Dayhaw-Barker P (2001) The role of the retinal pigment epithelium: topographical variation and ageing changes. Eye 15:384–389
9. Brown B, Tobin C, Roche N, Wolanowski A (1986) Cone adaptation in age-related maculopathy. Am J Optom Physiol Opt 63:450–454
10. Cruickshanks KJ, Klein R, Klein BEK (1993) Sunlight and age-related macular degeneration: the Beaver Dam Eye Study. Arch Ophthalmol 111:514–518
11. Deckert A, Schmitz-Valckenberg S, Jorzik J, Bindewald A, Holz FG, Mansmann U (2005) Automated analysis of digital fundus autofluorescence images of geographic atrophy in advanced age-related macular degeneration using confocal scanning laser ophthalmoscopy (cSLO). BMC Ophthalmol 5:8

12. De Jong PT, Klaver CC, Wolfs RC, Assink JJ, Hofman A (1997) Familial aggregation of age-related maculopathy. Am J Ophthalmol 124:862–863
13. Delori FC, Dorey CK, Staurenghi G, Arend O, Goger DG, Weiter JJ (1995) In vivo fluorescence of the ocular fundus exhibits RPE lipofuscin characteristics. Invest Ophthalmol Vis Sci 36:718–729
14. Edwards AO, Ritter III R, Kenneth JA, Manning A et al (2005) Complement factor H polymorphism and age-related macular degeneration. Science 308:421–424
15. Esparza-Gordillo J, Soria JM, Buil A et al. (2004) Genetic and environmental factors influencing the human factor H plasma levels. Immunogenetics 56:77–82
16. Freeman EE, Munoz B, West SK, Tielsch J, Schein OD (2003) Is there an association between cataract surgery and age-related macular degeneration? Data from three population-based studies. Am J Ophthalmol 135:849–856
17. Friedman DS, O'Colmain BJ, Munoz B et al (2004) Eye Diseases Prevalence Research Group. Prevalence of age-related macular degeneration in the United States. Arch Ophthalmol 122:564–572
18. Gass JDM (1973) Drusen and disciform macular degeneration. Arch Ophthalmol 90:206–217
19. Gold B, Merriam J, Zernant J et al (2006) Variation in factor b (BF) and complement component 2 (C2) genes is associated with age-related macular degeneration. Nat Genet 38:458–462
20. Green WR, Enger C (1993) Age-related macular degeneration histopathologic studies: the 1992 Lorenz E. Zimmermann Lecture. Ophthalmology 100:1519–1535
21. Grimm C, Wenzel A, Williams TP, Rol PO, Hafezi F, Reme CE (2001) Rhodopsin-mediated blue light damage to the rat retina: effect of photoreversal bleaching. Invest Ophthalmol Vis Sci 42:497–505
22. Hageman GS, Anderson DH, Johnson LV et al (2005) A common haplotype in the complement regulatory gene factor H (HF1/CFH) predisposes individuals to age-related macular degeneration. Proc Natl Acad Sci USA 102:7227–7232
23. Haines JL, Hauser MA, Schmidt S, Scott WK et al (2005) Complement factor H variant increases the risk of age-related macular degeneration. Science 308:419–421
24. Heiba IM, Elston RC, Klein BE, Klein R (1994) Sibling correlations and segregation analysis of age-related maculopathy: the Beaver Dam Eye Study. Genet Epidemiol 11:51–67
25. Holz FG, Wolfensberger TJ, Piguet B et al (1994) Bilateral drusen in age-related macular degeneration—prognosis and risk factors. Ophthalmology 101:1522–1528
26. Holz FG, Bellmann C, Staudt S, Schütt F, Völcker HE (2001) Fundus autofluorescence and development of geographic atrophy in age-related macular degeneration. Invest Ophthalmol Vis Sci 42:1051–1056
27. Holz FG, Bindewald-Wittich A, Fleckenstein M et al (2007) Progression of geographic atrophy and impact of fundus autofluorescence patterns in age-related macular degeneration. Am J Ophthalmol 143(3):463–472.e2
28. Klaver CC, Wolfs RC, Vingerling JR, Hofman A, de Jong PT (1998) Age-specific prevalence and causes of blindness and visual impairment in an older population: the Rotterdam Study. Arch Ophthalmol 116:653–658
29. Klein R, Klein BE, Tomany SC, Meuer SM, Huang GH (2002) Ten-year incidence and progression of age-related maculopathy: the Beaver Dam eye study. Ophthalmology 109:1767–1779
30. Klein RJ, Zeiss C, Chew EY, Tsaei JY et al (2005) Complement factor H polymorphism in age-related macular degeneration. Science 308:385–389
31. Macular Photocoagulation Study Group (1993) Five-year follow-up of fellow eyes of patients with age-related macular degeneration and unilateral extrafoveal choroidal neovascularisation. Arch Ophthalmol 111:1189–1199
32. Maguire P, Vine AK (1986) Geographic atrophy of the retinal pigment epithelium. Am J Ophthalmol 102:621–625
33. Marmor MF, McNamara JA (1996) Pattern dystrophy of the retinal pigment epithelium and geographic atrophy. Am J Opthalmol 122:382–392
34. Michaelides M, Hunt DM, Moore AT (2003) The genetics of inherited macular dystrophies. J Med Genet 40:641–650
35. Mitchell P, Smith W, Attebo K, Wang JJ (1995) Prevalence of age-related maculopathy in Australia. The Blue Mountains Eye Study. Ophthalmology 102:1450–1460

36. Muñoz B, Klein R, Rodriguez J, Synder R, West SK (2005) Prevalence of age-related macular degeneration in a population-based sample of Hispanic people in Arizona: Proyecto VER. Arch Ophthalmol 123:1575–1580
37. Pollack A, Marcovich A, Bukelman A, Oliver M (1996) Age-related macular degeneration after extracapsular cataract extraction with intraocular lens implantation. Ophthalmology 103:1546–1554
38. Pollack A, Marcovich A, Bukelman A, Zalish M, Oliver M (1997) Development of exudative age-related macular degeneration after cataract surgery. Eye 11:523–530
39. Rivera A, Fisher SA, Fritsche LG et al (2005) Hypothetical LOC387715 is a second major susceptibility gene for age-related macular degeneration, contributing independently of complement factor H to disease risk. Hum Mol Genet 14:3227–3236
40. Rohrschneider K, Fendrich T, Becker M, Krastel H, Kruse FE, Völcker HE (1995) Static fundus perimetry using the scanning laser ophthalmoscope with an automated threshold strategy. Graefes Arch Clin Exp Ophthalmol 233:743–749
41. Rückmann AV, Fitzke FW, Bird AC (1997) Fundus autofluorescence in age-related macular disease imaged with a laser scanning ophthalmoscope. Invest Ophthalmol Vis Sci 38:478–486
42. Sarks JP, Sarks SH, Killingsworth MC (1988) Evolution of geographic atrophy of the retinal pigment epithelium. Eye 2:552–577
43. Sarks SH (1976) Aging and degeneration in the macular region: a clinicopathological study. Br J Opthhalmol 60:324–341
44. Schatz H, McDonald HR (1989) Atrophic macular degeneration. Rate of spread of geographic atrophy and visual loss. Ophthalmology 96:1541–1551
45. Seddon JM, Ajani UA, Mitchell BD (1997) Familial aggregation of age-related maculopathy. Am J Ophthalmol 123:199–206
46. Schmitz-Valckenberg S, Jorzik J, Unnebrink K, Holz FG (2001) Analysis of digital scanning laser ophthalmoscopy fundus autofluorescence images of geographic atrophy in advanced age-related macular degeneration. Graefes Arch Clin Exp Ophthalmol 40:73–78
47. Schmitz-Valckenberg S, Bültmann S, Dreyhaupt J, Bindewald A, Holz FG, Rohrschneider K (2004) Fundus autofluorescence and fundus perimetry in the junctional zone of geographic atrophy in patients with age-related macular degeneration. Invest Ophthalmol Vis Sci 45:4470–4476
48. Schmitz-Valckenberg S, Bindwald-Wittich A, Dolar-Szczasny J et al (2006) Correlation between the area of increased autofluorescence surrounding geographic atrophy and disease progression in patients with AMD. Invest Ophthalmol Vis Sci 47:2648–2654
49. Scholl HP, Bellmann C, Dandekar SS, Bird AC, Fitzke FW (2004) Photopic and scotopic fine matrix mapping of retinal areas of increased fundus autofluorescence in patients with age-related maculopathy. Invest Ophthalmol Vis Sci 34:574–583
50. Schütt F, Sallyanne D, Kopitz J, Holz FG (2000) Photodamage to human RPE cells by A2-E, a retinoid component of lipofuscin. Invest Ophthalmol Vis Sci 41:2303–2308
51. Smith W, Assink J, Klein R et al (2001) Risk factors for age-related macular degeneration: pooled findings from three continents. Ophthalmology 108:697–704
52. Solbach U, Keilhauer C, Knabben H, Wolf S (1997) Imaging of retinal autofluorescence in patients with age-related macular degeneration. Retina 17:385–389
53. Sparrow JR, Nakanishi K, Parish CA (2000) The lipofuscin fluorophore A2E mediates blue light-induced damage to retinal pigmented epithelial cells. Invest Ophthalmol Vis Sci 41:1981–1989
54. Sunness JS, Applegate CA (2005) Long term follow-up of fixation patterns in eyes with central scotomas from geographic atrophy that is associated with age-related macular degeneration. Am J Ophthalmol 140:1085–1093
55. Sunness JS, Gonzales-Baron J, Applegate CA et al (1999) Enlargement of atrophy and visual acuity loss in the geographic atrophy form of age-related macular degeneration. Ophthalmology 106:1768–1779
56. Sunness JS, Gonzales-Baron J, Bressler NM et al (1999) The development of choroidal neovascularisation in eyes with the geographic atrophy form of age-related macular degeneration. Ophthalmology 106:910–919

57. Sunness J, Applegate CA, Gonzales-Baron J (2000) Improvement of visual acuity over time in patients with bilateral geographic atrophy from age-related macular degeneration. Retina 20:162–169
58. Taylor HR, West SK, Munoz B et al (1992) The long-term effects of visible light on the eye. Arch Ophthalmol 110:99–104
59. West SK, Rosenthal FS, Bressler NM et al (1989) Exposure to sunlight and other risk factors for age-related macular degeneration. Arch Ophthalmol 107:875–879
60. Yang Z, Camp NJ, Sun H et al (2006) A variant of the HTRA1 gene increases susceptibility to age-related macular degeneration. Science 314:992–993
61. Young RW (1988) Solar radiation and age-related macular degeneration. Surv Ophthalmol 32:252–269

Chapter 9

Diabetic Macular Edema: Current Treatments

Florian K.P. Sutter, Mark C. Gillies, Horst Helbig

Core Messages

- Diabetic macular edema is a common blinding disease that represents a significant burden with the increasing incidence and prevalence of diabetes worldwide and limited resources for public health systems.
- Screening is essential to detect vision-threatening stages prior to loss of visual function.
- Binocular stereoscopic ophthalmoscopy with the slit-lamp remains the most important diagnostic tool. Optical coherence tomography (OCT) has rapidly come to play an important role in diagnosis and follow-up and may further guide treatment strategies and research in the future. Fluorescein angiography is mandatory to show capillary nonperfusion; for other purposes its importance may decrease.
- Treatment strategies combine the optimization of systemic risk factors with systemic and local pharmacological therapies as well as laser interventions and surgical approaches.
- Ophthalmologists may play a key role in patient motivation and effective cooperation with general practitioners, primary care physicians, and endocrinologists is essential.
- Laser therapy is still based on the principles of the ETDRS (Early Treatment of Diabetic Retinopathy Study), but has been adapted so that lighter burns of longer duration are used. Intravitreal triamcinolone acetonide (IVTA) is an alternative to grid coagulation for diffuse edema, but steroid-related adverse effects represent a significant problem with long-term use of this treatment.
- The risks of diabetic macular edema worsening after uneventful modern cataract surgery seem to be small. Risks and potential benefits, however, should be weighed against each other based on the clinical situation.
- The use of novel anti-VEGF compounds is under investigation and not recommended outside experimental settings.

9.1 Introduction

Diabetic macular edema (DME), a microvascular complication of diabetes mellitus, accounts for about three-quarters of cases of visual loss due to diabetic eye disease, yet it is still an underestimated complication of diabetes [61]. Loss of vision from DME may be prevented with appropriate treatment in some but not all cases. Prevention of its development, however, should be the primary goal of management.

9.2 Epidemiology

Diabetic retinopathy is the leading cause of visual impairment in patients aged 20 to 74 in developed countries [6, 38]. The Wisconsin Epidemiologic Study of Diabetic Retinopathy (WESDR) reported that none of the patients with type I diabetes of less than 5 years' duration had macular edema compared with 32% of patients after 22–24 years with the disease. In another study, only 5% of people with type II diabetes showed macular edema 5 years after diagnosis compared with 28% after 21–22 years [41].

There seems to be a genetic predisposition for the development of diabetic retinopathy. Some polymorphisms of the aldose reductase gene have been found to be associated with an increased risk of diabetic retinopathy and other microvascular complications after controlling for independent risk factors [19, 83]. By contrast, there are individuals who do not develop retinopathy despite extended disease duration with mediocre glycemic control, suggesting the presence of an unknown protective factor.

Significant variations in the incidence and prevalence of diabetic macular edema have been reported by various epidemiologic studies depending on the type of diabetes (type I or II), the mode of treatment (insulin, oral hypoglycemic agents or diet only), and the mean duration of disease [84]. In general, the lifetime risk of developing a sight-threatening retinal complication (macular edema or proliferative retinopathy) is almost 50% for a patient with type I diabetes and one in three for a patient with type II diabetes [72].

With the inexorable increase in the incidence of type II diabetes, diabetic retinopathy including diabetic macular edema has become a major public health problem with significant socioeconomic implications, since an increasing number of affected patients are of working age. There are now approximately 200 million people with diabetes in the world with an increase of 10 million people per year [85].

Some racial groups are at higher risk of developing diabetes. The self-reported prevalence of diabetes in Latinos over 65 in Los Angeles was found to be as high as 25.7% [7]. The Los Angeles Latino Eye Study found a prevalence of macular edema of 10.4% of people with diabetes. The prevalence of visual impairment (best-corrected visual acuity worse than 20/40 in the better eye) in persons with diabetes was 6%, compared with 2% of those without diabetes [82]. Diabetic retinal disease (retinopathy and macular edema) was responsible for 18% of patients with low vision or blindness [14]. In view of these statistics, and taking into account the increase in diabetes in developing and developed countries around the world [85], a dramatic increase in patients with diabetic macular edema is anticipated in the years to come.

Summary for the Clinician

- Diabetic macular edema is a common cause of blindness due to the increasing number of diabetes patients worldwide and limited public health resources.

9.3 Pathophysiology

The development of macular edema is not limited to people with diabetes, but represents a common response to a range of retinal diseases. The macula has a significant predilection for the development of edema. This is probably due to the loose intercellular adhesion in this area, the absence of Müller cells in the fovea and possibly the higher susceptibility of the macula to both hypoxic and oxidative stress.

Vascular endothelial damage is a major contributor to diabetic retinopathy and diabetic macular edema. This results in the breakdown of the inner blood retina barrier and accumulation of fluid and serum macromolecules in the intercellular space. Macular edema is visible on fundoscopy as retinal thickening associated with exudates and usually microaneurysms. The latter are the result of microvascular damage and thought to be the consequence of loss of capillary pericytes, proliferation of endothelial cells, and outpouching of the vessel wall.

9.4 Diabetic Macular Edema and Laboratory Science

One of the fundamental problems in understanding diabetic macular edema is the limited information from laboratory science that is available on its pathogenesis and treatment. While some therapeutic strategies like laser coagulation or intravitreal steroids have been shown to be effective in clinical trials, the understanding of precisely how they work is rudimentary. One important reason for this is the shortage of appropriate and accessible animal models. While streptotocin-induced diabetic rats are easily available, they are not a good model for macular edema because rodents do not have a macula. Although it has been shown that there is increased leakage soon after the induction of diabetes, they do not develop retinal thickening but rather retinal thinning. Galactose-fed dogs are a better model, but the development of retinal changes takes up to 5 years [21]. Sub-human primates have macular structures similar to those of humans, but are not easily available as animal models due to obvious financial and ethical issues.

9.5 Quality of Life

The WESDR showed a reduced mean visual function questionnaire (VFQ) score of 83 in patients with macular edema compared with a mean score of 88 for all study participants [44]. This is consistent with results from studies assessing quality of live and reduced central vision due to other macular diseases. The effect of macular edema on quality of life and dependency of patients may be compounded by other complications such as peripheral vascular disease and neuropathy, which further affects patients' mobility in conjunction with reduced vision. Impaired vision may make achieving good glycemic control more difficult in people with insulin-dependent diabetes if it affects their ability to draw up an accurate dose of insulin in a syringe.

9.6 Diagnosis and Screening

For all types of diabetic retinopathy it is necessary to apply treatment in the vision-threatening stages before the eyes actually begin to lose vision. Diabetic microvascular disease is a chronic progressive process. The goal of therapy is rarely improvement of vision; in most cases it is preservation of vision and avoidance of further visual loss. How best to screen regularly for retinopathy the hundreds of millions of people with diabetes around the world is a controversial subject. While dilated stereoscopic fundus examination by an experienced examiner is highly sensitive and specific, it imposes a huge workload and requires a high density of experienced health care providers. This may be difficult to perform regularly in remote areas. Fluorescein angiography is helpful in detecting leaking points and ischemia prior to treatment, but it is an invasive intervention that is not appropriate for routine screening. Optical coherence tomography (OCT) allows noninvasive quantitative and examiner-independent examination of macular edema, as well as traction at the vitreoretinal interface, but may be unable to detect significant retinopathy if edema is absent [54]. The role of OCT in screening for diabetic retinopathy has not been adequately studied. Currently, there is considerable scientific interest in digital fundus photography with automated grading of diabetic changes [60] (e.g., microaneurysms counting). For patients in remote areas screening approaches using telemedicine are being developed [50, 62]. Screening techniques, however, do not completely replace a formal eye examination with patient counseling.

Summary for the Clinician

- Early screening is vital, prior to loss of visual function.
- Binocular stereoscopic ophthalmoscopy with the slit-lamp remains the most important diagnostic tool.
- Optical coherence tomography plays an important role in diagnosis and follow-up.
- Fluorescein angiography is essential for demonstrating capillary nonperfusion.

9.7 Types of Diabetic Macular Edema

9.7.1 Clinically Significant Macular Edema

The Early Treatment of Diabetic Retinopathy Study (ETDRS) was one of the first large clinical trials sponsored by the National Eye Institute (NEI). The ETDRS coined the term "clinically significant macular edema" (CSME) for macular edema that involves or threatens the center of the fovea [20]. The definition of CSME includes:
1. Thickening of the retina at or within 500 μm of the center of the macula
2. Hard exudates at or within 500 μm of the center of the macula, if associated with thickening of the adjacent retina (i.e., not residual hard exudates remaining after the disappearance of retinal thickening)
3. A zone or zones of retinal thickening 1 disc area or larger, any part of which is within 1 disc diameter of the center of the macula

9.7.2 Focal Diabetic Macular Edema

In addition to this spatial classification, diabetic macular edema can be clinically divided into focal edema and diffuse edema. In focal edema there are localized areas of retinal thickening caused by focal leakage from retinal capillaries or microaneurysms. These areas are frequently demarcated by partial or complete rings of hard exudate called circinate exudates.

9.7.3 Diffuse Diabetic Macular Edema

In diffuse macular edema there is more widespread thickening of the macula secondary to generalized abnormal permeability of the retinal capillaries. This generalized leakage is thought to be the result of compensatory dilation of perfused capillaries in the presence of occlusion in neighboring parts of the capillary bed. Risk factors for the progression to diffuse macular edema are increasing microaneurysm count [43], adult onset diabetes, hypertension, cardiovascular disease, vitreomacular adhesion, and advanced retinopathy [51].

In clinical practice, however, a wide variety of mixed forms may be encountered and there is no clear-cut scientific definition of focal and diffuse edema.

9.7.4 Cystoid Macular Edema

As mentioned above, macular edema is a nonspecific complication of many underlying pathological processes. In many of these conditions the formation of cystoid spaces (frequently radially oriented) filled with ophthalmoscopically clear fluid may be observed. This cystoid appearance may or may not be associated with diabetic macular edema. An attached posterior hyaloid surface seems to play a role in the pathogenesis of cystoid macular edema [31]. The presence or absence of this cystoid appearance, however, does not directly influence prognosis or management.

9.7.5 Ischemic Macular Edema

An important variant of diabetic macular edema is "nonperfused" or "ischemic" macular edema. Gradually increasing occlusion of macular capillaries is commonly present in the course of diabetic macular disease. Rarification of the perifoveal network and occlusion of the perifoveal capillary arcade is a poor prognostic indicator of central visual acuity. Eyes with capillary occlusion in the peripheral macula may still have good central visual function. Only angiography is able to show the degree of ischemia in diabetic retinopathy.

9.7.6 OCT Patterns of Diabetic Macular Edema

Optical coherence tomography is a fast and noninvasive tool for examining the retina in cross-sectional images that correlate well with retinal histology [78]. OCT allows not only a quantitative, but also a qualitative analysis of the important features of diabetic macular edema. Several different patterns of structural changes within the retina in diabetic macular edema have been reported and correlated with visual acuity [40]. It is likely that the analysis of these OCT patterns in the future will reduce the requirement for fluorescein angiography and guide therapeutic strategies. A novel OCT-based classification of diabetic macular edema has been proposed [59], which takes into account five parameters: retinal thickness, diffusion, volume, morphology, and presence of vitreous traction.

9.8 Treatment

Treatment of diabetic macular edema (and diabetic retinopathy) combines the optimization of systemic risk factors with systemic and local pharmacological treatment as well as laser intervention and surgical approaches.

Since diabetic retinopathy and macular edema are the result of microvascular damage and ischemia, all treatment concepts ideally should aim to improve vascular integrity and/or ocular oxygenation [73] in the long term.

9.8.1 Systemic Treatment

9.8.1.1 Glycemic Control

Tight blood glucose control is essential for the prevention of all types of diabetic end organ damage and complications including diabetic retinopathy and diabetic macular edema. The population-based WESDR showed a strong relationship between baseline glycosylated hemoglobin (HbA1c) values and the incidence of macular edema over a 10-year period [42]. The Diabetes Control and Complications Trial (DCCT) demonstrated a 26% reduction in the risk of developing macular edema in the intensive insulin treatment group compared with the conventional therapy group in people with type I diabetes. Tight glycemic control is therefore strongly recommended for all patients with diabetes. However, there is no specific figure to aim for. There is no level of HbA1c below which the risk of diabetic eye disease cannot be lowered any further. However, since with tighter control there is an increasing risk of hypoglycemic complications as well [16], an HbA1c level of 7.0% is the target level recommended by the American Diabetes Association's guidelines [1]. On the other hand, the National Health and Nutrition Examination Survey III demonstrates that only a few patients with diabetes reach this level of control [45]. In addition to being a risk factor for the development of macular edema, elevated levels of HbA1c have been found to be associated with poor response to focal laser treatment as well as with bilateral disease [18]. It is noteworthy that tight blood glucose control is cost effective because it substantially reduces the costs of complications [29].

9.8.1.2 Blood Pressure Control

People with type I diabetes with a diastolic blood pressure within the fourth quartile range had a 3.3-fold increased risk of developing macular edema compared with patients with diastolic blood pressure values in the first quartile range in the WESDR. The UK Prospective Diabetes Study (UKPDS) [79] reported a 47% reduction in loss of 3 or more lines of visual acuity (mainly due to macular edema) associated with tight blood pressure control [80] in people with type II diabetes. The Appropriate Blood Pressure Control in Diabetes (ABCD) study, however, failed to demonstrate a significant effect of intensified blood pressure control in people with type II diabetes [23]. This may be due to lower blood pressure values at baseline and poorer glycemic control in participants in the ABCD study compared with other trials.

It is important to note that a significant effort is often needed to reach and maintain tight blood pressure control. Many patients require three or more hypotensive medications in order to reach therapeutic goals, which is an additional burden for these patients, who may also have a number of other health problems.

9.8.1.3 Reducing Levels of Blood Lipids

In the ETDRS there was a positive correlation between serum lipid levels and an increased risk of developing hard exudates and decreased visual acuity [11]. Data from the Diabetes Control and

Complications Trial (DCCT) show a predictive value of total-to-HDL cholesterol ratio and LDL for the development of clinically significant macular edema in people with type I diabetes. However, there is little evidence so far for the efficacy of lipid-lowering medications in preventing the development of macular edema or visual loss.

9.8.1.4 Treatment of Renal Dysfunction and Anemia

There are some reports of improvement of diabetic macular edema after initiation of appropriate treatment in patients with diabetes with nephropathy [55] or anemia [25]. However, there are no controlled trials supporting these anecdotal observations.

9.8.1.5 Smoking

Smoking is a major and reproducible risk factor for diabetic microvascular and macrovascular complications. Even if there are no trials reporting the beneficial effects of smoking cessation on diabetic macular edema it is obvious to include this measure in the essential steps to reducing systemic risk factors in patients with diabetes.

9.8.2 Systemic Pharmacotherapy

9.8.2.1 PKC-ß Inhibitors

Protein kinase C is a group of isoenzymes involved in intracellular signal transduction that are activated in response to various stimuli. Hyperglycemia preferentially induces the activation of the PKC-ß isoform. Ruboxistaurin mesylate, a selective inhibitor of PKC-ß, has been shown to reduce the risk of vision loss (40% reduction), need for laser coagulation (26% reduction), and progression of macular edema (26% reduction) compared with placebo [63]; however this study did not achieve its primary endpoint. Further randomized clinical trials are underway to determine whether this class of drugs will find a role in the prevention of loss of vision in patients with diabetes.

9.8.2.2 Aldose Reductase and AGE Inhibitors

Hyperglycemia results in elevated levels of sorbitol secondary to an increase in the activity of the polyol pathway. Endothelial aldose reductase plays a key role in this pathway. The build-up of intracellular sorbitol that is produced as a result of this increased activity may result in cellular damage [27]. While clinical trials of aldose reductase inhibitors have reduced the number of nonperfused capillaries, fluorescein leakage, and microaneurysm counts, there was no significant effect on the progression of diabetic retinopathy [13].

Increased formation of advanced glycosylation end products (AGE) in diabetes has been proposed as another possible mechanism leading to vascular endothelial cell damage. In the diabetic dog model the AGE inhibitor aminoguanidine effectively inhibited the development of diabetic retinopathy [39]. Recently, a novel AGE inhibitor has been shown to be effective in the diabetic rat model [74]. A clinical trial demonstrating the efficacy of AGE inhibitors in the treatment of people with diabetes has not yet been reported.

9.8.2.3 Antioxidants

Hyperglycemia is followed by an increased production of free radicals (reactive oxygen species) by various mechanisms. Free radicals are thought to play a key role in the development of microvascular damage in diabetes. Reduction of free radicals should therefore have a beneficial effect on diabetic microvascular complications [57] like diabetic retinopathy and macular edema. Conclusive clinical trials in this area are lacking. Calcium dobesilate (Doxium), for example, is a potent antioxidant registered for the treatment of diabetic retinopathy in more than 20 countries [5]. While there are many reports of its beneficial effect on vascular permeability and erythrocyte membrane properties in vitro and in animal models [48, 58, 68], whether it is clinically efficacious remains controversial [64].

9.8.3 A Team Approach to the Prevention of Loss of Vision in People with Diabetes

It is an important function of eye care specialists in developed countries to screen people with diabetes in order to prevent diabetes-related blindness. Many patients seen will have some degree of retinopathy for which specific ophthalmic treatment is not yet needed. In many of these patients the development of the ocular complications of diabetes could be prevented with optimization of systemic risk factors as previously described. It has been shown that in many patients the fear of becoming blind is more important than the fear of dying. Modern digital photography documents retinal changes and allows their demonstration to the patient at the time of examination. By contrast, the systemic complications of diabetes, such as renal or vascular disease, remain invisible and to a certain extent theoretical for the asymptomatic patient. Ophthalmologists are therefore in a unique position to explain the importance of addressing systemic risk factors to the patient and to increase the patient's motivation and compliance. It is important, however, that this communication between eye care specialist and patient takes place in a constructive, friendly, and empowering way. The ophthalmologist should seek not to intimidate a patient with the prospect of blindness, but rather to explain the correlation of poor diabetes control and "worsening of sight." In cases in which systemic risk factors are poorly controlled it may be helpful to arrange an appointment with the primary care physician (general practitioner) or endocrinologist soon after the eye check, combined with an appropriate letter suggesting redoubling of efforts to control systemic risk factors. In our clinical experience cooperation, good communication among the GP, the endocrinologist, and the ophthalmologist is an invaluable tool to empower the patient's motivation and cooperation. All ophthalmologists should try to make use of this tool in the best interest of their patients with diabetes.

This sounds simple, but it obviously takes significant time and personal emphasis during busy clinics. It is important that each patient understands that it is not the ophthalmologist's role to maintain visual function by his treatments, but that the prognosis of his or her vision in the future mainly depends on control of systemic risk factors. This control is a day-to-day struggle for the individual patient and his primary care physician. Advanced ophthalmic diagnostic machinery, laser photocoagulation, and drugs may be of only marginal use if systemic risk factors remain uncontrolled.

Many patients do not understand the difference between random blood glucose levels (in mmol/l) that they measure themselves and glycosylated hemoglobin levels (HbA1c, presented as a percentage), which reflect glycemic control over a period of several months and which are closely correlated with visual outcomes. In our view it is essential that every patient with diabetes understands the difference between these two measures and is encouraged to be aware of the target and current HbA1c values, which they should report to their ophthalmologist at every visit.

The cooperation between ophthalmologist and primary care physician is of particular importance in patients with "early worsening." This phenomenon, which is a common cause of "florid diabetic retinopathy" [49], refers to cases in which acute tightening of glycemic control after long-standing severe hyperglycemia may trigger rapid progression. It has been linked to upregulation of insulin-like growth factor 1 (IGF-1). Laser treatment has been reported to be less successful in these cases, but restoration of poor metabolic control [10], as well as the administration of a somatostatin analogue [9], may be helpful. Most diabetologists now try to lower blood glucose slower, in order to prevent the "early worsening" of diabetic retinopathy. Furthermore, it is important to emphasize that the long-term benefits of intensive treatment outweigh the risks of early worsening [17].

Summary for the Clinician

- Ophthalmologists play an important part in patient motivation and in cooperating with general practitioners, primary care physicians, and endocrinologists.

9.8.4 Local Ophthalmic Treatment

Laser treatment has been the main intervention for diabetic macular edema for the past two decades and remains the cornerstone of management. The Early Treatment of Diabetic Retinopathy Study (ETDRS) was a large multicenter randomized clinical trial carried out between 1980 and 1989 and sponsored by the US National Eye Institute (NEI). Although completed almost 20 years ago, the principles of treatment of diabetic retinopathy and macular edema continue to be based on its findings. One goal of the study was to examine the efficacy of laser photocoagulation for macular edema guided by fluorescein angiography. Treatment was applied to "clinically significant macular edema" (CSME) as defined in Sect. 9.7.1. The ETDRS showed that the risk of moderate visual loss (3 or more lines on a LogMAR chart) was reduced by 50% in eyes treated with immediate laser coagulation compared with control eyes (12% vs. 24%) at 3 years.

9.8.4.1 Focal Macular Laser

The goal of focal laser treatment is to seal focal leaks. The preferred endpoint as described in the ETDRS was to obtain a whitening or darkening of the microaneurysms. Spot sizes from 50 to 200 µm could be used, although the 50- to 100-µm spot sizes were usually used. Within 500 µm of the centre of the macula, the 50-µm spot size was recommended. Clumps of microaneurysms could be treated with larger spot sizes (200–500 µm), but additional treatment with 50- to 100-µm spot sizes was necessary to obtain darkening or whitening of the individual microaneurysms. Exposure time was limited to 0.1 s or less. The 0.05-s exposure was suggested when treating within 500 µm of the center of the macula.

9.8.4.2 Grid Macular Laser

Grid photocoagulation is applied to areas of thickened retina showing diffuse fluorescein leakage and/or capillary drop-out, with any associated focal leak treated as outlined above. Retinal thickening associated with diffuse leakage or capillary drop-out identified by fluorescein angiography is treated with 100- to 200-µm burns of light intensity (above the threshold, but less intense than those applied for panretinal photocoagulation [PRP]) with constant attention to energy levels, since uptake in these areas can be variable. At least one burn width is left between burns. Areas of intense leakage are covered with grid spots placed one burn width apart, while areas of less intense leakage can be treated with a more widely spaced grid. The grid is not placed within 500 µm of the disc margin, but can be placed in the papillomacular bundle. It can extend in all directions up to 2 disc diameters from the center of the macula, or to the border of PRP treatment.

The exact treatment technique for both focal and grid coagulation is described in great detail in the ETDRS report number 2 [20].

9.8.4.3 Recent Trends in Macular Laser Therapy

Even though the principles of macular laser therapy have been established 20 years ago, these recommendations [20] still form the basis of the current treatment guidelines. However, laser photocoagulation of the macula is inherently destructive and creates a small area of irreversible damage to the retinal tissue. Furthermore, enlargement of the laser scars with progression into the central fovea and subsequent loss of vision has been reported [69]. Most laser surgeons these days have therefore adapted their laser techniques. There is a trend toward larger spot sizes, lower energy levels, and longer exposure times, especially for grid coagulation in cases of diffuse edema. Currently, much lighter intensities are used in order to obtain a barely discernible reaction of the RPE. There is an increasing number of retina specialists who do not "shoot aneurysms," as described by the ETDRS, any more since the color change requires too more energy and is not necessary. For focal leaks away from the center more visible effects are suggested, as this may be more effective with regard to the need for retreatment in these areas. For very central leaks observation combined with improved systemic disease control are preferred and treatment at the margin of the foveolar avascular zone is avoided.

The efficacy of the ring-like or "c"-like untargeted grid laser coagulation around the center of the macula is usually disappointing in clinical practice. Therefore, if there are no appropriate targets for focal laser coagulation demonstrated by fluorescein angiography we tend to withhold this treatment and to discuss other therapeutic options like intravitreal corticosteroids or vitrectomy.

9.8.4.4 Micropulsed, Sub-threshold "Selective" Laser Therapy

Histologic studies have shown that there may be a full thickness retinal reaction, even to barely visible laser burns [65]. In clinical pilot studies sub-threshold laser coagulation (using a green Nd:YLF micropulsed laser) was effective in eyes with diabetic macular edema, while minimizing chorioretinal damage [52, 66]. Randomized clinical trials examining the efficacy of sub-threshold laser therapy, however, are still under way.

> **Summary for the Clinician**
> - Laser therapy is still carried out in accordance with the ETDRS, but there is now a tendency toward applying lighter burns of longer duration.
> - Intravitreal triamcinolone acetonide is an alternative to grid coagulation for diffuse edema, but long-term use brings steroid-related adverse effects.

9.8.4.5 Vitrectomy

The absence of posterior vitreous detachment may be associated with cystoid macular edema in eyes of patients with diabetes [31]. Pars plana vitrectomy was reported to be associated with reduced diabetic macular edema and stabilizing or improving vision in eyes with diabetic macular edema by consecutive uncontrolled case series [32, 46]. Possible explanations for such an effect include the release of traction on the vitreoretinal interface due to macular traction, epiretinal membranes and taut posterior hyaloid surfaces, as well as the increased oxygenation that some authorities propose that vitrectomy may afford [73]. A feasibility study assessed the options and hurdles of a randomized clinical trial comparing vitrectomy and laser coagulation, but failed to demonstrate any evidence of efficacy [77]. Whether peeling of the inner limiting membrane is advisable in these cases needs further evaluation [71]. The advances in surgical technique as well as the possibility of evaluating subtle pathologies at the vitreoretinal interface using OCT may improve outcomes and identify a role for vitrectomy in the treatment of diabetic macular edema.

A major drawback of vitrectomy for diabetic macular edema is the fact that it reduces the efficacy and duration of intravitreal triamcinolone (Sect. 9.8.4.6), which may be a problem if the vitrectomy fails to be effective.

9.8.4.6 Intravitreal Steroids

Glucocorticoids have been widely used for the treatment of edema in the brain [24]. Their efficacy is possibly mediated through suppression of vascular endothelial growth factor [30]. Since the blood–brain barrier is similar to the blood–retinal barrier, corticosteroids have been evaluated for the treatment of macular edema. Furthermore, steroids have been found to reduce vascular leak [81] and to suppress the release of endothelial cell activators [2] in asthma, which is also characterized by increased vascular leakage.

Initially, uncontrolled interventional case series reported an unprecedented efficacy of intravitreal steroids (usually triamcinolone acetonide) in reducing diabetic macular edema, often accompanied by significant improvement of visual acuity [33, 34, 53]. These uncontrolled series were followed by randomized, placebo-controlled trials demonstrating the efficacy of IVTA compared with standard care, both short- [75] and long-term [28]. While these studies were generally performed in eyes with persistent macular edema, despite focal and/or grid coagulation, a recently published trial demonstrated the efficacy of IVTA vs. laser coagulation [4].

Although the efficacy of this treatment is generally accepted, there are some uncertainties regarding the optimal dosage of IVTA. A recently published randomized prospective study found no difference in efficacy and safety between 2 mg and 4 mg IVTA [3], while other studies comparing 4 mg, 6 mg, and 8 mg [47], as well as 2 mg, 5 mg, and 13 mg [70] found a more prolonged effect of higher dosage.

The beneficial effect of an intravitreal injection of triamcinolone in most cases lasts for 6–9 months. In the Intravitreal Triamcinolone for Clinically Significant Diabetic Macular Oedema That Persists After Laser Treatment (TDMO) study the mean number of injections was only 2.4 over 2 years with a total potential of five injections according to the study protocol [28]. It has been reported that repeated intravitreal injections may not be as effective as the initial treatment [8]; however, the TDMO study found that there was no difference in the reduction in central macular thickness and improvement in visual acuity in eyes receiving 4–5 injections, compared with the first injection (unpublished data).

The high incidence of steroid-related adverse events associated with intravitreal triamcinolone need to be weighed against the benefits of treatment. In the only randomized controlled trial (RCT)with 2 years' follow-up [28, 75] 54% of phakic treated eyes required cataract surgery. All cataract extractions were performed 1–2 years after beginning treatment. As modern minimally invasive cataract surgery is a relatively safe and efficacious intervention, the risk of developing cataract may not be an absolute contraindication to treatment with intravitreal triamcinolone in eyes that are otherwise losing vision despite conventional treatment.

The other significant steroid-related adverse event associated with IVTA is elevation of intraocular pressure, which may subsequently lead to the development of glaucomatous optic neuropathy, if not detected and promptly treated. In the 2-year study referred to above, 44% of treated eyes required glaucoma medication and 6% required trabeculectomy. Steroid-related pressure rise may be dramatic and resistant to medical treatment.

The introduction of IVTA has been a major advance in the treatment of refractory diabetic macular edema. The high risk of steroid-related adverse events, however, leaves room for improvement and innovation in treatment strategies. Macular laser photocoagulation after IVTA, for example, has been shown to maintain improved vision [36] and may reduce recurrent macular edema after IVTA.

9.8.4.7 Periocular Steroids

In order to avoid some of the adverse events associated with intravitreal therapy, particularly infectious endophthalmitis, some authors have studied the use of periocular steroids to treat diabetic macular edema. While some have found this approach to be effective [4a], but with a less pronounced effect than IVTA, some trials found no significant effect compared with placebo [22]. Further studies are needed to delineate the value of periocular steroid injections in clinical practice.

9.8.4.8 Intravitreal Anti-VEGF Antibodies

Patients with diabetic macular edema have been found to have increased levels of VEGF in the vitreous [26]. Thus, the potent and specific anti-VEGF drugs pegaptanib (Macugen), an anti-VEGF aptamer; bevacizumab (Avastin), an anti-VEGF antibody); and ranibizumab (Lucentis), an anti-VEGF antibody fragment are obvious candidates for the treatment of diabetic macular edema and prospective clinical trials are under way. A phase II RCT [15] of pegaptanib and some experimental pilot studies with ranibizumab have been published and report some efficacy [12, 18]. These new compounds may not be as effective as IVTA, but they do not cause the adverse events associated with corticosteroids. On the other hand, the frequent injections (every 4–6 weeks) for a presumably extended period that may be required with the currently available anti-VEGF compounds, make injection-related complications such as infectious endophthalmitis a major drawback.

A further important issue is the consideration that upregulation of VEGF in diabetic eye disease that will subsequently contribute to macular edema (and proliferative diabetic retinopathy) represents a physiologic response to the hypoxic stimulus that is the impetus for these pathophysiological processes. Intraretinal reperfusion of nonperfused areas has been demonstrated in longitudinal angiography studies [76], which is most likely dependent on VEGF upregulation. Inhibiting VEGF may counteract this mechanism and therefore worsen retinal ischemia. It is therefore from a theoretical point of view questionable whether therapeutic strategies decreasing VEGF directly without improving the oxygenation of the retina represent a valid long-term therapeutic principle for this disease. It is entirely possible that repeated injections of anti-VEGF compounds may decrease macular edema in the short term, but accelerate the development of ischemic diabetic eye disease in the long term. In our view, anti-VEGF remains an experimental treatment for diabetic macular edema at the moment.

Summary for the Clinician

- Therapeutic strategies for diabetic macular edema involve combating systemic risk factors and the use of systemic and local pharmacological therapies, laser treatments, and surgical approaches.
- Investigation of novel anti-VEGF compounds is underway. They are not recommended outside experimental settings.

9.8.4.9 Cataract Surgery

Cataract surgery appears to aggravate diabetic retinopathy and diabetic macular edema. While the progression of diabetic retinal disease is well documented after intracapsular and extracapsular cataract extraction, recent studies [37, 67] found only a limited influence of modern, uneventful, small-incision phacoemulsification. Disease progression was associated with systemic factors and stage of retinopathy, but less with surgery itself. The limitation of these studies, however, is the lack of adequate controls. On the other hand, even in diabetics without retinopathy, extracapsular cataract surgery induces macular edema more frequently than in nondiabetics [56], probably due to the more vulnerable blood–retina barrier in diabetics.

The potential benefits of cataract surgery in diabetic patients, therefore, always need to be weighed against the small but present risk of progression of retinopathy and macular edema.

However, if significant lens opacities are present in eyes with diabetic retinopathy or macular edema, cataract surgery seems to be a rather safe option to improve the vision of these patients. Still, it seems advisable to stabilize systemic control for some months prior to surgery. In cases of significant retinopathy or macular edema cataract surgery may be combined with an intraoperative injection of triamcinolone, even if well-performed studies showing its efficacy are still scarce [35].

9.9 Current Clinical Practice/Recommendations

Summarizing the previously given information, the following recommendations can be made:

1. The treatment of diabetic macular edema should combine the current standard of care and the new therapeutic options as appropriate for each individual patient.
2. It is essential to encourage patients with diabetic macular edema to optimize the control of their systemic risk factors. The first step in our recommended approach to the management of diabetic macular edema is a detailed conversation with the patient and his or her relatives about the importance of controlling systemic risk factors in order to reduce the risk of loss of vision. This is combined with a detailed report to the GP, primary care physician or endocrinologist. A detailed history (duration of diabetes, presence of other complications, current medication, glycemic and blood pressure control, history of eye surgery and laser, duration and speed of visual loss) is taken and each patient should be thoroughly examined with dilated fundus examination. OCT and/or fluorescein angiography is included in the work-up as needed in order to assess the extent and type of macular edema (focal, diffuse, cystoid, ischemic, macular traction or a com-

bination). Special attention should be paid to the vitreoretinal interface (traction, posterior vitreous detachment [PVD], taut or thickened posterior hyaloid, epiretinal membrane).

Depending on these findings one of the following treatment options may be offered to the patient:
1. In patients with poor and improvable systemic control (especially blood pressure) or diabetic renal disease and stable visual acuity or slow decrease in vision, initiation of better systemic treatment (blood glucose, blood pressure, hemodialysis, anemia) should be the first step. Specific ophthalmic treatment may be deferred if possible and ophthalmologic follow-up should be scheduled. Re-evaluation of ophthalmologic treatment may occur after improvement of systemic treatment.
2. For cases of focal edema without significant ischemia, focal laser is still the first choice of treatment. Compared with the ETDRS guidelines we recommend applying lighter burns of longer duration and to perform the treatment in more than one session in severe cases.
3. Intravitreal or (rarely) peribulbar steroids are recommended in cases in which laser treatment has not been effective, or seems unlikely to be. If the eye is phakic the risk of steroid-induced cataract must be discussed. If there are significant lens opacities at baseline cataract extraction may be combined with IVTA intraoperatively. Pre-existing glaucoma or family history of glaucoma should be taken into account. Intraocular pressure has to be followed closely.
4. After IVTA the situation should be re-evaluated and focal laser coagulation applied if appropriate.
5. Vitrectomy (combined with peeling of epiretinal membranes and the ILM) may be considered for eyes with pathology of the vitreoretinal interface. This procedure may be preceded by or combined with intravitreal steroids.
6. For all these options the other features of diabetic retinopathy should be taken into account and therapeutic approaches may be combined (focal laser followed by PRP, IVTA followed by PRP, vitrectomy combined with endolaser coagulation, etc.)
7. In individual cases of uncontrollable adverse steroid effects after IVTA and persistent or relapsing edema with further deterioration of vision treatment with VEGF antagonists on an experimental basis may be offered to the patients.
8. The efficacy of all these different therapeutic approaches should be monitored and evaluated and strategies may be varied depending on the development of visual acuity, clinical findings, and the onset of complications.

References

1. American Diabetes Association (2003) Standards of medical care for patients with diabetes mellitus. Diabetes Care 26 [Suppl 1]:S33–S50
2. Atsuta J, Sterbinsky SA, Plitt J, Schwiebert LM, Bochner BS, Schleimer RP (1997) Phenotyping and cytokine regulation of the BEAS-2B human bronchial epithelial cell: demonstration of inducible expression of the adhesion molecules VCAM-1 and ICAM-1. Am J Respir Cell Mol Biol 17(5):571–582
3. Audren F, Lecleire-Collet A, Erginay A, Haouchine B, Benosman R, Bergmann JF et al (2006) Intravitreal triamcinolone acetonide for diffuse diabetic macular edema: phase 2 trial comparing 4 mg vs 2 mg. Am J Ophthalmol 142(5):794–799
4. Avitabile T, Longo A, Reibaldi A (2005) Intravitreal triamcinolone compared with macular laser grid photocoagulation for the treatment of cystoid macular edema. Am J Ophthalmol 140(4):695–702
4a. Bakri SJ, Kaiser PK. Posterior subtenon triamcinolone acetonide for refractory diabetic macular edema. Am J Ophthamol 2005;139(2):290-4
5. Berthet P, Farine JC, Barras JP (1999) Calcium dobesilate: pharmacological profile related to its use in diabetic retinopathy. Int J Clin Pract 53(8):631–636
6. Centers for Disease Control and Prevention (1996) Blindness caused by diabetes—Massachusetts, 1987–1994. JAMA 276(23):1865–1866
7. Centers for Disease Control and Prevention (2003) Diabetes among Hispanics—Los Angeles County, California, 2002–2003. MMWR Morb Mortal Wkly Rep 52(47):1152–1155

8. Chan CK, Mohamed S, Shanmugam MP, Tsang CW, Lai TY, Lam DS (2006) Decreasing efficacy of repeated intravitreal triamcinolone injections in diabetic macular oedema. Br J Ophthalmol 90(9):1137–1141
9. Chantelau E, Frystyk J (2005) Progression of diabetic retinopathy during improved metabolic control may be treated with reduced insulin dosage and/or somatostatin analogue administration—a case report. Growth Horm IGF Res 15(2):130–135
10. Chantelau E, Meyer-Schwickerath R (2003) Reversion of 'early worsening' of diabetic retinopathy by deliberate restoration of poor metabolic control. Ophthalmologica 217(5):373–377
11. Chew EY, Klein ML, Ferris FL III, Remaley NA, Murphy RP, Chantry K et al (1996) Association of elevated serum lipid levels with retinal hard exudate in diabetic retinopathy. Early Treatment Diabetic Retinopathy Study (ETDRS) Report 22. Arch Ophthalmol 114(9):1079–1084
12. Chun DW, Heier JS, Topping TM, Duker JS, Bankert JM (2006) A pilot study of multiple intravitreal injections of ranibizumab in patients with center-involving clinically significant diabetic macular edema. Ophthalmology 113(10):1706–1712
13. Comer GM, Ciulla TA (2005) Current and future pharmacological intervention for diabetic retinopathy. Expert Opin Emerg Drugs 10(2):441–455
14. Cotter SA, Varma R, Ying-Lai M, Azen SP, Klein R. Causes of low vision and blindness in adult Latinos: the Los Angeles Latino Eye Study. Ophthalmology 113(9):1574–1582
15. Cunningham ET Jr, Adamis AP, Altaweel M, Aiello LP, Bressler NM, D'Amico DJ et al (2005) A phase II randomized double-masked trial of pegaptanib, an anti-vascular endothelial growth factor aptamer, for diabetic macular edema. Ophthalmology 112(10):1747–1757
16. Diabetes Control and Complications Trial Research Group (1993) The effect of intensive treatment of diabetes on the development and progression of long-term complications in insulin-dependent diabetes mellitus. The Diabetes Control and Complications Trial Research Group. N Engl J Med 329(14):977–986
17. Diabetes Control and Complications Trial (1998) Early worsening of diabetic retinopathy in the Diabetes Control and Complications Trial. Arch Ophthalmol 116(7):874–886
18. Do DV, Shah SM, Sung JU, Haller JA, Nguyen QD (2005) Persistent diabetic macular edema is associated with elevated hemoglobin A1c. Am J Ophthalmol 139(4):620–623
19. Dos Santos KG, Canani LH, Gross JL, Tschiedel B, Souto KE, Roisenberg I (2006) The -106CC genotype of the aldose reductase gene is associated with an increased risk of proliferative diabetic retinopathy in Caucasian-Brazilians with type 2 diabetes. Mol Genet Metab 88(3):280–284
20. Early Treatment Diabetic Retinopathy Study Research Group (1987) Treatment techniques and clinical guidelines for photocoagulation of diabetic macular edema. Early Treatment Diabetic Retinopathy Study Report Number 2. Ophthalmology 94(7):761–774
21. Engerman RL, Kern TS (1995) Retinopathy in animal models of diabetes. Diabetes Metab Rev 11(2):109–120
22. Entezari M, Ahmadieh H, Dehghan MH, Ramezani A, Bassirnia N, Anissian A (2005) Posterior sub-tenon triamcinolone for refractory diabetic macular edema: a randomized clinical trial. Eur J Ophthalmol 15(6):746–750
23. Estacio RO, Jeffers BW, Gifford N, Schrier RW (2000) Effect of blood pressure control on diabetic microvascular complications in patients with hypertension and type 2 diabetes. Diabetes Care 23 [Suppl 2]:B54–B64
24. Fishman RA (1975) Brain edema. N Engl J Med 293(14):706–711
25. Friedman EA, Brown CD, Berman DH (1995) Erythropoietin in diabetic macular edema and renal insufficiency. Am J Kidney Dis 26(1):202–208
26. Funatsu H, Yamashita H, Nakamura S, Mimura T, Eguchi S, Noma H et al (2006) Vitreous levels of pigment epithelium-derived factor and vascular endothelial growth factor are related to diabetic macular edema. Ophthalmology 113(2):294–301
27. Gabbay KH (1975) Hyperglycemia, polyol metabolism, and complications of diabetes mellitus. Annu Rev Med 26:521–536
28. Gillies MC, Sutter FK, Simpson JM, Larsson J, Ali H, Zhu M (2006) Intravitreal triamcinolone for refractory diabetic macular edema: two-year results of a double-masked, placebo-controlled, randomized clinical trial. Ophthalmology 113(9):1533–1538

29. Gray A, Raikou M, McGuire A, Fenn P, Stevens R, Cull C et al (2000) Cost effectiveness of an intensive blood glucose control policy in patients with type 2 diabetes: economic analysis alongside randomised controlled trial (UKPDS 41). United Kingdom Prospective Diabetes Study Group. BMJ 320(7246):1373–1378
30. Heiss JD, Papavassiliou E, Merrill MJ, Nieman L, Knightly JJ, Walbridge S et al (1996) Mechanism of dexamethasone suppression of brain tumor-associated vascular permeability in rats. Involvement of the glucocorticoid receptor and vascular permeability factor. J Clin Invest 98(6):1400–1408
31. Ikeda T, Sato K, Katano T, Hayashi Y (1999) Attached posterior hyaloid membrane and the pathogenesis of honeycombed cystoid macular edema in patients with diabetes. Am J Ophthalmol 127(4):478–479
32. Jahn CE, Topfner von Schutz K, Richter J, Boller J, Kron M (2004) Improvement of visual acuity in eyes with diabetic macular edema after treatment with pars plana vitrectomy. Ophthalmologica 218(6):378–384
33. Jonas JB, Sofker A (2001) Intraocular injection of crystalline cortisone as adjunctive treatment of diabetic macular edema. Am J Ophthalmol 132(3):425–457
34. Jonas JB, Kreissig I, Sofker A, Degenring RF (2003) Intravitreal injection of triamcinolone for diffuse diabetic macular edema. Arch Ophthalmol 121(1):57–61
35. Jonas JB, Kreissig I, Budde WM, Degenring RF (2005) Cataract surgery combined with intravitreal injection of triamcinolone acetonide. Eur J Ophthalmol 15(3):329–335
36. Kang SW, Sa HS, Cho HY, Kim JI (2006) Macular grid photocoagulation after intravitreal triamcinolone acetonide for diffuse diabetic macular edema. Arch Ophthalmol 124(5):653–658
37. Kato S, Fukada Y, Hori S, Tanaka Y, Oshika T (1999) Influence of phacoemulsification and intraocular lens implantation on the course of diabetic retinopathy. J Cataract Refract Surg 25(6):788–793
38. Kempen JH, O'Colmain BJ, Leske MC, Haffner SM, Klein R, Moss SE et al (2004) The prevalence of diabetic retinopathy among adults in the United States. Arch Ophthalmol 122(4):552–563
39. Kern TS, Engerman RL (2001) Pharmacological inhibition of diabetic retinopathy: aminoguanidine and aspirin. Diabetes 50(7):1636–1642
40. Kim BY, Smith SD, Kaiser PK (2006) Optical coherence tomographic patterns of diabetic macular edema. Am J Ophthalmol 142(3):405–412
41. Klein R, Klein BE, Moss SE, Davis MD, DeMets DL (1985) The Wisconsin Epidemiologic Study of Diabetic Retinopathy. IV. Diabetic macular edema. Ophthalmology 91(12):1464–1474
42. Klein R, Klein BE, Boss SE, Cruickshanks KJ (1995) The Wisconsin Epidemiologic Study of Diabetic Retinopathy. XV. The long-term incidence of macular edema. Ophthalmology 102(1):7–16
43. Klein R, Meuer SM, Moss SE, Klein BE (1995) Retinal microaneurysm counts and 10-year progression of diabetic retinopathy. Arch Ophthalmol 113(11):1386–1391
44. Klein R, Moss SE, Klein BE, Gutierrez P, Mangione CM (2001) The NEI-VFQ-25 in people with long-term type 1 diabetes mellitus: the Wisconsin Epidemiologic Study of Diabetic Retinopathy. Arch Ophthalmol 119(5):733–740
45. Koro CE, Bowlin SJ, Bourgeois N, Fedder DO. Glycemic control from 1988 to 2000 among U.S. adults diagnosed with type 2 diabetes: a preliminary report. Diabetes Care 27(1):17–20
46. Lai WW, Mohamed S, Lam DS (2005) Improvement of visual acuity in eyes with diabetic macular edema after treatment with pars plana vitrectomy. Ophthalmologica 219(3):189
47. Lam DS, Chan CK, Mohamed S, Lai TY, Tsang CW, Chan WM et al (2007) A prospective randomized trial of different doses of intravitreal triamcinolone for diabetic macular edema. Br J Ophthalmol 91(2):199–203
48. Lameynardie S, Chiavaroli C, Travo P, Garay RP, Pares-Herbute N (2005) Inhibition of choroidal angiogenesis by calcium dobesilate in normal Wistar and diabetic GK rats. Eur J Pharmacol 510(1–2):149–156
49. Lattanzio R, Brancato R, Bandello FM, Azzolini C, Malegori A, Maestranzi G (2001) Florid diabetic retinopathy (FDR): a long-term follow-up study. Graefes Arch Clin Exp Ophthalmol 239(3):182–187

50. Liesenfeld B, Kohner E, Piehlmeier W, Kluthe S, Aldington S, Porta M et al (2000) A telemedical approach to the screening of diabetic retinopathy: digital fundus photography. Diabetes Care 23(3):345–348
51. Lopes de Faria JM, Jalkh AE, Trempe CL, McMeel JW (1999) Diabetic macular edema: risk factors and concomitants. Acta Ophthalmol Scand 77(2):170–175
52. Luttrull JK, Musch DC, Mainster MA (2005) Subthreshold diode micropulse photocoagulation for the treatment of clinically significant diabetic macular oedema. Br J Ophthalmol 89(1):74–80
53. Martidis A, Duker JS, Greenberg PB, Rogers AH, Puliafito CA, Reichel E et al (2001) Intravitreal triamcinolone for refractory diabetic macular edema. Ophthalmology 109(5):920–927
54. Massin P, Girach A, Erginay A, Gaudric A (2006) Optical coherence tomography: a key to the future management of patients with diabetic macular oedema. Acta Ophthalmol Scand 84(4):466–474
55. Matsuo T (2006) Disappearance of diabetic macular hard exudates after hemodialysis introduction. Acta Med Okayama 60(3):201–205
56. Menchini U, Bandello F, Brancato R, Camesasca FI, Galdini M (1993) Cystoid macular oedema after extracapsular cataract extraction and intraocular lens implantation in diabetic patients without retinopathy. Br J Ophthalmol 77(4):208–211
57. Nishikawa T, Edelstein D, Du XL, Yamagishi S, Matsumura T, Kaneda Y et al (2000) Normalizing mitochondrial superoxide production blocks three pathways of hyperglycaemic damage. Nature 404(6779):787–790
58. Padilla E, Ganado P, Sanz M, Zeini M, Ruiz E, Trivino A et al (2005) Calcium dobesilate attenuates vascular injury and the progression of diabetic retinopathy in streptozotocin-induced diabetic rats. Diabetes Metab Res Rev 21(2):132–142
59. Panozzo G, Parolini B, Gusson E, Mercanti A, Pinackatt S, Bertoldo G et al (2004) Diabetic macular edema: an OCT-based classification. Semin Ophthalmol 19(1–2):13–20
60. Patton N, Aslam TM, MacGillivray T, Deary IJ, Dhillon B, Eikelboom RH et al (2006) Retinal image analysis: concepts, applications and potential. Prog Retin Eye Res 25(1):99–127
61. Patz A, Schatz H, Berkow JW, Gittelsohn AM, Ticho U (1973) Macular edema—an overlooked complication of diabetic retinopathy. Trans Am Acad Ophthalmol Otolaryngol 77(1):OP34–42
62. Peter J, Piantadosi J, Piantadosi C, Cooper P, Gehling N, Kaufmann C et al (2006) Use of real-time telemedicine in the detection of diabetic macular oedema: a pilot study. Clin Experiment Ophthalmol 34(4):312–316
63. PKC-DRS2 Group; Aiello LP, Davis MD, Girach A et al (2006) Effect of ruboxistaurin on visual loss in patients with diabetic retinopathy. Ophthalmology 113(12):2221–2230
64. Ribeiro ML, Seres AI, Carneiro AM, Stur M, Zourdani A, Caillon P et al (2006) Effect of calcium dobesilate on progression of early diabetic retinopathy: a randomised double-blind study. Graefes Arch Clin Exp Ophthalmol (published online, doi: 10.1007/s00417-006-0318-2)
65. Roider J (1999) Laser treatment of retinal diseases by subthreshold laser effects. Semin Ophthalmol 14(1):19–26
66. Roider J, Brinkmann R, Wirbelauer C, Laqua H, Birngruber R (2000) Subthreshold (retinal pigment epithelium) photocoagulation in macular diseases: a pilot study. Br J Ophthalmol 84(1):40–47
67. Romero-Aroca P, Fernandez-Ballart J, Almena-Garcia M, Mendez-Marin I, Salvat-Serra M, Buil-Calvo JA (2006) Nonproliferative diabetic retinopathy and macular edema progression after phacoemulsification: prospective study. J Cataract Refract Surg 32(9):1438–1444
68. Rota R, Chiavaroli C, Garay RP, Hannaert P (2004) Reduction of retinal albumin leakage by the antioxidant calcium dobesilate in streptozotocin-diabetic rats. Eur J Pharmacol 495(2–3):217–224
69. Schatz H, Madeira D, McDonald HR, Johnson RN (1991) Progressive enlargement of laser scars following grid laser photocoagulation for diffuse diabetic macular edema. Arch Ophthalmol 109(11):1549–1551
70. Spandau UH, Derse M, Schmitz-Valckenberg P, Papoulis C, Jonas JB (2005) Dosage dependency of intravitreal triamcinolone acetonide as treatment for diabetic macular oedema. Br J Ophthalmol 89(8):999–1003

71. Stefaniotou M, Aspiotis M, Kalogeropoulos C, Christodoulou A, Psylla M, Ioachim E et al (2004) Vitrectomy results for diffuse diabetic macular edema with and without inner limiting membrane removal. Eur J Ophthalmol 14(2):137–143
72. Stefansson E (2006) Why are diabetics still going blind? Ophthalmol Times Europe 2(4):36–37
73. Stefansson E (2006) Ocular oxygenation and the treatment of diabetic retinopathy. Surv Ophthalmol 51(4):364–380
74. Sun W, Oates PJ, Coutcher JB, Gerhardinger C, Lorenzi M (2006) A selective aldose reductase inhibitor of a new structural class prevents or reverses early retinal abnormalities in experimental diabetic retinopathy. Diabetes 55(10):2757–2762
75. Sutter FK, Simpson JM, Gillies MC (2004) Intravitreal triamcinolone for diabetic macular edema that persists after laser treatment: three-month efficacy and safety results of a prospective, randomized, double-masked, placebo-controlled clinical trial. Ophthalmology 111(11):2044–2049
76. Takahashi K, Kishi S, Muraoka K, Shimizu K (1998) Reperfusion of occluded capillary beds in diabetic retinopathy. Am J Ophthalmol 126(6):791–797
77. Thomas D, Bunce C, Moorman C, Laidlaw DA (2005) A randomised controlled feasibility trial of vitrectomy versus laser for diabetic macular oedema. Br J Ophthalmol 89(1):81–86
78. Toth CA, Narayan DG, Boppart SA, Hee MR, Fujimoto JG, Birngruber R et al (1997) A comparison of retinal morphology viewed by optical coherence tomography and by light microscopy. Arch Ophthalmol 115(11):1425–1428
79. UK Prospective Diabetes Study (UKPDS) (1991) VIII. Study design, progress and performance. Diabetologia 34(12):877–890
80. UK Prospective Diabetes Study (UKPDS) (1998) Tight blood pressure control and risk of macrovascular and microvascular complications in type 2 diabetes: UKPDS 38. UK Prospective Diabetes Study Group. BMJ 317(7160):703–713
81. Van de Graaf EA, Out TA, Roos CM, Jansen HM (1991) Respiratory membrane permeability and bronchial hyperreactivity in patients with stable asthma. Effects of therapy with inhaled steroids. Am Rev Respir Dis 143(2):362–368
82. Varma R, Torres M, Pena F, Klein R, Azen SP (2004) Prevalence of diabetic retinopathy in adult Latinos: the Los Angeles Latino eye study. Ophthalmology 111(7):1298–1306
83. Wang Y, Ng MC, Lee SC, So WY, Tong PC, Cockram CS et al (2003) Phenotypic heterogeneity and associations of two aldose reductase gene polymorphisms with nephropathy and retinopathy in type 2 diabetes. Diabetes Care 26(8):2410–2415
84. Williams R, Airey M, Baxter H, Forrester J, Kennedy-Martin T, Girach A (2004) Epidemiology of diabetic retinopathy and macular oedema: a systematic review. Eye 18(10):963–983
85. Zimmet P, Alberti KG, Shaw J (2001) Global and societal implications of the diabetes epidemic. Nature 414(6865):782–787

Chapter 10

Treatment of Retinal Vein Occlusions

Rajeev S. Ramchandran, R. Keith Shuler, Sharon Fekrat

Core Messages

- Despite the multitude of cases series and reports of various treatments for retinal vein occlusions, grid pattern laser photocoagulation is the only proven therapy to obtain visual improvement for a certain subset of eyes with branch retinal vein occlusion.
- Ocular and systemic risk factors for developing a retinal vein occlusion should be addressed.
- While medical therapies have primarily addressed the sequelae of a retinal vein occlusion, namely macular edema, many surgical therapies have generally focused on anatomically circumventing or resolving the vein occlusion.
- In developing more effective treatment strategies, a greater understanding of the histopathology and pathophysiology of retinal venous occlusive disease is necessary.
- A more thorough comprehension of the natural history of retinal venous occlusive disease is required in order to determine the actual benefit of proposed treatments.
- Adequately powered, well-designed, prospective clinical trials are needed to establish efficacy of any future treatment strategies for retinal venous occlusive disease.
- One such prospective trial, The Standard of Care vs. Corticosteroid for Retinal Vein Occlusion (SCORE) Study, is underway to determine the long-term effects of intravitreal injection of triamcinolone acetonide for, and the extended natural history of, central and branch retinal vein occlusions

10.1 Introduction

Retinal vein occlusion (RVO) has been reported to occur in 1–2% of the population and is the second most common retinal vascular disease after diabetic retinopathy. It is more common in individuals with underlying vascular disease who are older than 50 years and increases in incidence with age. Based on anatomic pathophysiology and extent of retinal involvement, RVO has been classified into three entities: branch, central, and hemi-retinal vein occlusion (BRVO, CRVO, and HRVO). Each type has its own natural history and management strategy (Table 10.1). Two multi-center, randomized controlled trials have demonstrated only limited visual improvement after laser therapy for macular edema and neovascularization, but they have formed the foundation for the way in which RVO has been managed. Since the completion of these trials, many more recent pharmacologic and surgical interventions have targeted the anatomic and cellular pathophysiology of RVO with varied success at improving vision.

Table 10.1 Current management strategies for vein occlusion. *rt-PA* recombinant tissue plasminogen activator, *VEGF* vascular endothelial growth factor, *ILM* internal limiting membrane

Branch retinal vein occlusion	Central retinal vein occlusion
Observation	Observation
Grid pattern laser photocoagulation	Systemic anticoagulation
Intravitreal triamcinolone or anti-VEGF	Grid pattern laser photocoagulation
Sustained steroid release devices	Intravitreal rt-PA
Vitrectomy ± ILM peeling	Intravitreal triamcinolone or anti-VEGF
Vitrectomy with arteriovenous sheathotomy	Sustained steroid release devices
	Laser chorioretinal venous anastomosis
	Vitrectomy ± ILM peeling
	Retinal vein cannulation
	Radial optic neurotomy

10.2 Pathophysiology

The precise pathophysiology of retinal vein occlusion is unknown.

Branch retinal vein occlusion primarily occurs at arteriovenous crossings, where arteries and veins course through the same adventitial sheath [23, 78, 87]. It is postulated that arterial changes, such as those seen in hypertensive disease, lead to compression of the underlying, relatively flaccid, venous vessel wall, which obstructs venous blood flow. This impedance of flow, as well as the turbulent nature of flow at the arteriovenous crossing points, may allow for the formation of a thrombus, as seen histopathologically [8, 22, 34, 53]. Whether an actual thrombus is present is unknown.

Central retinal vein occlusion, as the name implies, has been associated with thrombus formation in the central retinal vein at the level of the lamina cribrosa [39]. Inflammation of vascular endothelium with disruption of laminar flow through the central retinal vein in this region may also lead to venous obstruction [27, 39]. The visual prognosis is generally poorer for eyes with CRVO compared with that of BRVO. In approximately one-fifth of eyes, the venous systems draining the superior and inferior retinal regions each join a superior and inferior venous trunk that connect to form a single central vein posterior to the lamina cribrosa. Occlusion of the superior or inferior venous trunk in these eyes may lead to a hemiretinal vein occlusion, which has clinical features and an ocular prognosis similar to CRVO [21, 43]. However, in the currently ongoing Standard of Care vs. Corticosteroid for Retinal Vein Occlusion (SCORE) Study, sponsored by the National Eye Institute (NEI), HRVO is considered to be a subset of BRVO.

In spite of histopathological data on each retinal vein occlusion subgroup, the pathophysiology of this group of disorders has not been fully understood. Visual impairment is primarily due to two inter-related mechanisms, macular ischemia and macular edema, which result from the venous occlusion-induced-retinal hypoxia. Retinal and/or vitreous hemorrhage from vein occlusions can impair vision acutely, but these generally resolve over time and have rarely led to permanent vision loss.

10.3 Branch and Central Vein Occlusion Studies

10.3.1 Background

The current standard of care for treating BRVO and CRVO is based on findings from two multicenter, randomized, controlled studies initiated by the NEI in the 1970s. Named the Branch Vein Occlusion Study (BVOS) and Central Vein Occlusion Study (CVOS) respectively, these studies have evaluated the natural history and demonstrated the effectiveness of various treatments targeted at decreasing macular edema, improving vision, and decreasing retinal and anterior segment neovascularization [9, 10, 16–19].

10.3.2 Branch Vein Occlusion Study

In the Branch Vein Occlusion Study, one-third to one-half of eyes with BRVO regained a visual acuity of 20/40 or better without therapy at 1 year. For the remaining eyes, a history of hypertension or decrease in vision due to macular edema for more than 1 year made it less likely for vision to be gained without an intervention. Therefore, the BVOS suggested observing eyes for 3 months for spontaneous resolution of macular edema and improvement in vision. This time would also allow for the clearing of any intraretinal hemorrhage in the foveal center that could contribute to vision loss. A high-resolution fluorescein angiogram would then be performed to determine the perfusion status of the macula. If leakage on the fluorescein angiogram was seen with perfusion of vessels in the macula, grid pattern laser was recommended. Grid pattern laser is not indicated for eyes with macular ischemia (as seen on the fluorescein angiogram), which may have macular edema without leakage.

Specifically, the BVOS showed that, by 3 years, 63% of eyes treated with grid pattern laser photocoagulation gained about 2 lines of vision compared with 36% of untreated eyes. However, the mean visual gain for the treated group was only 1 Snellen line of acuity compared with untreated eyes [5, 9, 29].

Grid pattern laser photocoagulation was performed using a blue-green argon laser with a light-to-medium spot burn measuring 50–100 μm in diameter, at a 0.1-s duration, in the area of perfused angiographic leakage and outside the foveal avascular zone (Table 10.2). It is theorized that this laser stimulates the retinal pigment epithelial cells to reabsorb fluid from the edematous retina and thins the retina to allow for more oxygen diffusion from the choriocapillaris into the inner retina [84]. Increased oxygen concentration may allow for retinal vascular constriction and help limit vasogenic edema [78]. Currently, along with fluorescein angiography, optical coherence tomography (OCT) is used to follow macular edema over time, and if persistent edema is seen, additional grid pattern laser may be considered.

The BVOS demonstrated the benefit of scatter laser photocoagulation in eyes that had developed retinal neovascularization. Eyes with BRVO having more than 5 disc diameters of retinal nonperfusion on fluorescein angiography are at greater risk of developing retinal neovascularization. This usually occurs during the first 6–12 months. Although a rare event after BRVO, anterior segment neovascularization may also occur, particularly in individuals with diabetes, but it is independent of the presence of diabetic retinopathy. According to the BVOS, eyes treated with prophylactic scatter laser to the ischemic retina had an incidence of retinal neovascularization of only 20% compared with 40% in the untreated group. However, advocating prophylactic treatment of all ischemic eyes would result in applying scatter laser to many eyes that would never develop neovascular changes. Therefore, the BVOS has advocated the use of scatter laser photocoagulation only after retinal neovascularization has been clinically documented in order to prevent vitreous hemorrhage. Laser treatment in this fashion decreased the incidence of vitreous hemorrhage from 60% in untreated eyes to 36% in treated eyes [10].

Table 10.2 Grid laser specification for treating macular edema after branch retinal vein occlusion (BRVO) according to the Branch Vein Occlusion Study

Size	50–100 μm
Exposure	0.05–0.1 s
Intensity	Mild
Number	Cover areas of diffuse retinal thickening
Placement	1–2 burn widths apart (500–3,000 μm from fovea)
Wavelength	Green to yellow

10.3.3 Central Vein Occlusion Study

The Central Vein Occlusion Study classified eyes as having a perfused CRVO (less than 10 disc diameters of retinal ischemia) or a nonperfused CRVO (greater than 10 disc diameters of retinal ischemia) based on fluorescein angiographic characteristics. The ability to see clearly and perceive light acutely after CRVO were the strongest predictive factors for visual recovery [16]. After a period of 3 years, the majority (65%) of eyes with baseline vision of or better than 20/40 remained at this level, and nearly 20% of eyes with baseline vision 20/50–20/200 improved to better than 20/40. In contrast, during the same period, 80% of eyes with baseline vision worse than 20/200 did not improve. By the end of this study, almost 40% of eyes with baseline vision 20/50–20/200 were worse than 20/200. This is consistent with nearly 40% of eyes converting from a perfused to a nonperfused status over the same period [19].

Grid pattern laser was not effective in improving vision in eyes with non-ischemic macular edema. Although macular edema resolved in nearly 30% of treated eyes compared with 0% of untreated eyes at 1 year, mean visual acuity was 20/200 for treated eyes and 20/160 for untreated eyes at 3 years. Extensive damage to the perifoveal capillary bed was thought to be the reason for this poor visual outcome [16]. There was a clinical trend suggesting that photocoagulation may be more effective in the eyes of patients under the age of 65. Seventeen treated eyes (23%) had an improvement of 2 or more lines of visual acuity, and 11 of those were individuals who were less than 60 years old. The results, however, were not statistically significant.

For nonperfused eyes, the CVOS showed that it was better to delay panretinal photocoagulation (PRP) until neovascularization appeared, rather than performing prophylactic treatment. Early treatment of ischemic CRVO with PRP decreased the development of anterior segment neovascularization to 20% compared with 34% in untreated eyes. However, eyes treated *after* the development of anterior segment neovascularization demonstrated greater resolution of the new blood vessels at 1 month compared with eyes treated prophylactically. Ninety-percent of eyes treated after the development of anterior segment neovascularization showed marked regression of neovascularization by 2 months [19].

The current standard of care is to wait until neovascularization develops before performing PRP. In general, neovascularization of the iris or angle tends to occur more readily than neovascularization of the disc or retina in eyes with CRVO, but the treatment for these manifestations of neovascularization is the same. For eyes with extensive retinal ischemia, prophylactic treatment may be considered, especially if frequent follow-up is difficult.

Summary for Clinician

- To date, the BVOS and CVOS studies are the only published randomized controlled trials of the treatment of RVO.
- Grid pattern laser photocoagulation is only advocated for nonischemic macular edema in eyes with BRVO.
- It is prudent to wait until neovascularization is present before initiating scatter laser photocoagulation in eyes with BRVO or CRVO, although treatment may be initiated in eyes with extensive ischemic disease if follow-up is questionable.

10.4 Systemic Pharmacologic Treatments

Systemic medical therapies have demonstrated varied success in improving visual outcomes in eyes with RVO. Increased retinal perfusion after CRVO has been achieved with oral pentoxifylline. This vasodilator may promote collateral circulation development. Oral pentoxifylline combined with hemodilution, to decrease blood viscosity, has proven to significantly improve visual acuity after 12 months compared with ordinary saline infusions in a randomized, prospective trial [85]. However, anticoagulation with warfarin sodium (Coumadin) has not been effective in preventing or altering the consequent natural history of CRVO [57]. One case report has shown brief improvement in macular edema and vision after treatment with oral corticosteroids and another has shown similar improvement after intravenous steroids [74].

Summary for Clinician

- Currently, use of systemic pharmacologic therapies for treating RVO is not widely advocated.

10.5 Targeting Macular Edema

Animal studies have shown that venous occlusions result in retinal hypoxia of varying degrees depending on the location of the occlusion [45]. Retinal hypoxia triggers the release of proinflammatory mediators, such as platelet-derived growth factor and platelet-activating factor [63], that upregulate vascular endothelial growth factor (VEGF) production. VEGF has been shown to increase phosphorylation of occludin and zonula occluden 1, as well as other tight junction proteins, and thereby increase retinal capillary permeability [1, 3, 68, 77]. Ischemic retinal tissue also releases prostaglandins and interleukins that further increase vascular permeability. With the resulting leakage of vascular proteins into the extracellular space, an osmotic gradient is created that leads to vasogenic retinal edema. Retinal ischemia resulting from vein occlusion also results in localized shutdown of cell function, which leads to cytotoxic edema of the intra- and extracellular space [31]. From cellular analysis, vision loss is thought to be due to macular edema-associated retinal anatomic disorganization and atrophy, pigmentary changes, and photoreceptor cell death [58].

10.6 Intravitreal Pharmacotherapy

10.6.1 Background

Currently, intravitreal treatments, which are less likely to have systemic side effects and risks, have been promoted. These pharmacologic therapies, including intravitreal corticosteroids and anti-VEGF agents, presently target the increased vascular permeability and inflammation following RVO at the cellular and molecular level.

Experimental studies have shown that intravitreally injected corticosteroids, such as triamcinolone acetonide, counteract and limit the effects of intraocular vasogenic and inflammatory mediators, such as VEGF, and thus, help stabilize the blood–retina barrier and decrease vascular permeability (Table 10.3) [52]. Small retrospective and prospective interventional case series have shown the effectiveness of intravitreal triamcinolone acetonide at the 4-mg/ml dose in decreasing macular edema and improving visual acuity after RVO. One small case series has also shown similar effectiveness of intravitreal anti-VEGF in treating macular edema after RVO. In addition to the small number of cases (10–20 eyes) reviewed, the variation in time to treatment from onset of RVO (ranging from 2–15 months on average), the relatively short follow-up period of about 1 year for most studies, and the nonrandomized nature of these studies must be considered (Table 10.4) [6, 14, 15, 20, 47, 50–52, 58, 67, 75, 86].

Steps for intravitreal injection (Fig. 10.1):
1. Obtain written informed consent
2. Administer topical and/or subconjunctival anesthesia.
3. Perform betadine preparation of lids and lashes.
4. Insert sterile speculum.
5. Use sterile cotton-tipped applicator to displace the conjunctiva.

Downregulation of inflammatory markers
• Downregulation of VEGF
• Modulation of adhesion molecule expression
• Inhibition of arachidonic acid pathway
• Decrease in prostaglandin synthesis
• Reduction in intraluminal and periluminal lymphocytes
Reduction of blood–retina barrier/vascular permeability
• Reduction of optic disc edema
• Reabsorption of macular edema

Table 10.3 Triamcinolone acetonide mechanism of action [60, 83]

Table 10.4 Reported case series of intravitreal triamcinolone injections for retinal vein occlusion (RVO)

Reference	Number of eyes treated	Disease	Dose (mg/ml)	Anatomical improvement (%)	Mean baseline visual acuity	Mean visual acuity at endpoint	Mean follow-up (months)	Mean duration of RVO (months)
[86]	12	BRVO	4	12/12 (100)	20/160	20/60	15.3	1.5
[15]	13	BRVO	4	9/9[b] (100)	20/100	20/70	13	7.4
[75]	17	BRVO	10	14/17 (82)	20/110	20/50	12.1	3.5
[20]	18	BRVO	4	18/18 (100)	20/129	20/100	14	11.6
[67]	10	CRVO	4	10/10 (100)	20/80	20/32	4.8	15.4
[52]	10	CRVO	4	10/10 (100)	20/159	20/142	7.6	6
[47]	13	CRVO	4	13/13 (100)	20/500	20/180	6	8
[81]	18	CRVO	2	18/18 (100)	20/300	20/150	4.8	2
[6]	20	CRVO	4	15/20 (75)	20/132	20/37	11	3.5
[14][a]	24	CRVO	4	–	20/167	20/91	10	5.4

[a] 52% reduction in mean fovea thickness
[b] Central foveal thickness measurements only reported for 9 eyes

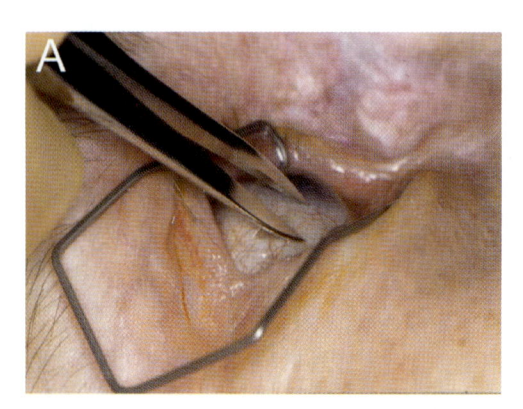

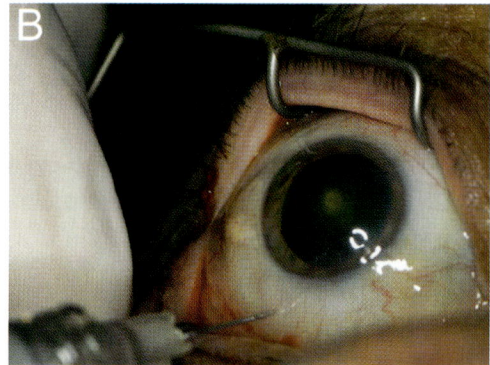

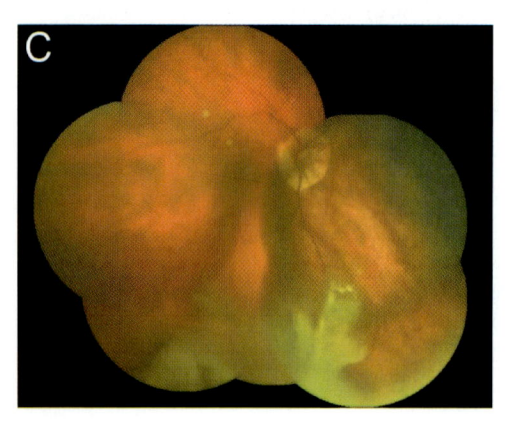

Fig. 10.1 A–C Technique for intravitreal injection. **A** Measurement 3.5 mm posterior to the limbus to mark the site of the injection. **B** Intravitreal injection. **C** Intravitreal triamcinolone acetonide seen in the inferior vitreous

6. Administer intravitreal injection 3.5 mm posterior to the limbus.
7. Place sterile cotton-tipped applicator over the injection site after needle removal.
8. Apply sterile topical antibiotic.
9. Perform indirect ophthalmoscopy to verify the placement of the medication and retinal arterial perfusion.
10. Measure intraocular pressure (IOP) to see if it is at an acceptable level.
11. Give a post-injection prescription for the topical antibiotic.

10.6.2 Intravitreal Triamcinolone: BRVO

For the majority of cases of BRVO treated with intravitreal triamcinolone that have been reviewed in the literature, mean macular edema and visual acuity improved nearly 50% by 3–6 months postinjection. Studies with shorter duration of BRVO showed more improvement, and one study of 13 eyes demonstrated no relationship between baseline and post-injection visual acuity [15, 20, 51, 59, 75, 86]. However, after 6 months, visual acuity and macular edema gradually worsened toward baseline levels in the majority of eyes, and many eyes required a repeat intravitreal triamcinolone injection. One study also suggested that previously vitrectomized eyes often require repeat steroid injection [86]. These findings parallel the pharmacokinetics of triamcinolone in the eye. The mean half-life of intravitreal triamcinolone has been shown to be about 19 days, with a measurable concentration lasting 3 months. The mean half-life has been shown to be even shorter for vitrectomized eyes, at about 3 days [7].

Although the visual and anatomic results after repeat injection were reported to be equal to those seen after the initial injection, repeated injections increased the risk of IOP rise. Thirty to 40% percent of treated eyes required IOP-lowering medications at 1 year. Significant cataract formation was also more common in eyes with repeated injections that were followed for greater than one year [15]. The risk of developing endophthalmitis, retinal detachment, and vitreous hemorrhage is also increased with repeated intravitreal injections [70].

10.6.3 Intravitreal Triamcinolone: CRVO

As reported in multiple small interventional cohort studies, the majority of eyes with CRVO gained significant visual acuity within a few months of an intravitreal triamcinolone injection. Eyes without significant retinal ischemia faired much better than those with substantial retinal ischemia. Macular edema also markedly improved within a few months of injection in many eyes with CRVO, and in one study, this improvement was similar for ischemic and non-ischemic occlusions [47]. However, by 6 months, the treatment effect had waned in many eyes, and vision and macular edema progressively became worse. Repeat injections were performed at this point, and although many eyes still gained substantial vision and had an improvement in their macular edema, each repeated injection carried the same risks as previously outlined, including IOP rise and progression of cataract. IOP elevation after intravitreal triamcinolone was more prevalent in the CRVO case series than in eyes with BRVO. This is consistent with the stronger association of glaucoma with CRVO. Nearly 60–70% of treated eyes with CRVO required treatment for IOP 1 year after treatment. Cataract progression in treated eyes was similar to that seen in the BRVO case series, with repeated injections associated with increased formation of cataracts. Moreover, few reports showed no significant relationship between baseline and post-treatment visual acuity, visual acuity and amount of macular edema, or the duration of RVO and visual acuity [6, 14, 46, 50, 52, 67, 75].

10.6.4 Fluocinolone Acetonide Intravitreal Implant

Since the effect of intravitreally injected triamcinolone is transient, a sustained steroid drug delivery system may be beneficial. This is especially true in cases of refractory macular edema where repeated injections are often necessary. Both non-biodegradable and biodegradable devices that are implanted surgically or in the office setting have been developed. Approved in 2005 by the Food and Drug Administration (FDA) for chronic noninfectious uveitis, a nonbiodegradable, surgically implanted fluocinolone acetonide intravitreal device (Retisert; Bausch and Lomb, Rochester, NY, USA) has been effective in treating macular edema and improving visual acuity in eyes with RVO. By releasing a sustained amount of drug (0.59 mg/day) for up to 3 years, this device has proven effective in resolving persistent macular edema and improving visual acuity over an extended period of time without the need for repeated intravitreal injections [49].

A small prospective case series of 19 eyes with BRVO and CRVO has shown this device to be effective throughout 12 months of treating selected cases of longstanding venous occlusive disease that was refractory to other therapies. Visual acuity was stabilized or improved by at least 2 Snellen lines in 70% of eyes at 12 months. The sustained steroid levels provided by the implant also improved central macular thickness to the normal range on OCT by 2 months in most eyes. At 2 months, the median central macular thickness improvement was 50% and was maintained at this level throughout 12 months (Fig. 10.2). However, as in eyes receiving repeated intravitreal steroid injections, careful monitoring of IOP and lens status was required. By 12 months post-implant, about 50% of eyes required IOP lowering medication, about 40% required glaucoma filtering surgery, and about 70% of previously phakic eyes required cataract surgery. In addition, one eye developed infectious endophthalmitis within 1 month of device implantation and subsequently had the device explanted [69].

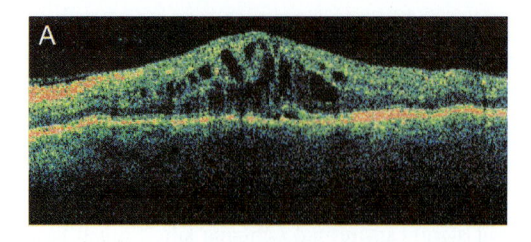

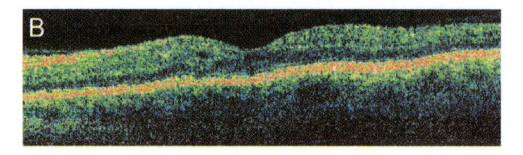

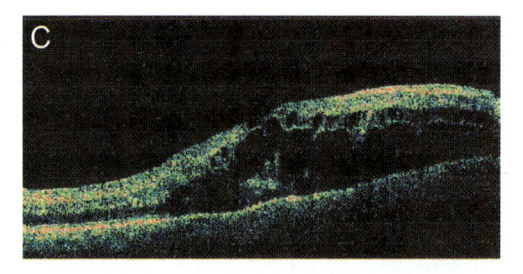

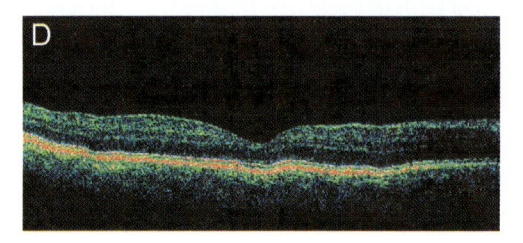

Fig. 10.2 A,B Improvement in macular edema after fluocinolone acetonide implant placement (0.59 mg/day) in an eye with central retinal vein occlusion (CRVO). **A** Pre-implant: best corrected visual acuity 20/80, central macular thickness 600 µm. **B** Two months post-implant: improvement in best corrected visual acuity to 20/25, central macular thickness improvement to 220 µm. Visual acuity and central macular thickness remained at this level throughout 12 months. **C, D** Improvement in macular edema after intravitreal bevacizumab (Avastin; 1.25 mg/0.05 ml) in an eye with CRVO. **C** Pre-injection best corrected visual acuity 20/100. **D** One month post-injection improvement of visual acuity to 20/20 with total resolution of macular edema

10.6.5 Standard of Care vs. Corticosteroid for Retinal Vein Occlusion Study

With the significant promise shown by intravitreal steroids of improving visual outcomes after RVO, its use among retinal specialists as first-line therapy, especially in eyes with CRVO, has dramatically increased, even though positive data from a clinical trial evaluating this approach are lacking. Therefore, the National Eye Institute has funded an ongoing multicenter, prospective, randomized clinical trial to compare 1 mg and 4 mg of intravitreal triamcinolone with grid pattern laser in BRVO and with observation in CRVO, the current standards of care. Known as the Standard of Care vs. Corticosteroid for Retinal Vein Occlusion (SCORE) Study, this project will follow about 1,200 eyes for up to 3 years (Table 10.5). At its conclusion, the SCORE study will provide a better insight into the natural history of RVO as well as systematically determining whether intravitreal triamcinolone is more effective in treating RVO than the current standard of care.

10.6.6 Intravitreal Anti-VEGF Therapy

In addition to corticosteroids, other immunologic agents that directly target the VEGF molecule are now being used to treat macular edema and improve vision after RVO. The published results of a recently completed phase II clinical trial of pegaptanib sodium (Macugen), a 28-base ribonucleic acid aptamer directed against the 165 isoform of VEGF, for the treatment of macular edema after CRVO are still awaited. The effectiveness of monthly intravitreal bevacizumab (Avastin), a full-length, humanized, murine monoclonal antibody to multiple biologically active forms of VEGF, has been studied in 16 eyes with refractory macular edema due to CRVO at a dose of 1.25 mg/0.05 ml [48]. Over 90% of these eyes demonstrated significant improvement in macular edema and gain in visual acuity over 3 months. These results parallel those seen for intravitreal triamcinolone, although with triamcinolone, increased cataract formation or a sustained increase in IOP were significant postinjection issues. However, the follow-up time for eyes treated with intravitreal bevacizumab was brief, and it is unclear whether intravitreal injections of anti-VEGF agents carry the risks of cardiovascular events and systemic hypertension similar to those associated with their systemic use.

> **Summary for Clinician**
>
> - Intravitreal steroid or anti-VEGF therapy is currently the treatment of choice for many ophthalmologists for eyes with RVO.
> - Ophthalmologists should be aware of potential ocular side-effects of intravitreal steroids and the potential systemic effects of intravitreal anti-VEGF agents.
> - Despite widespread use of intravitreal triamcinolone, long-term data are still needed. The results of the SCORE Study will determine the true efficacy and safety of intravitreal triamcinolone.

Table 10.5 SCORE study inclusion and exclusion criteria. *VA* visual acuity, *ETDRS* Early Treatment Diabetic Retinopathy Study, *CRVO* central retinal vein occlusion, *BRVO* branch retinal vein occlusion, *OCT* optical coherence tomography, *PRP* panretinal laser photocoagulation, *Nd-YAG* neodymium-yttrium-aluminum-garnet, *SCORE* standard of care vs. corticosteroid for retinal vein occlusion

SCORE inclusion criteria	SCORE exclusion criteria

• At least 18 years of age
• Center-involved macular edema due to CRVO or BRVO
  – no longer than 24 months
• Retinal thickness >250 µm on OCT
• ETDRS visual acuity score:
  – Lower limit: >19 letters (20/400)
  – Upper limit: <73 letters (20/40)
	• Oral corticosteroids within prior 4 months
	• Prior grid pattern laser photocoagulation
	• Other cause of macular edema
	• Other eye disease affecting VA
	• Prior intravitreal steroid
	• Periocular steroid within last 6 months
	• PRP within last 4 months or in next 4 months
	• Prior vitrectomy
	• Nd-YAG within the last 2 months
	• Intraocular surgery within the last 6 months or the next 6 months

10.7 Surgical Treatments

Because the primary cause of RVO may be an anatomic problem, a number of surgical treatments to target problematic posterior segment anatomic relationships have been explored.

10.7.1 BRVO

Pars plana vitrectomy with removal of the posterior hyaloid to relieve potential vitreomacular traction and to improve posterior segment oxygenation with and without gas tamponade has been shown in small case series to improve visual acuity and reduce macular edema as evidenced on exam and by fluorescein angiography [2, 54, 71]. In addition to vitrectomy, non-randomized studies have shown some benefit of arteriovenous sheathotomy in re-establishing retinal perfusion, reducing intra-retinal hemorrhage and macular edema, and improving visual acuity [61, 64, 66, 72, 73]. An arteriovenous sheathotomy entails using a bent microvitreoretinal (MVR) or other blade to section the common arteriovenous sheath and separate the artery from the underlying retinal vein at the site of occlusion [66, 73]. It is thought that decompressing the vein in this fashion allows for venous recanalization and thrombus displacement at the blockage site with the return of distal venous flow. This technique is not without complications as nerve fiber layer defects, hemorrhage, and retinal detachment, among others, have been reported. It is also unclear if a stable thrombus that forms in the compressed vein at the arteriovenous junction could be dislodged by potentially creating more space around the vessel. Moreover, given the relatively limited data, it is difficult to determine the actual benefit of this treatment for eyes with BRVO and arteriovenous sheathotomy has largely been abandoned.

10.7.2 CRVO

Multiple surgical treatments for CRVO have been suggested with limited evidence of effectiveness. Each strategy seeks to improve the vascular flow in the retina. Vitreous surgery is routinely performed to treat the sequelae of CRVO, including non-clearing vitreous hemorrhage and extensive fibrovascular proliferation. Pars plana vitrectomy with subsequent induction of a posterior hyaloid detachment alone may improve the visual outcome after CRVO by increasing the oxygenation of the retina by bathing it in aqueous. Simultaneous peeling of the internal limiting membrane may offer benefit, although this has not been well-studied.

10.7.2.1 Laser-Induced Venous Chorioretinal Anastomosis

By 3 years, approximately 30% of eyes with CRVO develop significant retinal ischemia, which carries a poor visual prognosis. In an attempt to prevent progression to ischemia, the creation of a chorioretinal anastomosis (CRA) has been tried. Through this method, the thrombosed central retinal vein is bypassed and retinal venous blood can then flow from the retina out through the choroidal circulation. This connection between the choroidal and retina circulations has been created surgically, through trans-retinal venipuncture [28], but has more often been accomplished with an argon and/or Nd-YAG laser to rupture the posterior wall of a branch retinal vein and adjacent Bruch's membrane. Studies have demonstrated a 10–54% success rate for CRA creation in eyes with perfused CRVO [30].

Creation of CRA is not without significant risk. Acutely, intraretinal, subretinal, and vitreous hemorrhage that may be non-clearing have all been reported. Venous thrombosis at the site of the CRA can occur and may lead to distal retinal ischemia and neovascular complications. Fibrovascular proliferation, choroidal, retinal, and anterior segment neovascularization, and tractional retinal detachment can also occur [11, 12, 28, 30]. Creation of CRA in eyes with an ischemic CRVO has met with limited success and is not recommended [55].

10.7.2.2 Recombinant Tissue Plasminogen Activator

Anatomically, the main histopathologic feature of CRVO is a central retinal vein thrombus that obstructs blood flow and perpetuates an ischemic environment in the macula. If a thrombus is indeed present, dissolving it may lead to improved visual outcome. Use of thrombolytic agents, such as recombinant tissue plasminogen activator, to improve vision after CRVO has shown some success. Recombinant tissue plasminogen activator (rt-PA) promotes the formation of plasmin from plasminogen, and thus initiates a cascade of events that leads to clot dissolution. Systemic, intravitreal, and endovascular rt-PA have all been reported in small series in the literature with varied outcomes.

Improvement in visual acuity ranging from 30 to 70% after systemic administration of rt-PA has been shown in a few studies [37, 41, 42, 56]. One prospective trial reported a mean improvement of 5 lines after receiving 50 μg of rt-PA systemically in about 40 out of 96 eyes. However, the subsequent death of one of the participants due to an intracranial hemorrhage, after receiving intravenous rt-PA in this trial, has discouraged use of this treatment for CRVO [56].

In an attempt to decrease systemic complications from rt-PA, intravitreal injections of 50 μg of rt-PA have been tried for both ischemic and non-ischemic CRVO. In a short follow-up of 6 months, three studies have shown 3 lines of improvement in 30–40% of eyes with CRVO of less than 21 days' duration [25, 36, 56]. Although visual improvement after intravitreal rt-PA was greater in eyes with perfused rather than nonperfused CRVO, improvement or change in venous perfusion was not seen in any of the treated eyes [68].

Injection of rt-PA (3.4 ml at a concentration of 200 μg/ml) into a cannulated branch retinal vein toward the optic nerve head after pars plana vitrectomy has also been performed in eyes with CRVO [79]. In this way, small quantities of rt-PA are delivered in close proximity to the thrombosed central retinal vein. In one study of eyes with CRVO of more than 1 month's duration and vision worse than 20/400, 14 out of 28 eyes recovered more than 3 lines of vision by 12 months post-treatment. However, complications, including vitreous hemorrhage and retinal detachment may occur more readily with the endovascular approach [79]. Further study is needed.

10.7.2.3 Radial Optic Neurotomy

It is thought that CRVO may occur in part from a decreased central retinal vein luminal diameter at the lamina cribrosa due to compression by a rigid scleral ring, which increases the risk of local thrombus formation. To relieve the presumed pressure on the central retinal vein at the scleral outlet, described as a "compartment syndrome," a radial optic neurotomy (RON) procedure has been proposed [65]. Following a pars plana vitrectomy, an MVR blade is pushed posteriorly through the outer optic disc and scleral junction with the tip placed at the nasal edge of the optic disc.

Small retrospective case series have shown visual improvement in eyes with CRVO and a baseline visual acuity of <20/400. Opremcak and colleagues reported 8 out of 11 eyes, 6 of which were nonperfused, to have improved visual acuity after a mean of 9 months following RON [65]. Weizer and co-workers reported quicker clearing of intraretinal hemorrhage and improvement of disc congestion after CRVO relative to the known natural history in 4 out of 5 patients, with mean visual acuity improving from 4/200 to 20/400 [80]. However, in both studies neovascular complications occurred in 2 eyes.

One prospective study demonstrated that RON may help to create a CRA at the surgical site, which favors improved visual acuity. In this study, 6 out of 14 eyes developed a CRA after RON. These eyes had a mean visual acuity of 20/60 compared with a mean visual acuity of 20/110 for eyes without CRA development. In addition, visual acuity improvement correlated with a decrease in macular edema after RON, and 8 out of 14 eyes gained at least 1 line of vision [35]. Presently, a large prospective, multicenter randomized clinical trial to evaluate the efficacy of RON after CRVO is underway in Europe, and findings from this study will more clearly delineate the effectiveness of RON in treating CRVO.

Although RON is thought to decompress the central retinal vein and increase venous outflow and thereby decrease macular edema and improve vision, external decompression of the optic nerve sheath and posterior scleral ring sectioning have not been shown to be effective treatments for CRVO [24, 58, 62, 76].

10.7.2.4 Intravitreal Triamcinolone: As Adjunctive Therapy

Two separate case series, one focusing on radial optic neurotomy (RON) and the other on endovascular recombinant tissue plasminogen activator (rt-PA), have looked at combining surgical treatments with intravitreal triamcinolone injection to treat CRVO. Another case series has evaluated grid pattern laser combined with intravitreal triamcinolone for both BRVO and CRVO. However, the outcomes of all of these studies mirror those of using intravitreal triamcinolone alone [4, 13].

> **Summary for Clinician**
> - Medical therapy should be considered before pursuing surgical options.
> - Currently, surgical therapies for RVO have not been well studied in randomized controlled trials. The results of a European study on RON for RVO are awaited to determine the suitability of this treatment.
> - Pars plana vitrectomy with endolaser treatment may be appropriate in eyes with a nonclearing vitreous hemorrhage due to RVO.
> - Combined medical and surgical therapies require more study before they are included in the standard of care.

10.8 Prevention—Systemic Factor Control

Prevention of RVO involves addressing the risk factors that contribute to its occurrence. It is important that ophthalmologists work with medical doctors to identify and appropriately treat systemic hypertension, hyperlipidemia, atherosclerotic disease, and diabetes, as these are the most common systemic factors associated with RVO as determined in the Eye Disease Case-Control Study [26, 27]. Systemic hypertension associated with macular edema after BRVO is also associated with a poor visual outcome [26].

While the above systemic factors are more commonly seen in RVO patients over the age of 60, hypercoagulable states and inflammatory vascular diseases have also been associated with RVO in younger patients [32, 40]. Coagulopathies including protein C and S deficiencies, activated protein C resistance, and the presence of Factor V Leiden, antiphospholipid antibodies, and abnormal fibrinogen levels, as well as increased blood viscosity due to dehydration, blood dyscrasias, and dysproteinemias may also increase the risk of RVO [33, 38, 44, 46, 82]. Therefore, these factors, which alter vascular flow, need to be managed appropriately when known.

Individuals suffering a CRVO in one eye have a 1% chance per year of developing a CRVO in the fellow eye [19]. Thus, a medical work-up to diagnose and treat the above systemic and hematologic factors predisposing the eyes to vein occlusion should be considered. Smoking cessation can also reduce the risk of developing an RVO by decreasing progression of vascular disease [26]. Finally, IOP monitoring and management are also important, as glaucoma is a known risk factor for RVO, especially CRVO.

> **Summary for Clinician**
> - It is important to document a thorough medical history in all patients with RVO that elicits the known risk factors for developing an RVO.
> - Communication and cooperation with the patient and their primary care team are crucial to ensure effective control of systemic risk factors for RVO.

10.9 Conclusion

In light of the multitude of available data, but limited rigorously proven data, evidence-based treatment strategies are scarce. First and foremost, a thorough history and physical examination for all patients who have experienced an RVO may facilitate the appropriate treatment of systemic and ocular factors that may predispose an eye to RVO development. Baseline fundus photography, fluorescein angiography, and OCT to better characterize the venous occlusion and macular edema can also be performed.

The visual outcome of BRVO is generally favorable with 30% having 20/40 or better vision. As shown by the BVOS, the grid pattern laser can be used in cases of perfused BRVO with persistent vision loss to treat any macular edema, albeit with only moderate visual gain expected. If retinal neovascularization is present, scatter laser in the affected area can limit the occurrence of vitreous hemorrhage. CRVO carries a worse visual prognosis. Observation and grid pattern laser have not been shown to be beneficial in most individuals. If NVA/NVI develops, performing PRP is the only proven management option. After the initial baseline vision, IOP measurement, anterior segment examination, undilated gonioscopy, dilated fundus examination and subsequent fluorescein angiography, and OCT of the macula can be obtained. Affected eyes can be followed monthly at least for the first 6 months, if observation is elected. At these visits, visual acuity and IOP measurements as well as undilated gonioscopy and dilated fundus examination can be performed to look for neovascularization, as neovascular glaucoma occurs in 40–60% of eyes with nonperfusion greater than 10 disc diameters, often by 3 months post-occlusion.

10.10 Current Practice and Future Trends

To date, surgical therapies that aim to improve venous perfusion and vascular flow in the retina have not been effective in improving retinal oxygenation and vision. Pending results of the RON trial in Europe may refute this fact. However, current practice is aimed at treating macular edema resulting from RVO. According to the 2005 ASRS Preferences and Trends Survey, perfused BRVO with macular edema and an initial vision of 20/40 that worsened to 20/250, was treated initially with grid laser by 50% of respondents. The other 50% would use intravitreal triamcinolone injections alone or in combination with the grid pattern laser as first-line therapy. In fact, 75% of those surveyed would offer intravitreal triamcinolone for refractory macular edema after grid pattern laser in BRVO. In addition, nearly 60% were apt to give intravitreal triamcinolone as first-line therapy to eyes with CRVO and at least 20/80 vision for 2 months (Fig. 10.3) In light of this trend toward using intravitreal triamcinolone as a first-line of treatment for macular edema after RVO, results from the SCORE study are awaited to determine the long-term efficacy and safety of this treatment regimen. Moreover, although both macular edema and visual acuity improve after intravitreal triamcinolone, there is limited correlation between a reduction in foveal thickness on OCT and gain in visual acuity. Thus, the mechanism behind how steroid treatment leads to improved vision after RVO is still unclear.

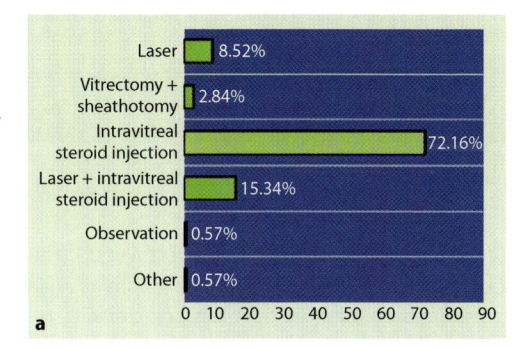

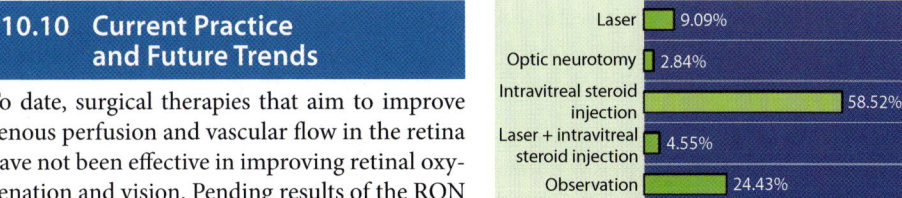

Fig. 10.3a,b Results of the 2005 ASRS Preferences and Trends Survey. **a** Percentage of respondents using each treatment as next line of therapy for macular edema associated with branch retinal vein occlusion (BRVO), an initial visual acuity of 20/40 that worsened to 20/250 after one grid pattern laser treatment. **b** Percentage of respondents using each treatment as primary therapy for macular edema associated with CRVO and at least 20/80 vision for 2 months

Better understanding of the exact etiology, pathophysiology, and natural history of RVO can help formulate treatment strategies that offer neuroprotection, improve retinal perfusion and oxygenation, decrease retinal oxygen demand and macular edema, prevent retinal atrophy, and thereby improve visual outcomes after RVO. Whether it is surgical, pharmacologic, or a combination of the two, carefully designed, well-powered, prospective, randomized clinical trials are needed to determine the efficacy and safety of any treatment for RVO.

References

1. Aiello LP, Bursell SE, Clermont A et al (1997) Vascular endothelial growth factor-induced retinal permeability is mediated by protein kinase C in vivo and suppressed by an orally effective beta-isoform-selective inhibitor. Diabetes 46:1473–1480
2. Amirikia A, Scott IU, Murray TG et al (2001) Outcomes of vitreoretinal surgery for complications of branch retinal vein occlusion. Ophthalmology 108:372
3. Antoneti DA, Barber AJ, Hollinger LA et al (1999) Vascular endothelial growth factor induced rapid phosphorylation of tight junction proteins occludin and zonula occluden 1. J Biol Chem 274:23463–23467
4. Avitabile T, Longo A, Reibaldi A (2005) Intravitreal triamcinolone compared with macular laser grid photocoagulation for the treatment of cystoid macular edema. Am J Ophthalmol 140(4):695.e1–e8
5. Bearelly S, Fekrat S (2004) Controversy in the management of retinal venous occlusive disease. Int Ophthalmol Clin 44(4):85–102
6. Bashshur ZF, Ma'luf RN, Allam S et al (2004) Intravitreal triamcinolone for the management of macular edema due to nonischemic central retinal vein occlusion. Arch Ophthalmol 122(8):1137–1140
7. Beer PM, Bakri SJ, Singh RJ et al (2003) Intraocular concentration and pharmacokinetics of triamcinolone acetonide after a single intravitreal injection. Ophthalmology 110(4):681–686
8. Bowers DK, Finkelstein D, Wolff SM et al (1987) Branch retinal vein occlusion: a clinicopathological case report. Retina 7:252–259
9. Branch Vein Occlusion Study Group (1984) Argon laser photocoagulation for macular edema in branch vein occlusion. Am J Ophthalmol 98:271
10. Branch Vein Occlusion Study Group (1986) Argon laser scatter photocoagulation for prevention of neovascularization and vitreous hemorrhage in branch vein occlusion. A randomized clinical trial. Arch Ophthalmol 104:34
11. Browning DJ, Antoszyk AN (1998) Laser chorioretinal venous anastomosis for nonischemic central retinal vein occlusion. Ophthalmology 105(4):670–677; discussion 7–9
12. Browning D, Rotberg M (1996) Vitreous hemorrhage complicating laser-induced chorioretinal anastomosis for central retinal vein occlusion. Am J Ophthalmol 122(4):588–589
13. Bynoe LA, Weiss JN (2003) Retinal endovascular surgery and intravitreal triamcinolone acetonide for central vein occlusion in young adults. Am J Ophthalmol 135(3):382–384
14. Cekic O, Chang S, Tseng J et al (2005) Intravitreal triamcinolone treatment for macular edema associated with central retinal vein occlusion and hemiretinal vein occlusion. Retina 25(7):846–850
15. Cekic O, Chang S, Tseng J et al (2005) Intravitreal triamcinolone injection for treatment of macular edema secondary to branch retinal vein occlusion. Retina 25(7):851–855
16. Central Vein Occlusion Study Group (1993) Baseline and early natural history report: the Central Vein Occlusion Study. Arch Ophthalmol 111:1087
17. Central Vein Occlusion Study Group (1995) Evaluation of grid pattern photocoagulation for macular edema in central vein occlusion: The Central Vein Occlusion Study Group M report. Ophthalmology 102: 1425
18. Central Vein Occlusion Study Group (1995) A randomized clinical trial of early panretinal photocoagulation for ischemic central vein occlusion: the Central Vein Occlusion Study Group N report. Ophthalmology 102:1434
19. Central Vein Occlusion Study Group (1997) Natural history and clinical management of central retinal vein occlusion: the Central Vein Occlusion Study Group. Arch Ophthalmol 115:486
20. Chen S, Sundaram V, Lochhead J, Patel C (2006) Intravitreal triamcinolone for treatment of ischemic macular edema associated with branch retinal vein occlusion. Am J Ophthalmol 141(5):876–883

21. Chopdar A (1984) Dual trunk central retinal vein incidence in clinical practice. Arch Ophthalmol 102:85
22. Clemett RS (1974) Retinal branch vein occlusion: changes at the site of obstruction. Br J Ophthalmol 58:548–554
23. Duker JS, Brown GC (1989) Anterior location of the crossing artery in branch retinal vein occlusion. Arch Ophthalmol 107:998
24. Dev S, Buckley EG (1999) Optic nerve sheath decompression for progressive central retinal vein occlusion. Ophthalmic Surg Lasers 30(3):181–184
25. Elman MJ, Raden RZ, Carrigan A (2001) Intravitreal injection of tissue plasminogen activator for central retinal vein occlusion. Trans Am Ophthalmol Soc 99:219–221; discussion 22–23
26. Eye Disease Case-Control Study Group (1993) Risk factors for branch retinal vein occlusion. Am J Ophthalmol 116:286–296
27. Eye Disease Case-Control Study Group (1996) Risk factors for central retinal vein occlusion. Arch Ophthalmol 114:545
28. Fekrat S, de Juan E Jr (1999) Chorioretinal venous anastomosis for central retinal vein occlusion: transvitreal venipuncture. Ophthalmic Surg Lasers 30(1):52–55
29. Fekrat S, Finkelstein D (2001) Branch retinal vein occlusion disease. In: Schachat AP (2001) Retina, 3rd edn. Mosby, St. Louis
30. Fekrat S, Goldberg MF, Finkelstein D (1998) Laser-induced chorioretinal venous anastomosis for nonischemic central or branch retinal vein occlusion. Arch Ophthalmol 116(1):43–52
31. Finkelstein D (1992) Ischemic macular edema: recognition and favorable natural history in branch vein occlusion. Arch Ophthalmol 119:1427–1434
32. Fong AC, Schatz H (1993) Central retinal vein occlusion in young adults. Surv Ophthalmol 38:88
33. Francis PJ, Stanford MR, Graham EM (2003) Dehydration is a risk factor for central retinal vein occlusion in young patients. Acta Ophthalmol Scand 81(4):415–416
34. Frangieh GT, Green WR, Barraquer-Somers E et al (1982) Histopathologic study of nine branch retinal vein occlusions. Arch Ophthalmol 100:1132
35. Garcia-Arumi J, Boixadera A, Martinez-Castillo V et al (2003) Chorioretinal anastomosis after radial optic neurotomy for central retinal vein occlusion. Arch Ophthalmol 121:1385–1391
36. Glacet-Bernard A, Kuhn D, Vine AK et al (2000) Treatment of recent onset central retinal vein occlusion with intravitreal tissue plasminogen activator: a pilot study. Br J Ophthalmol 84(6):609–613
37. Ghazi NG, Noureddine BN, Haddad RS et al (2003) Intravitreal tissue plasminogen activator in the management of central retinal vein occlusion. Retina 23:780–784
38. Gottlieb JL, Blice JP, Mestichelli B et al (1998) Activated protein C resistance, factor V Leiden, and central retinal vein occlusion in young adults. Arch Ophthalmol 116:577–579
39. Green W, Chan C, Hutchins G et al (1981) Central retinal vein occlusions: a prospective histopathologic study of 29 eyes in 28 cases. Retina 1:27
40. Gutman FA (1983) Evaluation of a patient with central retinal vein occlusion. Ophthalmology 90(5):481–483
41. Hattenbach LO, Steinkamp G, Scharrer I et al (1998) Fibrinolytic therapy with low-dose recombinant tissue plasminogen activator in retinal vein occlusion. Ophthalmologica 212(6):394–398
42. Hattenbach LO, Wellermann G, Steinkamp GW et al (1999) Visual outcome after treatment with low-dose recombinant tissue plasminogen activator or hemodilution in ischemic central retinal vein occlusion. Ophthalmologica 213(6):360–366
43. Hayreh SS, Hayreh MS (1980) Hemi-central retinal vein occlusion: pathogenesis, clinical features, and natural history. Arch Ophthalmol 98:1600
44. Hayreh SS, Zimmerman MB, Podhajsky P (2002) Hematologic abnormalities associated with various types of retinal vein occlusion. Graefes Arch Clin Exp Ophthalmol 240(3):180–196
45. Hockley DJ, Tripathi RC, Ashton N (1979) Experimental branch vein occlusion in the rhesus monkeys. III. Br J Ophthalmol 63:393–411
46. Hvarfner C, Hillarp A, Larsson J (2003) Influence of factor V Leiden on the development of neovascularisation secondary to central retinal vein occlusion. Br J Ophthalmol 87(3):305–306
47. Ip MS, Gottlieb JL, Kahana A et al (2004) Intravitreal triamcinolone for the treatment of macular edema associated with central retinal vein occlusion. Arch Ophthalmol 122(8):1131–1136
48. Iturralde D, Spaide RF, Meyerle CB et al (2006) Intravitreal bevacizumab (Avastin) treatment of macular edema in central retinal vein occlusion. Retina 26(3):279–284

49. Jaffe GJ et al (2005) Long-term follow-up results of a pilot trial of a fluocinolone acetonide implant to treat posterior uveitis. Ophthalmology 112(7):1192–1198
50. Jonas JB (2002) Intravitreal triamcinolone acetonide as treatment of macular edema in central retinal vein occlusion. Graefes Arch Clin and Exp Ophthalmol 240(9):782–783
51. Jonas JB, Akkoyun I, Kamppeter B et al (2005) Branch retinal vein occlusion treated by intravitreal triamcinolone acetonide. Eye 19(1):65–71
52. Krepler K, Ergun E, Sacu S et al (2005) Intravitreal triamcinolone acetonide in patients with macular oedema due to central vein occlusion. Acta Ophthalmol Scand 83(1):71–75
53. Kumar B, Yu DY, Morgan WH et al (1998) The distribution of angioarchitectural changes within the vicinity of the arteriovenous crossing in branch retinal vein occlusion. Ophthalmology 105:424–427
54. Kurimoto M, Takagi H, Suzuma K (1999) Vitrectomy for macular edema secondary to retinal vein occlusion: evaluation by retinal thickness analyzer. Jpn J Ophthalmol 53:717
55. Kwok AK, Lee VY, Lai TY et al (2003) Laser induced chorioretinal venous anastomosis in ischaemic central retinal vein occlusion. Br J Ophthalmol 87(8):1043–1044
56. Lahey JM, Fong DS, Kearney J (1999) Intravitreal tissue plasminogen activator for acute central retinal vein occlusion. Ophthalmic Surg Lasers 30(6):427–434
57. Lai JC, Mruthyunjaya P, Fekrat S (2002) Central retinal vein occlusion in patients on chronic Coumadin® anticoagulation. Invest Ophthalmol Vis Sci 42:ARVO E-Abstract 519
58. Lardenoye CWTA, Probst K, DeLint PJ et al (2000) Photoreceptor function in eyes with macular edema. Invest Ophthalmol Vis Sci 41(12):4048–4053
59. Lee H, Shah GK (2005) Intravitreal triamcinolone as primary treatment of cystoid macular edema secondary to branch retinal vein occlusion. Retina 25(5):551–555
60. McCuen BW Jr, Bessler M, Tano Y et al (1981) The lack of toxicity of intravitreally administered triamcinolone acetonide. Am J Ophthalmol 91(6):785–788
61. Mester U, Dillinger P (2000) Vitrectomy with decompression in branch retinal vein occlusion. Club Jules Gonin Meeting, Sicily
62. Nauck M, Karaklulakis G, Perruchoud AP et al (1998) Corticosteroids inhibit the expression of the vascular endothelial growth factor gene in human vascular smooth muscle cells. Eur J Pharmacol 341:309–315
63. Nauck M, Roth M, Tamm M et al (1997) Induction of vascular endothelial growth factor by platelet-activating factor and platelet-derived growth factor is downregulated by corticosteroids. Am J Respir Cell Mol Biol 16:398–406
64. Opremcak EM, Bruce RA (1999) Surgical decompression of branch retinal vein occlusion via arteriovenous crossing sheathotomy: a prospective review of 15 cases. Retina 19:1
65. Opremcak EM, Rehmar AJ, Ridenour CD et al (2006) Radial optic neurotomy with adjunctive intraocular triamcinolone for central retinal vein occlusion. Retina 26:306–313
66. Osterloh MD, Charles S (1988) Surgical decompression of branch retinal vein occlusions. Arch Ophthalmol 106:1469
67. Park CH, Jaffe GJ, Fekrat S (2003) Intravitreal triamcinolone acetonide in eyes with cystoid macular edema associated with central retinal vein occlusion. Am J Ophthalmol 136(3):419–425
68. Pe'er J, Folberg R, Itin A et al (1998) Vascular endothelial growth factor upregulation in human central retinal vein occlusion. Ophthalmology 105:412–416
69. Ramchandran RS, Jaffe GJ, Fekrat S et al (2006) Fluocinolone acetonide sustained drug delivery device for chronic retinal venous occlusive disease: 12 month results. ARVO Abstract
70. Roth DB, Chieh J, Spirn MJ et al (2003) Noninfectious endophthalmitis associated with intravitreal triamcinolone injection. Arch Ophthalmol 121(9):1279–1282
71. Saika S, Tanaka T, Miyamoto T (2001) Surgical posterior vitreous detachment combined with gas/air tamponade for treating macular edema associated with branch retinal vein occlusion: retinal tomography and visual outcome. Graefes Arch Clin Exp Ophthalmol 239:729
72. Shah GK (2000) Adventitial sheathotomy for treatment of macular edema associated with branch retinal vein occlusion. Curr Opin Ophthalmol 11:171
73. Shah GK, Sharma S, Fineman MS et al (2000) Arteriovenous adventitial sheathotomy for the treatment of macular edema associated with branch retinal vein occlusion. Am J Ophthalmol 129:104

74. Shaikh S, Blumenkranz MS (2001) Transient improvement in visual acuity and macular edema in central retinal vein occlusion accompanied by inflammatory features after pulse steroid and anti-inflammatory therapy. Retina 21(2):176–178
75. Tsujikawa A, Fujihara M, Iwawaki T et al (2005) Triamcinolone acetonide with vitrectomy for treatment of macular edema associated with branch retinal vein occlusion. Retina 25(7):861–867
76. Vasco-Posada J (1972) Modification of the circulation in the posterior pole of the eye. Ann Ophthalmol 4(1):48–59
77. Vinores SA, Youssri AL, Luna JD et al (1997) Upregulation of vascular endothelial growth factor in ischemic and non-ischemic human and experimental retinal disease. Histol Histopathol 12:99–109
78. Weinberg D, Dodwell DG, Fern SA (1990) Anatomy of arteriovenous crossings in branch retinal vein occlusion. Am J Ophthalmol 109:298–302
79. Weiss JN, Bynoe LA (2001) Injection of tissue plasminogen activator into a branch retinal vein in eyes with central retinal vein occlusion. Ophthalmology 108(12):2249–2257
80. Weizer JS, Stinnett SS, Fekrat S (2003) Radial optic neurotomy as treatment for central retinal vein occlusion. Am J Ophthalmol 136(5):814–819
81. Williamson TH, O'Donnell A (2005) Intravitreal triamcinolone acetonide for cystoid macular edema in nonischemic central retinal vein occlusion. Am J Ophthalmol 139(5):860–866
82. Williamson TH, Rumley A, Lowe GD (1996) Blood viscosity, coagulation, and activated protein C resistance in central retinal vein occlusion: a population controlled study. Br J Ophthalmol 80(3):203–208
83. Wilson CA, Berkowitz BA, Sato Y et al (1992) Treatment with intravitreal steroid reduces blood-retinal barrier breakdown due to retinal photocoagulation. Arch Ophthalmol 110(8):1155–1159
84. Wilson DJ, Finkelstein D, Quigley HA et al (1998) Macular grid photocoagulation: an experimental study on the primate retina. Arch Ophthalmol 106:100
85. Wolf S, Arend O, Bertram B et al (1994) Hemodilution therapy in central retinal vein occlusion: one-year results of a prospective randomized study. Graefes Arch Clin Exp Ophthalmol 232(1):33–39
86. Yepremyan, M et al (2005) Early treatment of cystoid macular edema secondary to branch retinal vein occlusion with intravitreal triamcinolone acetonide. Ophthalmic Surg Lasers Imaging 36(1):30–36
87. Zhao J, Sastry SM, Sperduto RD et al (1993) Arteriovenous crossing patterns in branch retinal vein occlusion. The Eye Disease Case-Control Study Group. Ophthalmology 100:423–428

Chapter 11

New Perspectives in Stargardt's Disease

Noemi Lois

Core Messages

- The onset of Stargardt's disease (STGD) can occur at any age, from early childhood to adulthood, and there is a wide variation in visual acuity, clinical appearance, and severity of the disease.
- Visual acuity varies from 20/20 to 20/400; only rarely does it drop below 20/400.
- Fundus examination discloses, typically, a central area of atrophy surrounded by a ring of flecks. Flecks can be also seen extending to the midperipheral retina. Early on in the course of the disease, however, fundus examination may be normal.
- Invasive imaging techniques, including fluorescein angiography (FFA) and indocyanine green angiography (ICG), are rarely needed to evaluate patients with STGD. Fundus autofluorescence (AF), a noninvasive imaging technique, can be used for this purpose.
- Patients with STGD may have one of three patterns of functional loss: macular dysfunction alone, macular and peripheral cone dysfunction, or macular and peripheral cone and rod dysfunction. These patterns of functional loss cannot usually be predicted based on fundus appearance.
- Imaging and histopathology studies have demonstrated increased levels of lipofuscin in the retinal pigment epithelium (RPE) in the majority of patients with STGD.
- STGD is inherited as an autosomal recessive trait and is caused by mutations in the ABCA4 gene, located in the short arm of chromosome 1 (1p).
- The protein codified by the ABCA4 gene, expressed in cone and rod photoreceptor cells, appears to play a role in the transport of retinoids, specifically N-retinylidene-phosphatidylethanolamine and all-trans-retinal, in photoreceptor outer segment disc membranes.
- Although the mechanism by which photoreceptors degenerate in STGD is not known. Accumulation of N-retinylidene-N-retinyl-ethanolamine (A2E), the major component of lipofuscin, seems to play an important role in the RPE cell degeneration and loss seen in STGD. Photoreceptor cell loss could occur in this disease subsequent to RPE cell degeneration.
- An animal model of STGD is now available, the abcr-/- knockout mice.
- Currently, there is no treatment for patients with STGD. However, laboratory studies suggest that patients with this retinal dystrophy may slow the progression of their disease by protecting their eyes from light exposure.
- New treatment strategies to reduce or prevent A2E accumulation in the RPE are being investigated.

11.1 Introduction

In 1909 Stargardt [51] described a form of recessive inherited macular dystrophy characterized by the presence of an atrophic macular lesion, which was eventually surrounded by irregular, white-yellow deep retinal lesions. Early on in the course of the disease, there appeared to be a disproportional loss of visual acuity when compared with clinical findings. Later on, in 1962, Franceschetti [21] proposed the term "fundus flavimaculatus" to designate a peculiar fundus affection in which the hallmark was the presence of yellow-white deep "fishlike" retinal lesions, now known as "flecks," varying in size, shape, opaqueness, and density, and limited to the posterior pole or extending to the equatorial region. In some patients described by Franceschetti atrophic macular lesions were also present and, thus, the disease was indistinguishable from that described earlier by Stargardt.

After the initial descriptions by Stargardt and Franceschetti, there was controversy in the literature as to whether or not Stargardt's disease (STGD) and fundus flavimaculatus (FFM) were representing different clinical entities. It is now widely accepted by clinicians and researchers that STGD and FFM are not separate diseases but different spectrums of the same disorder.

11.2 Epidemiology and Clinical Findings

Stargardt's disease is the most common form of recessively inherited macular dystrophy. It has been estimated that it affects approximately 1 person in 10,000 [6]. There seems to be no gender or race predilection [3, 21, 25, 32, 48, 51] and there is a wide variation in the age at onset of the disease, which can occur from early childhood to adulthood [1, 21, 25, 32, 38, 51], visual acuity [1, 38, 48], clinical appearance [1, 25, 38], and severity of the disease [1, 38].

Patients with STGD may be asymptomatic or complain, most frequently, of visual acuity loss, photophobia, and, less commonly, nictalopia [25]. Visual acuity usually ranges from 20/20 to 20/400 [23, 25, 48]. In very few patients visual acuity may fall to a counting finger or hand motion level [1, 25, 48]. It seems that the prognosis for patients who are seen initially with vision of 20/40 or better is dependent upon their age at presentation [48]. Thus, it was estimated that patients of 20 years of age or younger presenting with visual acuity of 20/40 or better would reach a visual acuity of 20/200 or worse at a median time of 7 years [48]. In comparison, older patients, aged 21 to 40 or 41 to 60, presenting with a visual acuity of 20/40 or better, would experience a deterioration in vision to 20/200 in a median time of 22 and 29 years respectively [48]. However, once vision has deteriorated to below 20/40, it usually decreases rapidly to 20/200 or worse and this occurs independently of the age of the patient [18, 48].

Early on in the course of the disease fundus examination may be normal, even when the visual acuity is already reduced [51]. Under these circumstances and when the disease affects young children or teenagers the diagnosis of STGD may be missed and patients may be thought to have functional visual loss. In adults, malingering may be suspected [28]. In these patients, pattern electroretinogram (PERG) will be helpful in establishing the diagnosis of STGD-FFM (see Sect. 11.4) since it would demonstrate a very reduced or absent macular function (i.e. very reduced or flat PERG) [36, 38]. Macular abnormalities are seen later on, including pigment mottling, a "bull's eye" appearance, frank macular atrophy, and fundus flecks (Fig. 11.1) [1, 17, 21, 25, 32].

Fundus flecks may be present at the macula only or may extend to the mid-peripheral retina. Characteristically, fundus flecks have a pisciform (fish-like) appearance, but they can also be round, like dots, and appear either as individual lesions or joined together in a confluent pattern [22, 32]. Mild pigmentation can occasionally be seen around them [22, 32]. Although flecks are often present when the first visual symptoms are detected, in some patients flecks may not appear initially, but present at a later date, once other overt macular changes have developed [1, 25, 28]. However, fundus flecks should be seen at one point during the follow-up in order to establish the diagnosis of STGD [21, 51]. Flecks may

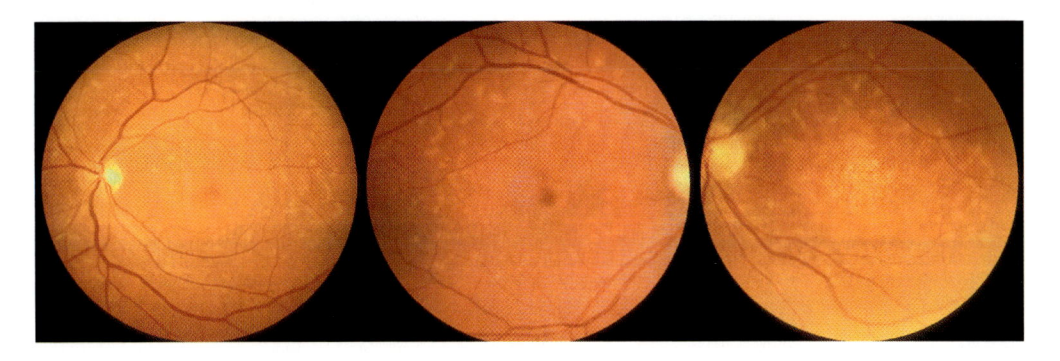

Fig. 11.1 Color fundus photographs of three patients with STGD showing active flecks and a normal appearance of the fovea (*left*), a bull's eye appearance (*center*), and foveal atrophy (*right*)

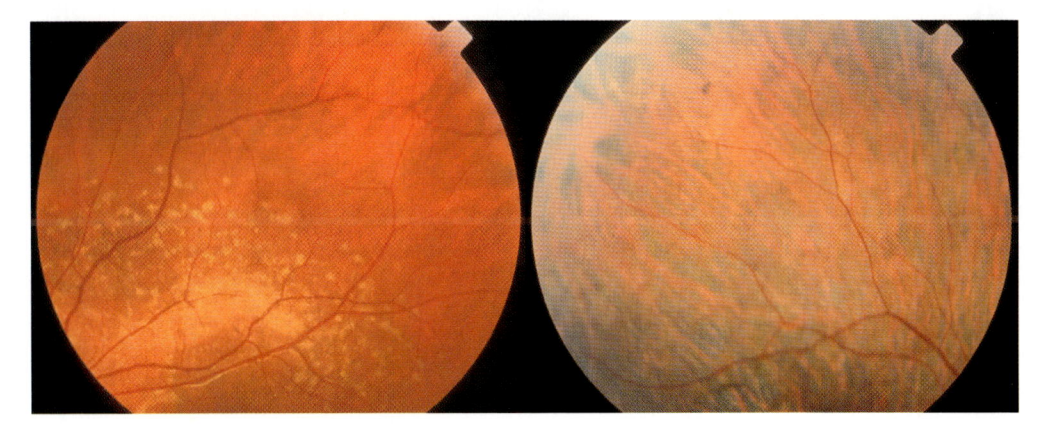

Fig. 11.2 Color fundus photographs of the midperipheral retina obtained from two patients with STGD showing active (*left*) and resorbed (*right*) flecks. Resorbed flecks are less clearly detected and appear as multiple and diffuse areas of depigmentation

be formed by the accumulation of yellow-white material in the RPE, known to be lipofuscin (see Sects. 11.3.3 and 11.5), or represent areas of depigmentation and atrophy of the RPE (Fig. 11.2). The former, usually called "active" flecks, are easily seen by slit-lamp biomicroscopy or indirect ophthalmoscopy. The latter, often termed "resorbed" flecks, are more difficult to visualize and are often missed by the examining ophthalmologist. "Resorbed" flecks occurred at sites previously occupied by "active" flecks and seem to be the result of the damage caused by the increased lipofuscin in the RPE at the site of the fleck [39].

Given that "resorbed" flecks may be present in patients with advanced disease and atrophic macular lesions, but no "active" flecks, the diagnosis of STGD may represent a challenge under these circumstances. Fundus autofluorescence (AF; see Sect. 11.3.3) has been shown to be very helpful in establishing the diagnosis of STGD in these cases, since resolved flecks are easily visualized on AF images as foci of decreased AF signal [39].

Different clinical classifications of STGD have been proposed based on the presence or absence and distribution of the fundus lesions, including

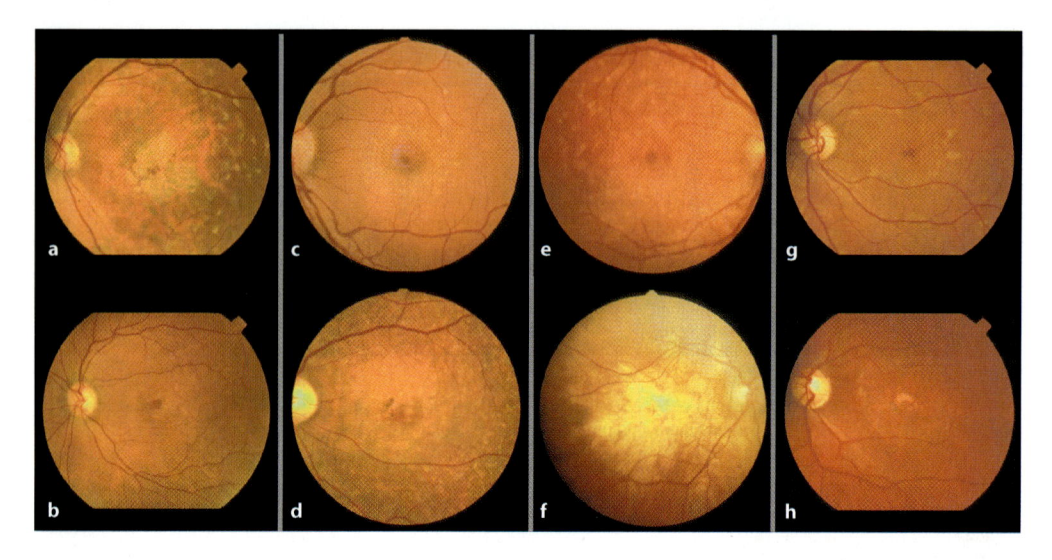

Fig. 11.3a–h Color fundus photographs of four sibling pairs (**a + b**, **c + d**, **e + f**, and **g + h**) showing intrafamilial variation in fundus features. However, siblings shared the same qualitative electrophysiological functional abnormalities

atrophy and "active" and "resorbed" flecks [1, 17, 32]. However, none of these classifications have been widely accepted. This is possibly related to the fact that the distribution of the fundus lesions may change over time [1, 3], do not correlate well with the functional loss observed in these patients [1, 25, 38], and that there seems to be no good intrafamilial concordance of these clinical attributes (Fig. 11.3) [1, 36].

It has been noted that in STGD there is a typical peripapillary sparing characterized by a lack of flecks and atrophy in this region, even in those cases with diffuse RPE abnormalities and atrophy (Fig. 11.4, top left) [11, 31, 39, 63]. This finding may also be helpful when establishing the diagnosis of STGD in patients with advanced disease in whom fundus flecks are no longer visible [39].

Rarely, patients with STGD may develop small or large areas of subretinal fibrosis (Fig. 11.4, top right) [11, 12, 38, 44]. In some of these cases, a previous history of trauma can be elucidated [12, 38]. The occurrence of choroidal neovascularization in STGD has also been reported (Fig. 11.4, bottom) [3, 31–33].

Summary for the Clinician

- Stargardt's disease can affect individuals of any gender and race and there is wide variability in age at onset, visual acuity, fundus appearance, and severity of the disease.
- Visual acuity may vary between 20/20 and 20/400. In only few patients will visual acuity drop below 20/400.
- Fundus examination can be normal in patients with STGD early on in the course of the disease. This should be taken into account when functional visual loss or malingering is being considered in a patient with reduced vision and normal fundus. PERG may be useful in the diagnosis of these cases since it will demonstrate very reduced macular function.
- Fundus examination may disclose RPE mottling, a bull's eye appearance, active or resorbed flecks or atrophy at the macula. Atrophy and flecks can also be observed in the midperipheral retina. Flecks should be seen at some point during the follow-up of the patient to confirm the diagnosis of STGD.

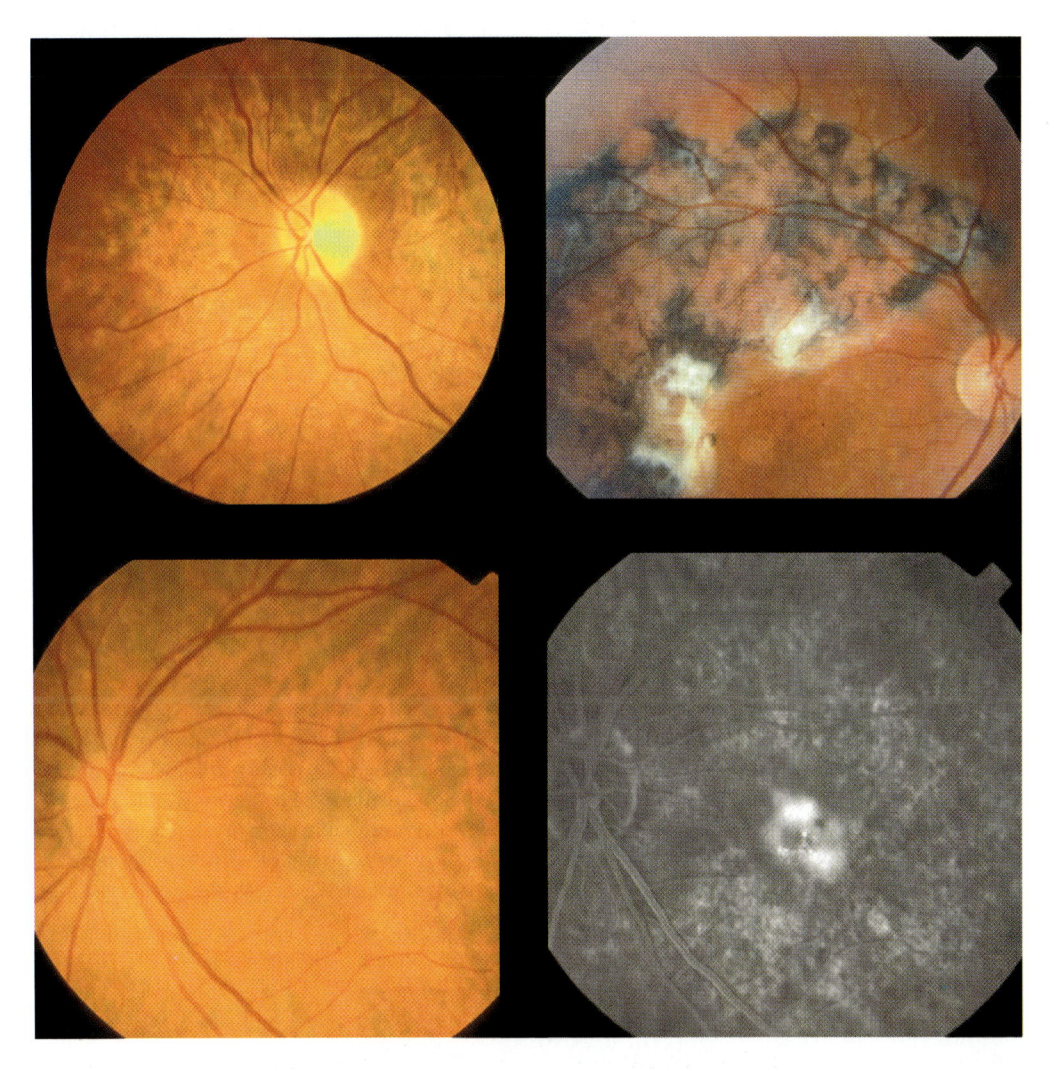

Fig. 11.4 Color fundus photographs (*top left and right, bottom left*) and fluorescein angiogram (*bottom right*) obtained from three patients with Stargardt's disease (STGD). Peripapillary sparing is observed in a patient with severe disease and confluent resorbed flecks in the midperipheral retina (*top left*). Marked subretinal fibrosis and retinal pigment epithelium (RPE) hyperplasia is shown in a large area of the retina in a young patient with STGD (*top right*). A history of contusive trauma was elucidated. Choroidal neovascularization was detected in a patient with STGD on slit-lamp biomicroscopy (*bottom left*) and fluorescein angiography (*bottom right*)

11.3 Imaging Studies

11.3.1 Fluorescein Angiography

Patients with STGD may have what has been referred to as the sign of "choroidal silence," or "dark choroid" (Fig. 11.5) [7]. FFA in these patients will reveal a lack of early hyperfluorescence coming from the choroid, so that the retinal blood vessels, even the small capillaries, are easily seen over a very dark background where no choroidal fluorescence is apparent. This sign is often best appreciated in the peripapillary region. However, not all patients with STGD will demonstrate "choroidal silence." In fact, in a recent study of a large cohort of patients with this disease, only 62% of patients had this FFA sign [48]. Similarly, "choroidal silence" is not exclusively seen in patients with STGD and it has also been observed in patients with cone dystrophy [57].

"Active" flecks appear hypofluorescent in the early and late frames of the FFA [25]. "Resorbed" flecks may appear hypo- [25] or hyperfluorescent [1]. Areas of frank macular atrophy are seen as areas where no choriocapillaris is present, but where only large choroidal vessels are seen.

11.3.2 Indocyanine Green Angiography

With ICG it is possible to see the choroidal details even in those patients with "dark choroid" on FFA [63]. This suggests that the "choroidal silence" or "dark choroid" on FFA relates to an obscuration of the view of the choroidal circulation by the accumulation of material beneath the retina, rather than being related to a lack of perfusion through the choroid. Choroidal vascular closure, however, can be detected in patients with STGD and atrophic macular lesions. Fundus flecks appear hypofluorescent on ICG, and are usually best detected on late frames of the angiogram [63].

Although FFA and ICG are safe, they are nonetheless invasive imaging techniques. Given that the information gathered by FFA and ICG is usually not required for diagnostic or prognostic purposes. These tests should be reserved for selected cases of STGD.

11.3.3 Fundus Autofluorescence

Fundus autofluorescence (AF) is a relatively new imaging technique that allows the evaluation of the RPE in vivo and, indirectly, of the photoreceptors. It has been shown that the AF signal is predominantly derived from lipofuscin in the RPE [13]. Lipofuscin is formed and accumulates in the RPE as a result of the incomplete digestion of photoreceptor outer segment discs by these cells. On fundus AF images areas of increased RPE lipofuscin will appear as areas of increased AF signal. In contrast, areas of decreased RPE lipofuscin (for instance, at sites of damaged or lost RPE) will appear as areas of decreased AF signal.

Using a confocal scanning laser ophthalmoscope (cSLO), high-quality fundus AF images can be obtained [59]. Furthermore, it is also possible to reproducibly measure levels of AF [35] and study the topographic distribution of quantitative values of AF across the entire macular region [37].

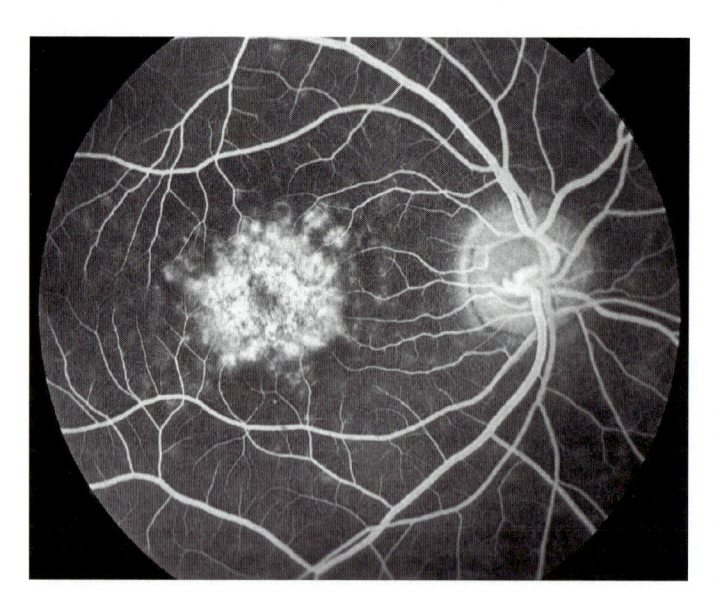

Fig. 11.5 Fluorescein angiogram from a patient with STGD demonstrating the sign of "choroidal silence" or "dark choroid." In the full venous phase of the angiogram retinal capillaries can be visualized over a very dark background where no choroidal fluorescence is apparent. Hyperfluorescence at the centre of the macula, corresponding to a relatively atrophic central macular lesion, is also observed

In patients with STGD areas of retinal atrophy detected clinically at the macula or in the midperipheral retina appear as areas of low AF signal on AF images[39]. Areas of atrophy not detected clinically are easily visualized using AF imaging [38]. "Active" flecks appear as foci of high AF signal, whereas "resorbed" flecks have a low signal on AF imaging (Fig. 11.6). Although "resorbed" flecks are usually difficult to see on slit-lamp biomicroscopy and indirect ophthalmoscopy, they are easily identified on fundus AF. This imaging technique can be very useful in the diagnosis of patients with STGD and advanced disease, where "active" fundus flecks are no longer visible.

Quantitative evaluation of levels of AF in patients with STGD has demonstrated high levels of AF in the majority of them [13, 39, 60], independently of whether or not "choroidal silence" was present on FFA [60]. Recent data evaluating levels of AF across the entire macula have shown that some patients with STGD may have low or even normal levels of AF compared with age-matched normal volunteers [39]. In patients with advanced or severe disease low levels of AF were detected, indicating that the RPE in these cases is severely affected [39]. In patients with normal levels of AF, an abnormal distribution of AF and an abnormal macular function, as determined by PERG, were found [39]. This may suggest that the threshold for RPE damage caused by lipofuscin may vary among patients and that, in some cases, RPE damage could occur with relatively "normal" levels of lipofuscin within the cell. Alternatively, normal levels of AF could be the result of the loss

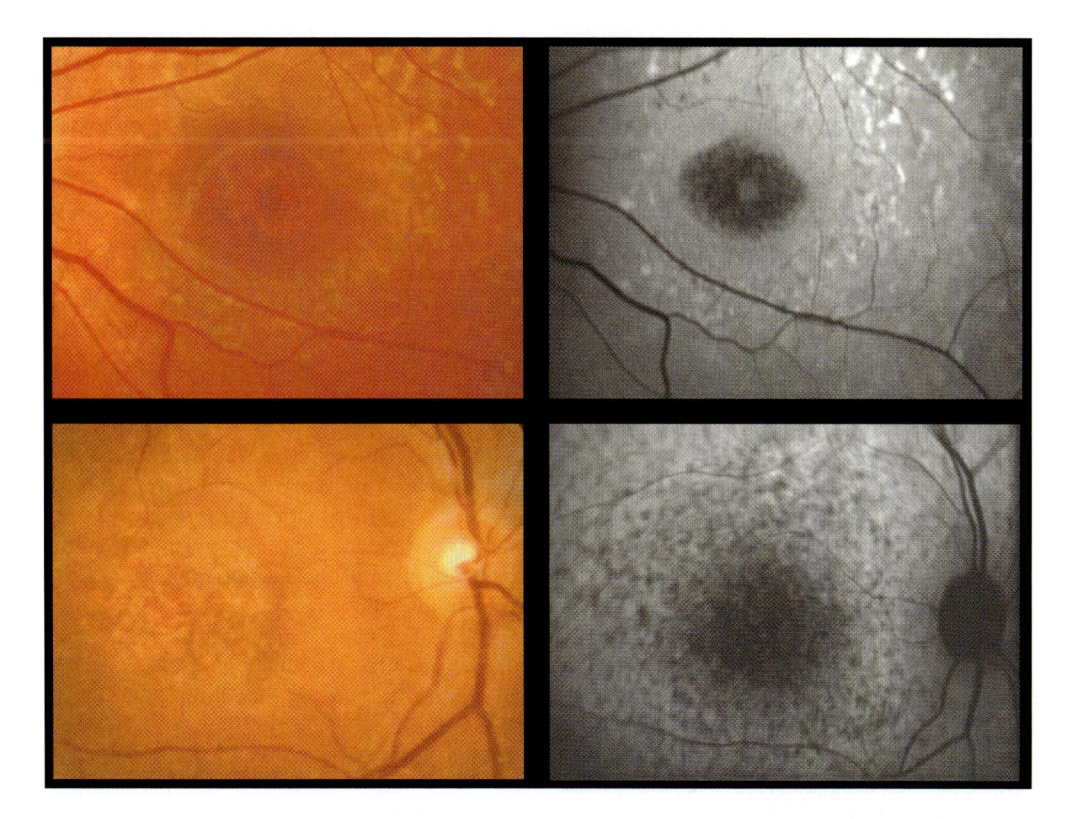

Fig. 11.6 Color fundus photographs (*left, top and bottom*) and fundus autofluorescence (AF) images (*right, top and bottom*) obtained from two patients with STGD showing active (*top*) and resorbed (*bottom*) flecks. Active flecks (*top left*) appear, on slit-lamp examination, as white-yellowish lesions formed by accumulation of material in the outer retina. On AF images (*top right*) active flecks are seen as foci of high AF signal. Resorbed flecks (*bottom left*), difficult to detect on slit-lamp biomicroscopy and appearing as small areas of depigmentation in the RPE, are easily visualized on AF images as multiple foci of low AF signal (*bottom right*)

of photoreceptors or RPE cells without noticeable atrophy. Moreover, it would be possible that these patients with normal AF levels might represent a different phenotype within STGD [41].

11.3.4 Optical Coherence Tomography

Optical coherence tomography (OCT), including ultrahigh-resolution OCT (UHR-OCT) has been very recently used to evaluate patients with STGD [16, 45]. The value of this imaging technique in facilitating the diagnosis or establishing the prognosis of patients with this condition, to date, remains to be elucidated.

> **Summary for the Clinician**
>
> - Fluorescein angiography and ICG are invasive imaging techniques that are not usually required for the diagnosis or evaluation of patients with STGD.
> - The typical sign of "choroidal silence" or "dark choroid" on FFA is not present in all patients with STGD and is not specific to this condition.
> - Fundus AF allows the evaluation of the RPE and, indirectly, of the photoreceptors, in patients with STGD and is a very useful noninvasive imaging technique to assess patients with this retinal dystrophy.
> - Fundus AF is very helpful in the diagnosis of patients with advanced disease, in whom "active" fundus flecks are no longer present.

11.4 Electrophysiology and Psychophysics

Patients with STGD may have different degrees of functional loss, as detected by PERG, full-field electroretinogram (ERG), and electro-oculogram (EOG) [1, 10, 17, 22, 25, 32, 36, 39, 52]. Marked functional abnormalities at the macula, with severely reduced or abolished PERG, are characteristic of STGD [38], even when the visual acuity is still good (20/40 or better). Scotopic and photopic full-field ERG responses may be normal or subnormal. Similarly, the EOG may be normal or subnormal, even in the presence of a normal full-field ERG [25, 38].

Patients with STGD may have one of three patterns of functional loss including macular dysfunction alone (abnormal PERG with normal full-field ERG), macular and peripheral cone dysfunction (abnormal PERG and photopic responses) or macular and peripheral cone and rod dysfunction (abnormal PERG and scotopic and photopic responses; Fig. 11.7) [38]. It appears that, in most families with this macular dystrophy, there is intrafamilial homogeneity in the qualitative pattern of functional loss present, with families having functional loss restricted to the macula and others experiencing, in addition, loss of peripheral cone or cone and rod function [1, 36]. This suggests that electrophysiological tests may have a prognostic value, i.e., patients with early peripheral cone and rod dysfunction would have higher chance of developing peripheral visual loss and, thus, a more severe form of the disease. Given that there seems to be no reliable way of predicting which type of functional visual loss would be found in patients with STGD based on the fundus appearance alone [17, 25, 38], electrodiagnostic tests are essential in the evaluation of patients with this retinal disorder. The only exception to this would be the finding of extensive chorioretinal atrophy throughout the fundus, as observed either on fundus examination [17] or AF imaging [39], which only seems to be present in patients with peripheral rod and cone dysfunction [17, 39].

In STGD there is a prolonged period of dark adaptation after illumination that bleaches a substantial fraction of rhodopsin [32], which affects, specifically, the later portion of the rod dark-adaptation curve [20, 29]. However, it has been recently shown that these patients may have similar responses to those observed in normal participants after exposure to weak bleaching illumination [29]. Abnormal recovery of macular cone photoreceptors after bleaching has also been detected in patients with STGD, even in

11.4 Electrophysiology and Psychophysics

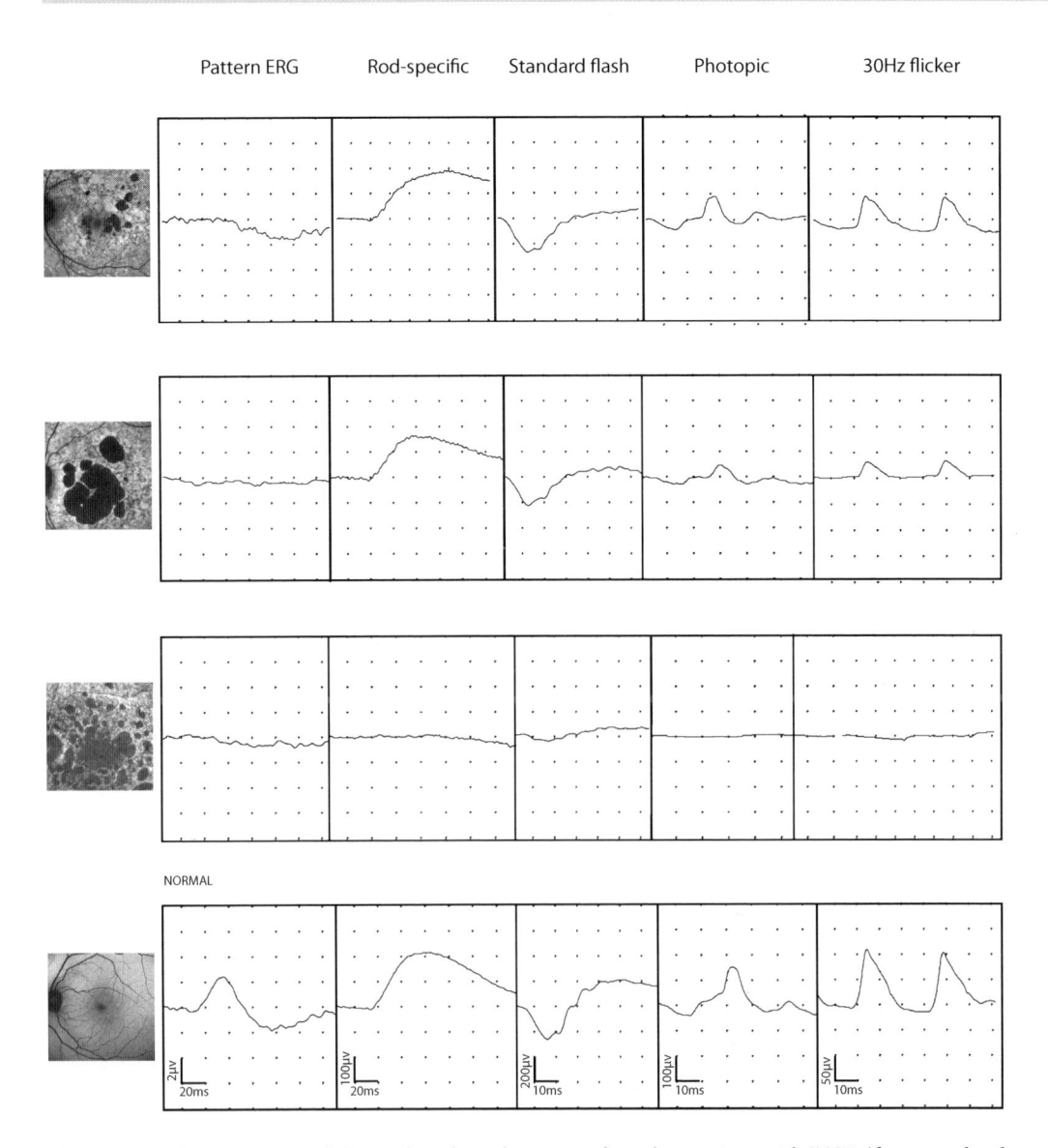

Fig. 11.7 Fundus AF images and electrophysiological responses from three patients with STGD (*first, second and third row*) and from an age-matched normal volunteer (*bottom*), from comparison purposes. Small areas of focal increased and decreased AF signal were seen in all patients at the macula and extending into the midperipheral retina. Well-defined larger areas of low AF signal were also detected at the macula in all patients. Despite the relatively similar pattern of distribution of AF changes, electrophysiology responses differed among patients and demonstrated macular dysfunction alone (abolished pattern electroretinogram [PERG]) with normal peripheral rod and cone responses (normal rod-specific, standard flash, photopic, and 30-Hz flicker responses; *first row*), macular (abolished PERG) and peripheral cone dysfunction (reduced photopic and 30-Hz flicker responses; *second row*) and severe macular and peripheral cone and rod dysfunction (flat electroretinogram for all stimuli; *third row*)

those cases of relatively preserved central visual field and visual acuity [43]. This abnormal recovery of macular cone photoreceptors could be the result of a reduced foveal cone pigment density and delayed pigment regeneration [58].

Color vision deficits are common in STGD, although in a few patients color vision can be normal [3, 38]. Elevation in the tritan axis is most frequently observed [1, 38]. However, when increased thresholds for all axes (protan, deutan and tritan) are present, there is usually a more severe elevation of protan and deutan axis [36, 38].

Visual field testing may be normal or show relative or absolute central or paracentral scotomas [3, 17, 19, 25, 32]. In severe cases of widespread retinal atrophy peripheral visual field constriction can occur [1, 3, 17, 19].

Summary for the Clinician

- There are different degrees of severity in STGD. Although the majority of patients have a disease restricted to the macula, some patients may have additional loss of peripheral cone or cone and rod function. The latter cases have the worst prognosis.
- Electrophysiology studies, including PERG and full-field ERG, are very helpful in the evaluation of patients with STGD, since they allow the recognition of patients with different degrees of severity (macular dysfunction alone, macular and peripheral cone dysfunction, and macular and peripheral cone and rod dysfunction). Electrophysiology is of particular importance since in STGD the functional loss cannot be predicted based on the fundus appearance.
- Patients with STGD have delayed dark adaptation, which specifically affects the later portion of the rod dark-adaptation curve.
- Color vision deficits and central and paracentral scotomas are commonly found in patients with STGD. Peripheral visual field defects can also be detected in patients with the severe form of the disease.

11.5 Histopathology

Histopathological evaluation of eyes from patients with STGD has shown RPE cells engorged and densely packed with a substance with ultrastructural, autofluorescent and histochemical characteristics consistent with lipofuscin [5, 14]. This appears to be the major and typical abnormality of the disease. One histopathology study, however, failed to detect increased lipofuscin in the RPE in a case of STGD without maculopathy [41]. Histopathology findings, thus, support those from in vivo autofluorescence studies (see Sect. 11.3.3).

Subretinal desquamated RPE cells, some of which had undergone cell lysis with spillage of their contents into the subretinal space, macrophages engorged with melanolipofuscin in the outer retina, RPE and choriocapillaris atrophy at the fovea, and photoreceptor cell loss at the fovea have also been observed [5, 14].

11.6 Differential Diagnosis

The differential diagnosis of STGD should include autosomal dominant Stargardt-like macular dystrophy, Best's disease, pattern dystrophies, cone dystrophy, central areolar choroidal dystrophy, retinitis pigmentosa, age-related macular degeneration, and maculopathy associated with 15257 mitochondrial DNA mutation.

11.7 Genetics and Molecular Biology

Stargardt's disease is inherited as an autosomal recessive trait and occurs as a result of mutations in a gene that was initially mapped to the short arm of chromosome 1 (1p) [30] and subsequently identified as the *ABCA4* gene [2]. The *ABCA4* gene belongs to the ABC (ATP Binding Cassette) superfamily of genes. The proteins codified by ABC genes are transmembrane proteins responsible for the transport of a wide variety of substances across membranes. It was initially thought that the protein codified by the *ABCA4* gene (in this chapter referred to as ABCR, or ATP Binding Cassette transporter of the Retina) was only expressed in rod photoreceptor cells [2] and localized to the rim region of the disc membrane of rod outer segments [27, 53]. However, it was later clearly established that ABCR was present in both rod and cone photoreceptor cells (Fig. 11.8) [42].

The *ABCA4* is a large gene composed of 50 exons. It is extremely polymorphic, making it difficult to elucidate which variations in this gene should be considered disease-causing mutations [61]. In this respect, disease-causing variations in the *ABCA4* gene had been found in only a relatively small proportion of alleles searched (31–60%) [8, 19, 34, 61]. Furthermore, disease-causing variations are uncommonly found in the two *ABCA4* alleles of each patient investigated [19, 34]. Most sequence changes thought to be pathogenic in STGD patients are missense mutations [2, 8, 34].

Despite the current technical difficulties in detecting disease-causing *ABCA4* variations, phenotype–genotype correlations have been attempted [19]. Thus, the Gly1961Glu change in exon 42 seemed to be associated with a milder form of the disease characterized by the presence of small atrophic macular lesions surrounded by a ring of flecks, most commonly with normal full-field cone and rod responses and absence of a choroidal silence [19]. It has also been shown that missense amino acid substitutions located in the *ABCA4* gene region encoding the amino-terminal one-third of the protein are associated with an earlier age of onset of the disease [34]. Similarly, patients homozygous or compound heterozygous for variations considered to be null mutations in the *ABCA4* gene develop a very severe form of the disease with macular and peripheral cone and rod dysfunction [24].

Laboratory evidence suggests that the function of the ABCR protein is the transport of retinoids in photoreceptor outer segments [55], preferentially N-retinylidene-phosphatidylethanolamine (N-retinylidene-PE) and all-trans-retinal [4, 55].

In normal circumstances, following photoactivation of rhodopsin it is presumed that all-trans-retinal is released into the hydrophobic environment of the disc membrane of the photoreceptor outer segments (Fig. 11.9, top). All-trans-retinal can then react with phosphatidylethanolamine (PE) and form N-retinylidene-PE, and free all-trans-retinal and

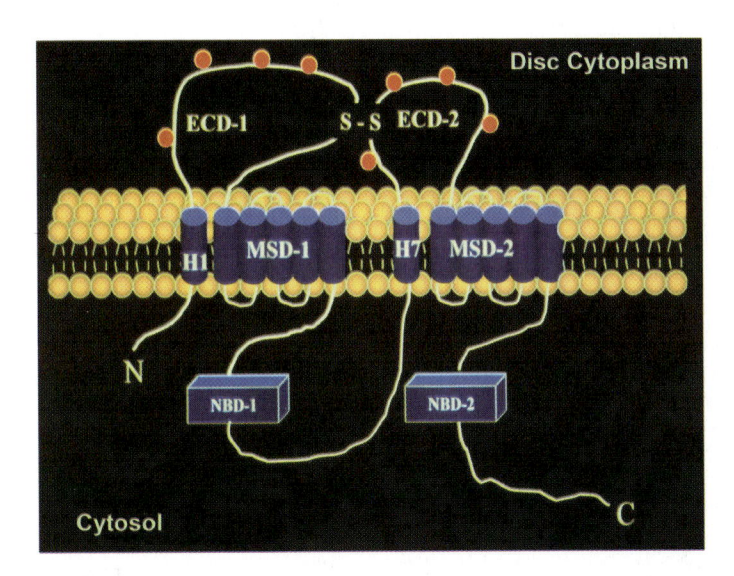

Fig. 11.8 Cartoon representing the structure of the ABCR protein. ABCR is organized into two tandemly arranged halves, each containing a membrane-spanning domain (MSD) followed by a nucleotide-binding domain (NBD). The N-terminal half contains a transmembrane segment designated as H1 and a large exocytoplasmic domain (ECD-1) preceding the MSD-1, which consists of five transmembrane segments. The C-terminal half has a similar arrangement, with a transmembrane segment designated as H7 and a large exocytoplasmic domain (ECD-2) preceding the MSD-2, which is also formed by five transmembrane segments. ABCR has eight glycosylation sites (*red circles*), four in each ECD, and disulfide linkage between ECD-1 and ECD-2 (S-S) [9]

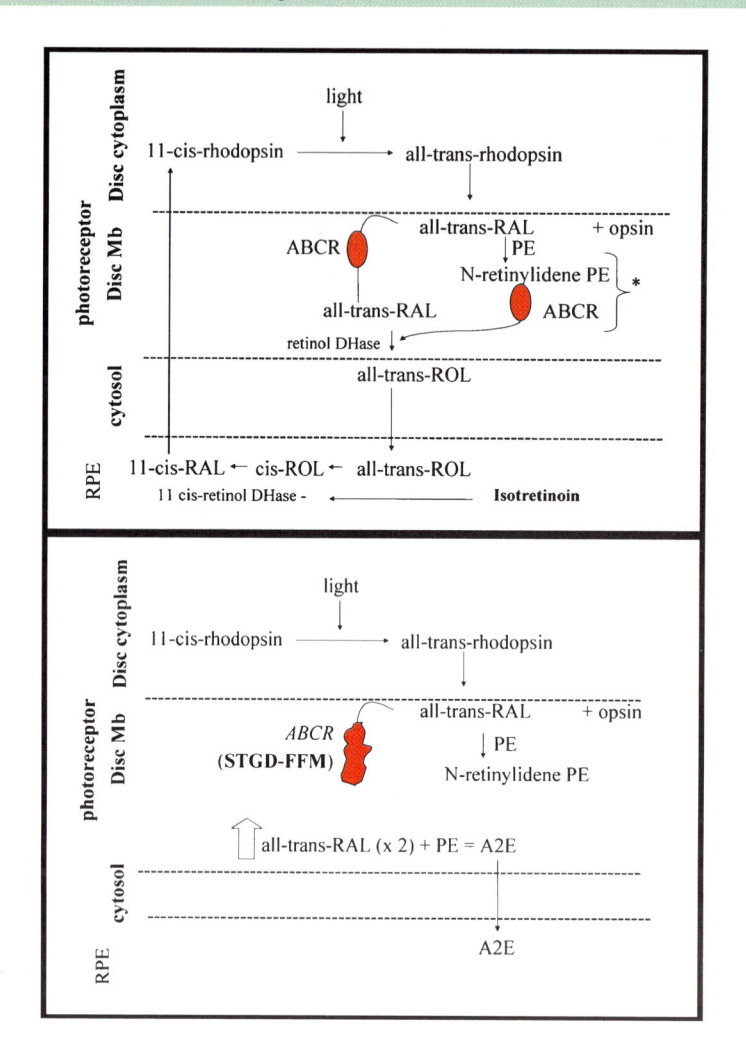

Fig. 11.9 *Top*: All-trans-retinal (*all-trans-RAL*), released following photoactivation of rhodopsin, can react with phosphatidylethanolamine (*PE*) and form N-retinylidene-PE. Free all-trans-RAL and all-trans-RAL contained in N-retinylidene-PE is then reduced to all-trans-retinol (*all-trans-ROL*) by the all-trans-retinol dehydrogenase (*retinol DHase*), localized to the cytosolic side of the disc membrane (*Mb*) of the photoreceptor outer segment. Evidence suggests that ABCR transports N-retinylidene-PE and all-trans-RAL from the cytoplasmic side of the disc membrane to the cytosolic side of the disc membrane, where they could be reduced to all trans-ROL by the retinol DHase. The *asterisk* denotes the preferred substrate for ABCR. *Bottom*: In patients with Stargardt's disease there is impaired transport of all-trans-RAL and N-retinylidene-PE with a subsequent accumulation of both molecules in the photoreceptor outer segment disc membrane. Condensation of all-trans-RAL and PE would then give rise to N-retinylidene-N-retinyl-ethanolamine (*A2E*) formation. A2E, the major component of lipofuscin, would then accumulate in the RPE cells following photoreceptor outer segment disc shedding.

all-trans-retinal contained in N-retinylidene-PE are then reduced to all-trans-retinol by the all-trans-retinol dehydrogenase. Since the latter enzyme is localized to the cytosolic side of the disc membrane of the photoreceptor's outer segment, it is required that N-retinylidene-PE and all-trans-retinal cross the disc membrane from the cytoplasmic to the cytosolic side of the disc. All-trans-retinol is transported to the RPE to be transformed into 11-cis-retinal, which will then return to the outer segment of the photoreceptor to re-enter the visual cycle.

It appears that ABCR may act as a "flippase," flipping N-retinylidene-PE and all-trans-retinal from the cytoplasmic side of the disc membrane to the cytosolic side, where all-trans-retinol dehydrogenase resides [55, 62]. Thus, the effect of ABCR would be to efficiently deliver all-trans-retinal to all-trans-retinol dehydrogenase, facilitating its conversion into all-trans-retinol and, thus, assisting with the rapid recovery of the photoreceptor cell following light exposure, reducing photoreceptor cell noise (the latter seems to be the result of an increase in all-trans-retinal and opsin, which, combined, can activate the visual transduction cascade) and reducing the accumulation of all-trans-retinal and N-retinylidene-PE within the disc membranes [55]. The latter, would, in its turn, give rise to increased production of N-retinylidene-N-retinyl-ethanolamine (A2E), the major fluorophore of lipofuscin, in the RPE. A2E has potentially cytotoxic effects on RPE cells, including inhibiting lysosomal enzymes [15, 26], causing blue light-mediated RPE cell damage [49] and releasing pro-apoptotic proteins from mitochondria in the RPE [56]. RPE cell damage and loss would possibly then be followed by photoreceptor cell degeneration and visual loss.

Based on the above postulated mechanism of action of ABCR [55, 62], patients with STGD would be expected to have increased levels of all-trans-retinal following light exposure (Fig. 11.9, bottom). Increased all-trans-retinal would facilitate the formation of noncovalent complexes between all-trans-retinal and opsin that are able to stimulate the phototransduction cascade and lead to a prolonged period of dark adaptation following light exposure. Furthermore, increased all-trans-retinal levels would facilitate the association of two molecules of all-trans-retinal with PE with the subsequent increased formation of A2E. A2E, the major component of lipofuscin, would then accumulate in the RPE cells following photoreceptor outer segment disc shedding (Fig. 11.9, right). Since both prolonged dark adaptation and increased levels of lipofuscin in the RPE have been detected in patients with STGD, it appears that the above proposed hypothesis of the mechanism of action of ABCR is likely to be correct.

Summary for the Clinician

- Mutations in the *ABCA4* gene are responsible for STGD.
- The product of *ABCA4* is ABCR. It appears that the function of ABCR is the transport of retinoids, specifically N-retinylidene-PE and all-trans-retinal, in photoreceptor outer segment disc membranes. Thus, ABCR acts to reduce the accumulation of N-retinylidene-PE and all-trans-retinal in outer segment disc membranes, which, in its turn, would cause increased A2E formation in the RPE.
- Accumulation of A2E in the RPE seems to be one of the major events leading to RPE cell damage and loss in STGD. Loss of RPE cells may be followed by degeneration and loss of photoreceptor cells and vision.

11.8 Animal Models of STGD-FFM

It has been shown that mice generated with null mutations in the *ABCA4* gene (abcr$^{-/-}$) develop a phenotype closely resembling that observed in patients with STGD [62]. Specifically, delayed rod dark adaptation, increased levels of all-trans-retinal, PE, and protonated N-retinylidene-PE and reduced levels of all-trans-retinol in photoreceptors following a photobleach, and accumulation of A2E in the RPE have been detected in this knockout rodent model [62]. These findings further support the hypothesized flippase function of ABCR in photoreceptor outer segments outlined above.

11.9 Current and Future Treatments

There is currently no treatment available for patients with STGD. However, several lines of evidence seem to support the recommendation that patients with STGD should protect their eyes from light exposure by using dark sunglasses or contact lenses. Thus, it has been shown that

ABCR is unusually sensitive to the photo-oxidative damage mediated by all-trans-retinal [54]. Irradiation of ABCR in the presence of all-trans-retinal and oxygen in vitro led to its functional inactivation [54]. Given that patients with STGD have an already impaired ABCR function and have increased levels of all-trans-retinal in their photoreceptors, it would be expected that these patients would be extremely susceptible to the effect of light exposure. Furthermore, accumulation of A2E in the RPE in abcr$^{-/-}$ mice has been demonstrated to be strongly light dependent, being almost completely suppressed in abcr$^{-/-}$ mice raised in total darkness [40]. Moreover, light exposure stimulates the formation of A2E oxiranes in abcr$^{-/-}$ mice [47], which have been shown to induce DNA fragmentation in cultured RPE cells and represent an important mechanism of A2E cytotoxicity [50].

A randomized, double-masked, controlled, crossover study, sponsored by the National Eye Institute in the USA, has been organized to evaluate the possible beneficial effect of docosahexaenoic acid (DHA) in patients with Stargardt-like macular dystrophy and patients with STGD. The rationale for this trial is as follows. Mutations in *ELOVL4* (ELOngation of Very Long chain fatty acid 4) have been found in patients with Stargardt-like macular dystrophy, which unlike STGD, is inherited as an autosomal dominant trait. The protein codified by *ELOVL4* plays a role in the synthesis of very long chain polyunsaturated fatty acids of the retina, of which DHA is the major one. The benefit of DHA in STGD, however, is questionable, given that mutations in *ABCA4* and not in *ELOVL4* are responsible for all cases of STGD, as stated above (Sect. 11.7).

It is likely that the increasing knowledge in the structure and mechanism of action of ABCR and the development of an animal model of the disease (abcr$^{-/-}$ mice) may lead to the discovery of possible treatment strategies for patients with STGD. One of these strategies could be to inhibit the formation of A2E (and lipofuscin) in the RPE, reducing subsequent RPE cell damage and RPE and secondary photoreceptor cell loss. This has already been attempted in the rodent model of STGD (abcr$^{-/-}$ mice) by using isotretinoin. Isotretinoin (13-cis-retinoic acid, or Accutane), a drug commonly used to treat patients with acne, has an inhibitory effect on 11-cis-retinol dehydrogenase in RPE cells (Fig. 11.9, bottom). This enzyme converts 11-cis-retinol into 11-cis-retinal, which is then used in the regeneration of rhodopsin in photoreceptors. Inhibition of 11-cis-retinol dehydrogenase would be expected to inhibit the regeneration of rhodopsin and would potentially reduce the formation of all-trans-retinal and N-retinylidene-PE in the disc membranes of photoreceptor outer segments and the formation of A2E in RPE cells. In abcr$^{-/-}$ mice isotretinoin suppressed the accumulation of A2E in the RPE biochemically and inhibited the accumulation of lipofuscin granules in the RPE as detected by electron microscopy [46]. The dose of isotretinoin used to achieve this effect, however, was much higher (20–40 mg/kg/day) than the dose used in humans to treat acne (0.5–2.0 mg/kg/day). Isotretinoin has also been shown to reduce the production of A2E oxiranes in abcr$^{-/-}$ mice [47].

Summary for the Clinician

- There is no treatment for patients with STGD.
- Based on current laboratory evidence, the recommendation to patients with STGD should be to reduce light exposure as much as possible. This could be achieved by using dark sunglasses or contact lenses.

References

1. Aaberg TM (1986) Stargardt's disease and fundus flavimaculatus: evaluation of morphologic progression and intrafamilial co-existence. Trans Am Ophthalmol Soc 84:453–487
2. Allikmets R et al (1997) A photoreceptor cell-specific ATP-binding transporter gene (ABCR) is mutated in recessive Stargardt macular dystrophy. Nat Genet 15:236–246
3. Armstrong JD et al (1998) Ophthalmology 105:448–458

4. Beharry S, Zhong M, Molday RS (2004) N-Retinylidene-phosphatidylethanolamine is the preferred retinoid substrate for the photoreceptor-specific ABC transporter ABCA4 (ABCR). J Biol Chem 52:53972–53979
5. Birnbach CD et al (1994) Histopathology and immunocytochemistry of the neurosensory retina in fundus flavimaculatus. Ophthalmology 101:1211–1219
6. Blacharski PA (1988) Fundus flavimaculatus. In: Newsome DA (ed) Retinal dystrophies and degenerations. Raven, New York, pp 135–159
7. Bonnin P (1971) Le signe du silence choroidien dans les degenerescences tapeto-retiniennes centrales examinees sous fluoresceine. Bull Soc Ophthalmol Fr 71:1423–1427
8. Briggs CE et al (2001) Mutations in ABCR (ABCA4) in patients with Stargardt macular degeneration or cone-rod degeneration. Invest Ophthalmol Vis Sci 42:2229–2236
9. Bungert S, Molday LL, Molday RS (2001) Membrane topology of the ATP binding cassette transporter ABCR and its relationship to ABC1 and related ABCA transporters: identification of N-linked glycosylation sites. J Biol Chem 276:23539–23546
10. Carr RE (1965) Fundus flavimaculatus. Arch Ophthalmol 74:163–168
11. De Laey JJ, Verougstraete C (1995) Hyperlipofuscinosis and subretinal fibrosis in Stargardt's disease. Retina 15:399–406
12. Del Buey ME et al (1993) Posttraumatic reaction in a case of fundus flavimaculatus with atrophic macular degeneration. Ann Ophthalmol 25:219–221
13. Delori FC et al (1995) In vivo measurement of lipofuscin in Stargardt's disease-Fundus flavimaculatus. Invest Ophthalmol Vis Sci 36:2327–2331
14. Eagle RCJ et al (1980) Retinal pigment epithelial abnormalities in fundus flavimaculatus: a light and electron microscopic study. Ophthalmology 87:1189–1200
15. Eldred GE, Lasky MR (1998) Retinal age pigments generated by self-assembling lysosomotropic detergents. Nature 361:724–726
16. Ergun E et al (2005) Assessment of central visual function in Stargardt's disease/fundus flavimaculatus with ultrahigh-resolution optical coherence tomography. Invest Ophthalmol Vis Sci, 46:310–316
17. Fishman GA (1976) Fundus flavimaculatus. Arch Ophthalmol 94:2061–2067
18. Fishman GA et al (1987) Visual acuity loss in patients with Stargardt's macular dystrophy. Ophthalmology 94:809–814
19. Fishman GA et al (1999) Variation of clinical expression in patients with Stargardt dystrophy and sequence variations in the ABCR gene. Arch Ophthalmol 117:504–510
20. Fishman GA, Farbman JS, Alexander KR (1991) Delayed rod dark adaptation in patients with Stargardt's disease. Ophthalmology 98:957–962
21. Franceschetti A. (1963) Über tapeto-retinale Degenerationen im Kindesalter (Kongenitale Form (Leber), amaurotische Idiotie, rezessivegeschlechtsgebundene tapeto-retinale Degenerationen, Fundus albipunctatus cum Hemeralopia, Fundus flavimaculatus). Dritter Fortbildungskurs der Deutschen Ophthalmologischen Gesellschaft, Hamburg 1962, herausgegeben von Prof. Dr. H. Sautter., in Entwicklung und Fortschritt in der Augenheilkunde. Funke, Stuttgart, pp 107–120
22. Franceschetti A (1965) A special form of tapetoretinal degeneration: fundus flavimaculatus. Trans Am Acad Ophthalmol Otolaryngol 69:1048–1053
23. Franceschetti A, Francois J (1965) Fundus flavimaculatus. Arch Ophthalmol 25:505–530
24. Fukui T et al (2002) ABCA4 gene mutations in Japanese patients with Stargardt's disease and retinitis pigmentosa. Invest Ophthalmol Vis Sci 43:2819–2824
25. Hadden OB, Gass JDM (1976) Fundus flavimaculatus and Stargardt's disease. Am J Ophthalmol 82:527–539
26. Holz FG et al (1999) Inhibition of lysosomal degradative functions in RPE cells by a retinoid component of lipofuscin. Invest Ophthalmol Vis Sci 40:737–743
27. Illing M, Molday LL, Molday RS (1997) The 220-kDa rim protein of retinal rod outer segments is a member of the ABC transporter superfamily. J Biol Chem 272:10303–10310
28. Irvine AR, Wergeland FLJ (1972) Stargardt's hereditary progressive macular degeneration. Br J Ophthalmol 56:817–826
29. Kang Derwent JJ et al (2004) Dark adaptation of rod photoreceptors in normal subjects, and in patients with Stargardt's disease and an ABCA4 mutation. Invest Ophthalmol Vis Sci 45:2447–2456

30. Kaplan J et al (1993) A gene for Stargardt's disease (fundus flavimaculatus) maps to the short arm of chromosome 1. Nat Genet 5:308–311
31. Klein R et al (1978) Subretinal neovascularization associated with fundus flavimaculatus. Arch Ophthalmol 96:2054–2057
32. Klien BA, Krill AE (1967) Fundus flavimaculatus. Clinical, functional, and histopathologic observations. Am J Ophthalmol 64:3–23
33. Leveille AS, Morse PH, Burch JV (1982) Fundus flavimaculatus and subretinal neovascularization. Ann Ophthalmol 14:331–334
34. Lewis RA et al (1999) Genotype/phenotype analysis of a photoreceptor-specific ATP-binding cassette transporter gene, ABCR, in Stargardt's disease. Am J Hum Genet 64:422–434
35. Lois N et al (1999) Reproducibility of fundus autofluorescence measurements obtained using a confocal scanning laser ophthalmoscope. Br J Ophthalmol 83:276–279
36. Lois N et al (1999) Intrafamilial variation of phenotype in Stargardt macular dystrophy—fundus flavimaculatus. Invest Ophthalmol Vis Sci 40:2668–2675
37. Lois N et al (2000) Quantitative evaluation of fundus autofluorescence "in vivo" in eyes with retinal disease. Br J Ophthalmol 84:741–745
38. Lois N et al (2001) Phenotypic subtypes of Stargardt macular dystrophy—fundus flavimaculatus. Arch Ophthalmol 119:359–369
39. Lois N et al (2004) Fundus autofluorescence in Stargardt macular dystrophy—fundus flavimaculatus. Am J Ophthalmol 138:55–63
40. Mata NL, Weng J, Travis GH (2000) Biosynthesis of a major lipofuscin fluorophore in mice and humans with ABCR-mediated retinal and macular degeneration. Proc Natl Acad Sci USA 97:7154–7159
41. McDonnell PJ et al (1986) Fundus flavimaculatus without maculopathy. A clinicopathologic study. Ophthalmology 93:116–119
42. Molday LL, Rabin AR, Molday RS (2000) ABCR expression in foveal cone photoreceptors and its role in Stargardt macular dystrophy. Nat Genet 25:257–258
43. Parisi V et al (2002) Altered recovery of macular function after bleaching in Stargardt's disease-fundus flavimaculatus: pattern VEP evidence. Invest Ophthalmol Vis Sci 43:2741–2748
44. Parodi MB (1994) Progressive subretinal fibrosis in fundus flavimaculatus. Acta Ophthalmol 72:260–264
45. Querques G et al (2006) Analysis of retinal flecks in fundus flavimaculatus using optical coherence tomography. Br J Ophthalmol 90:1157–1162
46. Radu RA et al (2003) Treatment with isotretinoin inhibits lipofuscin accumulation in a mouse model of recessive Stargardt's macular degeneration. Proc Natl Acad Sci USA 100:4742–4747
47. Radu RA et al (2004) Light exposure stimulates formation of A2E oxiranes in a mouse model of Stargardt's macular degeneration. Proc Natl Acad Sci USA 101:5928–5933
48. Rotenstreich Y, Fishman GA, Anderson RJ (2003) Visual acuity loss and clinical observations in a large series of patients with Stargardt's disease. Ophthalmology 110:1151–1158
49. Sparrow JR, Nakanishi K, Parish CA (2000) The lipofuscin fluorophore A2E mediates blue light-induced damage to retinal pigmented epithelial cells. Invest Ophthalmol Vis Sci 41:1981–1989
50. Sparrow JR et al (2003) A2E-epoxides damage DNA in retinal pigment epithelial cells. Vitamin E and other antioxidants inhibit A2E-epoxide formation. J Biol Chem 278:18207–18213
51. Stargardt K (1909) Über familiäre progressive Degeneration in der Makulagegend des Auges. Graefes Arch Klin Ophthalmol 71:534–550
52. Stavrou P et al (1998) Electrophysiological findings in Stargardt's—fundus flavimaculatus. Eye 12:953–958
53. Sun H, Nathans J (1997) Stargardt's ABCR is localized to the disc membrane of retinal rod outer segments. Nat Genet 17:15–16
54. Sun H, Nathans J (2001) ABCR, the ATP-binding cassette transporter responsible for Stargardt macular dystrophy, is an efficient target of all-trans-retinal-mediated photooxidative damage in vitro. Implications for retinal disease. J Biol Chem 276:11766–11774
55. Sun H, Molday RS, Nathans J (1999) Retinal stimulates ATP hydrolysis by purified and reconstituted ABCR, the photoreceptor-specific ATP-binding cassette transporter responsible for Stargardt's disease. J Biol Chem 274:8269–8281

56. Suter M et al (2000) Age-related macular degeneration. The lipofuscin component N-retinyl-N-retinylidene ethanolamine detaches proapoptotic proteins from mitochondria and induces apoptosis in mammalian retinal pigment epithelial cells. J Biol Chem 275:39625–39630
57. Uliss AE, Moore AT, Bird AC (1987) The dark choroid in posterior retinal dystrophies. Ophthalmology 94:1423–1427
58. Van Meel GJ, Van Norren D (1986) Foveal densitometry as a diagnostic technique in Stargardt's disease. Am J Ophthalmol 102:353–362
59. Von Rückmann A, Fitzke FW, Bird AC (1995) Distribution of fundus autofluorescence with a scanning laser ophthalmoscope. Br J Ophthalmol 79:407–412
60. Von Rückmann A, Fitzke FW, Bird AC (1997) In vivo fundus autofluorescence in macular dystrophies. Arch Ophthalmol 115:609–615
61. Webster AR et al (2001) An analysis of allelic variation in the ABCA4 gene. Invest Ophthalmol Vis Sci 42:1179–1189
62. Weng J et al (1999) Insights into the function of Rim protein in photoreceptors and etiology of Stargardt's disease from the phenotype in abcr knockout mice. Cell 98:13–23
63. Wroblewski JJ et al (1995) Indocyanine green angiography in Stargardt's flavimaculatus. Am J Ophthalmol 120:208–218

Chapter 12

Idiopathic Macular Telangiectasia

Peter Charbel Issa, Hendrik P.N. Scholl, Hans-Martin Helb, Frank G. Holz

Core Messages

- Idiopathic macular telangiectasia, (initially described by J.D.M. Gass as idiopathic parafoveolar telangiectasis) is a descriptive term for different disease entities presenting with telangiectatic alterations of the juxtafoveolar capillary network.
- Type 1 idiopathic macular telangiectasia ("aneurysmatic telangiectasia") occurs unilaterally, predominantly in males and is characterized by retinal exudation. It is considered to be a less severe variant of Coats' syndrome with a fair visual prognosis.
- Type 2 idiopathic macular telangiectasia (perifoveal telangiectasia) typically occurs bilaterally and is associated with foveal atrophy, loss of retinal transparency, superficial retinal crystalline deposits, blunted dilated parafoveal venules, and intraretinal pigment proliferation. There is no gender predisposition. Ocular complications include intraretinal and choroidal neovascularizations.
- The etiology of the various types of telangiectasia is unknown.

12.1 Introduction

The term "retinal telangiectasis" was first proposed by Reese to describe retinopathies characterized by dilated and incompetent vessels [45]. They differ from similar vascular alterations that may develop secondary to retinal vein occlusion, vasculitis, diabetes, carotid occlusive disease, and radiation therapy. Retinal telangiectasis occurring in the parafoveal region without a known cause has been termed "idiopathic juxtafoveolar telangiectasis." The ectatic-appearing juxtafoveolar capillaries predominantly occur in the temporal area of the macula with a similar distribution superior and inferior to the horizontal raphe [18, 19, 50].

Gass and Oyakawa (1982) were the first to categorize the condition based on ophthalmoscopic and fluorescein angiographic findings [19]. The classification was updated by Gass and Blodi in 1993, each category having a suggested pathophysiology (Table 12.1) [18]. This largest case series to date (140 patients) included patients from the previous case series on which the classification was based. Type 1 has been considered a developmental anomaly and presents with unilateral telangiectasia predominantly in males. It has been interpreted as a variant of Coats' disease by some authors. In contrast, type 2 presents with a bilateral manifestation involving the temporal parafoveal area. In type 3, there is progressive obliteration of the perifoveal capillary network and optic nerve pallor. Gass and Blodi considered types 2 and 3 to be acquired diseases.

12.2 Type 1 Idiopathic Macular Telangiectasia

12.2.1 Epidemiology

Data on the prevalence of the disease are lacking. In their series of consecutive cases Gass and Blodi classified 28% of patients with IMT as type 1, of whom 90% were males [18]. Other smaller case series reported a proportion of type 1 IMT between 38 and 57% of all patients with IMT and

Table 12.1 Summary of the classification of idiopathic juxtafoveolar telangiectasis established by Gass and Blodi [18]

Group	Clinical findings	Gender predominance	Mean age	Sub type	
1	Unilateral, visible telangiectasis, macular edema, hard exudates	Males	40	A	Involved area >2 clock hours
				B	Involved area ≤2 clock hours
2	Bilateral, occult telangiectasis, minimal exudation, foveolar atrophy, superficial retinal crystalline deposits	Males = females	50–60	A	Stage 1 Diffuse hyperfluorescence in late phase fluorescein angiography
					Stage 2 Reduced retinal transparency parafoveally
					Stage 3 Dilated right-angled venules
					Stage 4 Intraretinal pigment clumping
					Stage 5 Vascular membranes
			~10	B	Juvenile familial
3	Bilateral, visible telangiectasis, minimal exudation, capillary occlusion, optic disc pallor	Inconclusive	50	A	
				B	associated CNS vasculopathy

a male predominance of 61–70% [1, 7, 50]. The mean age was reported to be 37–56 years (range 7–74 years).

12.2.2 Diagnostic Approach and Clinical Findings

Typical funduscopic findings are visible telangiectasia surrounded by retinal edema and deposition of intraretinal lipid exudates [1, 18, 50]. The vascular changes typically involve an irregular or oval zone which is centered temporal to the fovea. The affected area is typically 1–2 disc diameters in size, but may also encompass larger extramacular areas and rarely, even involvement of areas in the peripheral fundus has been described [18, 50]. Larger aneurysms may be associated with retinal hemorrhage [50]. Microaneurysms and hard exudates appear in the early stages of the disease, but seem to regress after years [49].

Early-phase fluorescein angiography (Fig. 12.1) reveals aneurysmal and telangiectatic abnormalities, with diffuse leakage in late phase angiography [1, 50]. The aneurysms involve the deep and superficial capillary network and some patients have minimal capillary ischemia [50]. Optical coherence tomography (OCT) shows retinal thickening in the presence of cystoid macular edema. Localized neurosensory detachment may also occur [50]. OCT imaging may be useful for documentation and for the evaluation of treatment effects.

12.2.3 Functional Implications

The most frequent presenting complaints are impaired visual acuity and blurred vision. Less frequently, patients complained of metamorphopsia or a negative scotoma [1, 19]. Type 1 IMT was found to be unilateral in 90–100% [1, 18, 50].

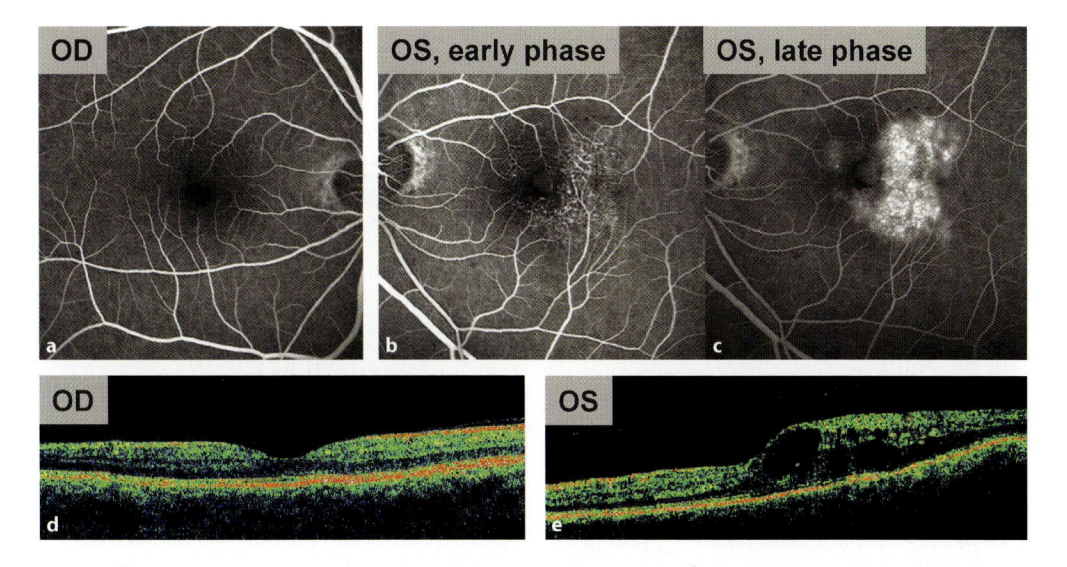

Fig. 12.1 a–c Fluorescein angiography and optical coherence tomography (OCT) imaging in a 54-year-old man with type 1 idiopathic macular telangiectasia in the left eye (OS). Visual acuity in the right eye (OD) was 20/20 and in the OS 20/40. **a** OD shows normal fluorescein angiography. **b, c** Fluorescein angiography in the early phase reveals capillary aneurysms temporal to the fovea (**b**) that show leakage in the late phase (**c**). **d, e** A horizontal OCT scan shows normal retinal configuration in OD and cystoid macular edema mainly located temporal to the fovea in OS

Gass and Blodi found a median visual acuity of 20/40 (range 20/20–1/200) in type 1A and rarely less than 20/25 in type 1B [18]. Abujamra and co-workers examined 8 patients who had a visual acuity between 20/50 and 20/80 in 75% and 20/100 and 20/200 in 25% of eyes [1].

Visual impairment is usually associated with a prominent cystoid macular edema [18, 19]. Progressive functional deterioration as well as rare spontaneous resolution of the intraretinal edema has been reported during a review period of up to 33 years [18]. In a retrospective study vision loss was associated with an increase in the extent of telangiectasia and intraretinal cystoid edema [49]. There have been no reports of functional deficits within the extrafoveal area of telangiectatic vessels. Recent preliminary individual microperimetric assessments show only slightly decreased retinal sensitivity in the area involved (Fig. 12.2).

12.2.4 Pathophysiological Considerations

Various links with systemic diseases have been described. However, no clear association with any systemic or other ocular disease has been found.

It has been proposed that type 1 IMT is a developmental disorder that represents a variant of Coats' syndrome and Leber's miliary aneurysms, with Coats' disease at one end of the spectrum and type 1 IMT at the other [5, 18]. The pathogenesis so far remains unclear.

12.2.5 Therapy

Focal laser photocoagulation [10, 18, 19] of the affected area, as well as intravitreal administration of triamcinolone [30], have been shown to result in a decrease of the macular edema and an improvement in visual acuity in type 1 IMT in small case series. However, spontaneous resolution has also been reported in some cases [18, 19]. From our own experience, rebound phenomena seem to be common after intravitreal triamcinolone injections (Fig. 12.3). At the same time, repeated injections carry potential risks, particularly with regard to steroid glaucoma. Information from prospective trials to systematically address the natural history and potential long-term treatment effects in this rare condition is lacking.

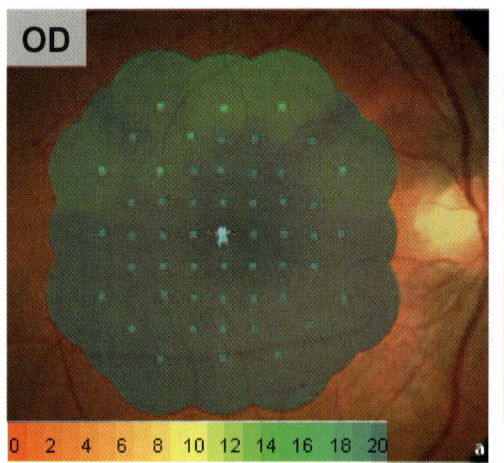

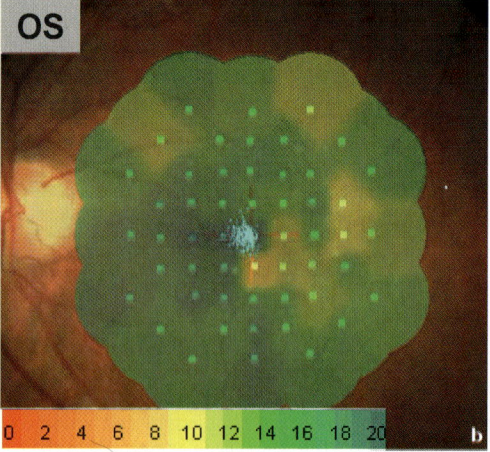

Fig. 12.2a,b Microperimetric examination with the MP 1 (Nidek). Interpolated sensitivity map of the patient with type 1 macular telangiectasia presented in Fig. 12.1. The blue dots demonstrate fixation stability during the examination time. **a** OD shows normal sensitivity. **b** OS shows only a minor decrease in retinal sensitivity temporal and inferior to the fovea

Summary for the Clinician

- Biomicroscopy, fluorescein angiography, and optical coherence tomography are essential for the diagnosis of typ 1 IMT.
- Fluorescein angiography reveals telangiectatic capillaries temporal to the fovea in the early phase with leakage of fluorescein dye in the late phase.
- Optical coherence tomography demonstrates intraretinal edema.
- The majority of patients maintain reading visual acuity.
- Focal laser photocoagulation and intravitreal triamcinolone have been described as potential treatment options.

12.3 Type 2 Idiopathic Macular Telangiectasia

This most common form of IMT was originally characterized as a distinct clinical entity by Hutton et al. in 1978 [24]. The vascular changes are bilateral, but may be asymmetric [50]. The major vascular abnormality appears to affect the deeper capillary network rather than the inner retinal capillaries. However, Yannuzzi and co-workers identified telangiectatic vessels, both in the inner and outer retinal circulation [50].

Gass and Blodi [18] described five stages (Table 12.1) and suggested a temporal sequence. Stage 1 is ophthalmoscopically unconspicious and vascular incompetence is only seen angiographically by diffuse hyperfluorescence in late-phase fluorescein angiography. At stage 2, minimal macular edema becomes evident by a reduction of parafoveal retinal transparency. Stage 3 is characterized by dilated right-angled

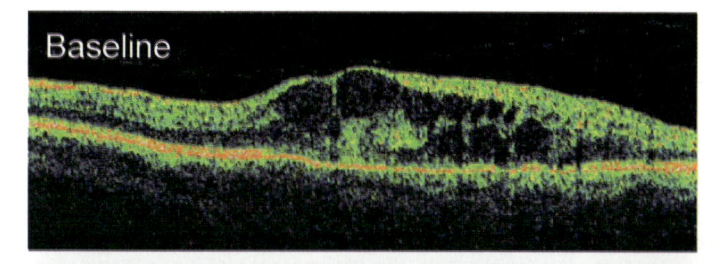

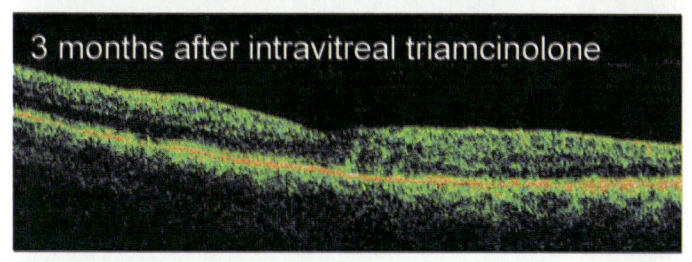

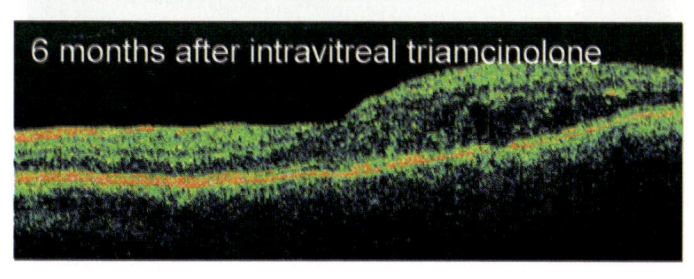

Fig. 12.3 Effect of intravitreal triamcinolone injection in type 1 macular telangiectasia. Left eye of the patient presented in Fig. 12.1. Three months following injection, the cystoid macular edema with marked retinal thickening has resolved. Note recurrence of macular edema 6 months after treatment

vessels and stage 4 by intraretinal proliferation of pigment epithelial cells typically along right-angled vessels. Stage 5 is characterized by a secondary neovascularization.

Further sequelae of type 2 IMT may be lamellar or full thickness macular holes, presumably due to progressive degeneration and atrophy of neurosensory retinal cell elements [18, 19, 38, 42]. Furthermore, retinal–retinal anastomosis was described [50].

12.3.1 Epidemiology

There are no data on the incidence or prevalence of type 2 IMT. The disease appears to occur without gender predilection [18, 50]. However, smaller case series suggested a higher prevalence in females [1] or in males [7].

The disease typically becomes symptomatic in the fifth or sixth decade. The mean age in different studies was between 52 and 59 years with a range from 33 to 82 years [1, 7, 18, 50].

Bilaterality has been reported in 90–100% of all cases [1, 18, 50], which, together with the occurrence in monozygotic twins as well as in families, suggests that genetic factors are involved in the pathogenesis of type 2 IMT [9, 24, 25, 29, 33, 37, 47].

12.3.2 Diagnostic Approach and Clinical Findings

The most frequent complaint was reported to be a loss in visual acuity in at least one eye. However, metamorphopsia or a positive scotoma may be present in individual patients [1, 19].

Ophthalmoscopically, vascular telangiectasia may not be readily identifiable, although visualization is facilitated using red-free light. The involved area is predominantly temporal to the fovea, but may encompass the entire perifoveal capillary network (Fig. 12.4a) [1, 18, 50]. Abujamra and co-workers reported a slight parafoveal retinal graying to be present in 100%, dilated right-angled venules in 82% and intraretinal stellar-shaped pigment plaques in 64% of affected patients [1]. Retinal crystalline deposits may be present in early and late stages [35] and were reported to occur in 38–68% [1, 18, 35]. They tend to aggregate temporal to the fovea. Foveal thinning or atrophy may be seen at any stage. In individual patients, development a central vitelliform

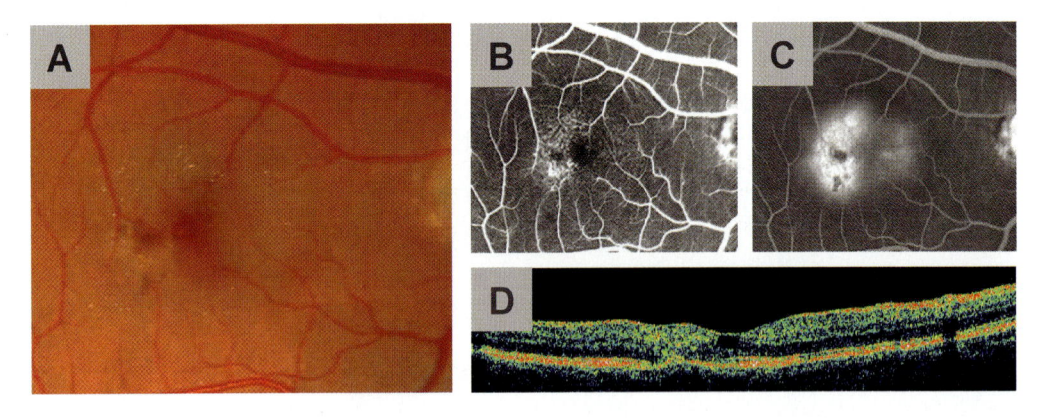

Fig. 12.4A–D Right eye of a 54-year-old man with type 2 macular telangiectasis. **A** Fundus color photograph shows perifoveal loss, retinal transparency, crystalline retinal deposits, and the impression of a lamellar macular hole. Temporal to the fovea, there is intraretinal pigment clumping and dilated right angled venules that end in the area of the pigmentation. **B, C** Fluorescein angiography shows telangiectatic parafoveal capillaries in the early phase (**B**) with leakage in the late phase (**C**), both predominantly temporal to the fovea. **D** OCT scan showing foveal atrophy in the superficial neurosensory layer with a covering internal limiting membrane drape, intraretinal pigment clumping to the left of the fovea. and adjacent disruption of the inner segment/outer segment photoreceptor junction line

lesion measuring a ¼ of disc diameter has been described [19]. Dilated right-angled venules and perivascular stellar intraretinal pigment hyperplasia was frequently [14, 17, 18], but not invariably [50], observed in eyes that subsequently developed neovascularization.

Fluorescein angiography has been the gold standard for confirmation of the diagnosis. It readily shows telangiectatic capillaries predominantly temporal to the fovea in the early phase (Fig. 12.4b) and an increasing diffuse hyperfluorescence in the late phase (Fig. 12.4c). Leakage in all four quadrants of the macula was reported to occur in 29–47% [1, 18].

On OCT imaging, very small to more prominent foveal hyporeflective or cystoid spaces that may occur in all neurosensory layers are present in most eyes (Fig. 12.4d) [20, 43]. The clinical correlate may be the impression of lamellar macular holes or foveal atrophy. Hyporeflective spaces in OCT imaging seem to be slightly decentered temporally and accordingly are sometimes only detected on horizontal scans. Interestingly, there is a lack of correlation between retinal thickening on OCT and leakage on fluorescein angiography [20, 43]. Further OCT findings may be a disruption of the inner segment/outer segment photoreceptor junction line, a unique internal limiting membrane draping across the foveola related to an underlying loss of tissue, intraretinal hyperreflectivity due to intraretinal pigmentary proliferation and/or neovascularization, neurosensory atrophy, and sometimes foveal detachment without subretinal new vessels. Despite these abnormalities, neurosensory thickness as measured by OCT is usually below or within the range of reference values due to neurosensory atrophy [6, 20].

As recently demonstrated with novel imaging techniques, a further phenotypic characteristic of type 2 IMT appears to be the abnormal distribution of luteal pigment in the macula (Fig. 12.5). Our group showed that macular pigment distribution reveals a consistent pattern in patients with type 2 IMT: corresponding to the parafoveal late hyperfluorescent area revealed by fluorescein angiography, macular pigment density was significantly reduced in the central macula with a preserved macular pigment density at the peripheral border (Fig. 12.5a–c). In contrast, in type 1 IMT normal macular pigment distribution is present with the highest density of macular pigment in the fovea and a decrease toward the periphery (Fig. 12.5d, e). The findings point toward an abnormal transport and/or storage of lutein and zeaxanthin in type 2 disease. Macular pigment mapping may be helpful in the differntial diagnosis.

Summary for the Clinician

- Fluorescein angiography in type 2 IMT shows telangiectatic capillaries parafoveally in the early phase and leakage in the late phase. These changes occur predominantly temporally, but may also encompass the entire juxtafoveal area.
- Despite visible leakage on fluorescein angiography, no intraretinal edema and thickening, but rather atrophic changes, are seen on OCT.
- OCT typically shows hyporeflective spaces in the foveal neurosensory retina.

12.3.3 Functional Implications

In the largest case series to date, Gass and Blodi reported a visual acuity of 20/20 or better in 32 eyes and a median visual acuity of 20/40 (range 20/15 to hand motions). None of the patients had a visual acuity of 20/200 or worse in either eye [18]. They stated that most patients would become symptomatic only after the occurrence of stage 3 changes. In a case series of 11 patients, visual acuity was 20/40 or better in 22.7%, 20/50–20/80 in 40.9%, 20/100–20/200 in 27.2%, and 20/400 or less in 9.2% of eyes [1].

In the early stages, functional impairment may be mild with no or only slight reduction in best-corrected central visual acuity. Mild metamorphopsia [19], predominantly located nasally to the fixation point, may be an early symptom that is most easily detected by examination with the Amsler grid. Visual acuity may decline gradually.

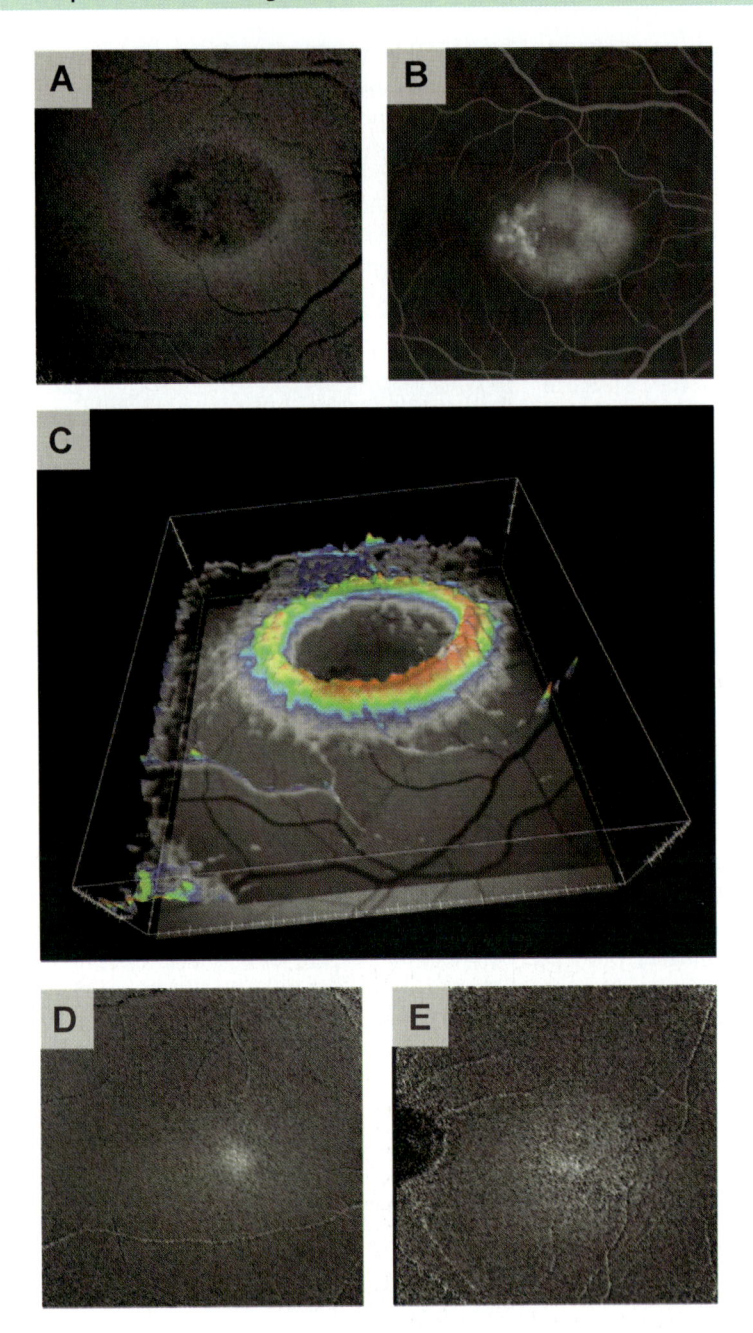

Fig. 12.5A–E Right eye of a 48-year-old woman with type 2 macular telangiectasis. **A, B** Macular pigment distribution and late phase fluorescein image. Corresponding to the late hyperfluorescent areas revealed by fluorescein angiography, macular pigment density was significantly reduced, while there was a marked area of preserved macular pigment density at the peripheral border at 5–7° eccentricity. **C** 3D macular pigment optical density image of the same eye. **D, E** Macular pigment density in OD (**D**) and OS (**E**) of the patient with type 1 IMT presented in Fig. 12.1 shows a normal distribution in OD with the highest density of macular pigment in the fovea and a regular pattern with a slightly washed out appearance in OS

However, Watzke and co-workers reported 25% of eyes to remain stable during a review period of 10–17 years [49]. Visual acuity less than 20/200 is rarely observed, but there may be a marked functional impairment due to progressive foveal atrophy or due to the development of intraretinal or choroidal neovascularization [14, 18, 49, 50].

Engelbrecht et al. [14] retrospectively studied the natural visual outcome in 26 eyes that developed stage 5 disease. Eighty percent of the eyes had a final visual acuity of 20/100 or worse. However, no prospective studies have yet been undertaken to more accurately determine the natural history of type 2 IMT and its progression over time, although such a multicenter study has recently been initiated by the MacTel consortium (see Sect. 12.5). Casswell and co-workers suggested the risk of developing bilateral disciform lesions to be high if one eye is already affected [7].

We recently used a microperimetric approach to record functional deficits in type 2 IMT [8].

Early disease stages usually show a preserved retinal sensitivity (Fig. 12.6a). In later stages, parafoveal sensitivity declines in topographic correlation to the area of late angiographic leakage (Fig. 12.6b). The main defect was found to be located temporal to the fovea. Stages 4 and 5 always showed an absolute scotoma. This sensitivity decrease was topographically related to either retinal pigment clumping or to the vascular membrane. Further causes of the development of deep scotomas were loss of outer neurosensory structures as seen on OCT imaging or atrophy of the pigment epithelium–neuroretina complex. Visual acuity was correlated with foveal light sensitivity, but not with the light sensitivity temporal to the fovea.

Assessment of fixation stability and reading acuity and speed revealed a functional impairment of reading in later disease stages, despite relatively stable central fixation, suggesting that the reduced parafoveal retinal sensitivity affect reading performance (unpublished observation).

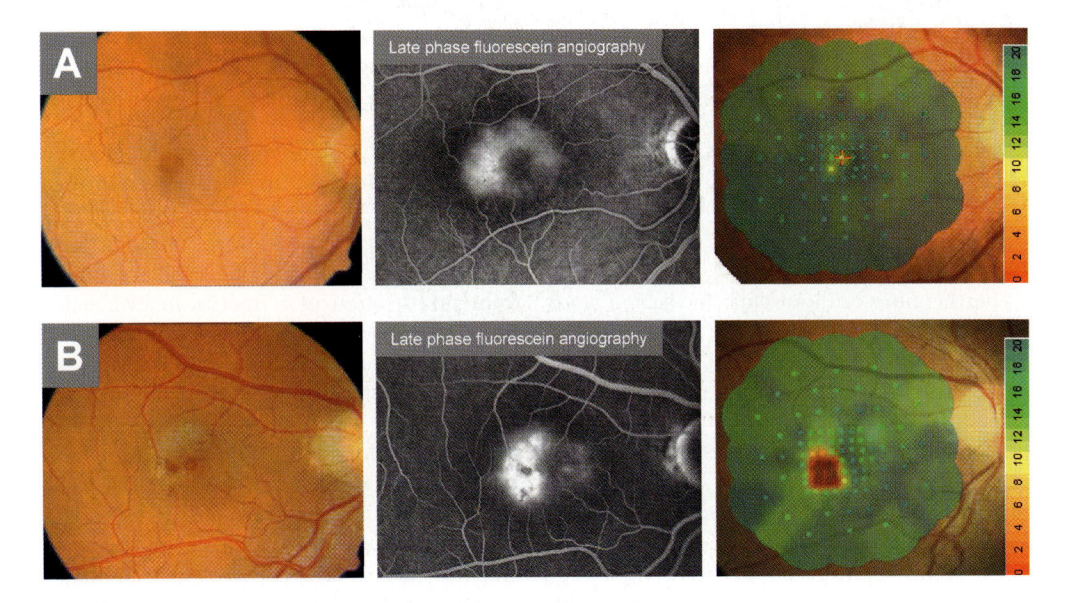

Fig. 12.6A,B Microperimetric examinations of eyes with type 2 macular telangiectasia. **A** Right eye of a 63-year-old male with stage 2 disease according to the classification by Gass and Blodi. Retinal graying is seen funduscopically, and small crystalline deposits are located temporal to the fovea. In the late angiographic phase, there is parafoveal leakage predominantly temporal to the fovea. Microperimetry shows only a minor decrease in retinal sensitivity foveal and temporally inferior to the fovea. **B** The same eye as in Fig. 12.4 with stage 4 disease. Microperimetry shows a total and sharply demarcated scotoma in the parafoveal quadrant temporal and inferior to the fovea

> **Summary for the Clinician**
>
> - Median visual acuity has been reported to be 20/40 in large case series, but the development of secondary neovascularization (stage 5 disease) may cause severe visual loss.
> - In later stages, parafoveal scotomas may be present due to atrophic changes located temporal to the fovea.

12.3.4 Associated Diseases

In larger studies, systemic arterial hypertension and diabetes mellitus were found in a proportion of patients with type 2 IMT [1, 18, 50]. A histopathological study revealed similar retinal capillary changes to those seen in diabetic patients [21]. Against this background, two groups further studied the potential role of diabetes mellitus in type 2 IMT. Maberley and co-workers [31] found abnormal glucose metabolism in 35% of 28 patients and Chew et al. described 5 patients with long-standing diabetes mellitus and type 2 IMT [9]. However, the prevalence of diabetes mellitus in other larger series was not found to be greater than expected in an age-matched population [31, 50, 50] and, therefore, larger studies are needed to determine whether or not there is a true association between the two diseases.

Furthermore, cardiovascular and heart disease [18, 50], polycythemia vera [18], Alport's disease [18], breast and prostate cancer [50], stroke [50], celiac sprue [28], spastic paraplegia [29], pseudoxanthoma elasticum [41], and facioscapulohumeral muscular dystrophy [15, 22] have been reported in individual patients. Single cases of different associated ocular diseases (hyperopia, keratoconus and congenital cataract, iris microhemangiomas) have been reported [3, 19]. In the authors' experience, hyperopia and synchysis scintillans seem to occur more often than in an average population. However, such associations are difficult to confirm due to the rarity of the disease, and clarification is awaited from larger studies.

12.3.5 Pathophysiological Considerations

The spatial predilection of the vascular abnormalities temporal to the fovea has been attributed by Gass and Oyakawa [19] to the presence of more numerous arteriovenous crossings temporal to the fovea compared with nasally. It was speculated that this might give rise to a chronic low-grade congestion or venous stasis of the temporal paramacular capillaries.

Watzke et al. [49] suggested a developmental origin based on findings by Nishimura and Taniguchi [36]. They found that the vessels in the temporal paramacular area were formed by anastomoses of superior and inferior vessels and not by extension, like all the other retinal vessels. This could cause structural abnormalities with subsequent decompensation of these vessels in adult life.

The dilated right-angled venules are considered to drain telangiectatic capillaries. The vascular membranes in stage 5 are most commonly located temporal to the fovea [14] and are believed to originate in the retinal vasculature, but may later also include connections to the choroidal vasculature or choroidal neovascularization [11, 14, 18].

Green et al. published a light and electron microscopic study of an eye with confirmed type 2 IMT [21]. Interestingly, they did not find telangiectatic vessels within the macular area, but rather narrowing of the capillary lumen from proliferation of a multilaminated endothelial cell basement membrane. Furthermore, they reported a partial loss of pericytes, accumulation of lipids within the capillary walls and localized areas with disrupted endothelial cells. The neurosensory retina showed intracellular and intercellular edema in the temporal parafoveal area with granular material in the extracellular spaces. Some ganglion cells and cells in the inner nuclear layer appeared to be undergoing degeneration. The outer nuclear layer was less affected. Similar changes were observed in the peripheral retina. The retinal pigment epithelium appeared normal. They postulated that the angiographic appearance of telangiectasia could be due to rapid diffusion of the dye into the thickened wall of the capillary sites of endothelial cell degeneration, subsequent diffusion within the wall, and eventual leakage into the surrounding tissue.

The clinical and pathologic resemblance of type 2 IMT to radiation retinopathy led to a case-control study with 65 cases and 175 controls. The group identified a history of therapeutic head or neck irradiation (odds ratio 4.06) and environmental radiation exposure (odds ratio 6.73) to be risk factors for type 2 IMT [31].

12.3.6 Therapeutic Approaches

In disease stages without neovascular membranes (*nonproliferative stage*), argon laser photocoagulation (ALP) [18, 40], the largest series reported by Park and co-workers [40], as well as photodynamic therapy [12], have not shown any beneficial effects. Argon laser photocoagulation in type 2 IMT may be complicated by subretinal hemorrhage [16] and by potential induction of neovascular menbranes [14, 39]. Long-term data on the outcome following argon laser photocoagulation in type 2 IMT are not available.

Intravitreal application of triamcinolone was performed in some patients [2, 6, 32], and a reduction of the late-phase hyperfluorescence in fluorescein angiography with [32] or without [2, 6] significant improvement in visual acuity was reported. The longest review period was 6 months in the study by Cakir and co-workers and showed a waning effect within that time period [6]. A recent study reported the effect of posterior juxtascleral administration of anecortave acetate, an angiostatic synthetic cortisol derivative without corticosteroid bioactivity [13]. It was found that visual acuity was stabilized over 24 months. However, no data were provided with regard to the natural history in the fellow eye, the angiographic effects, or alterations on OCT imaging.

A new pharmacological approach may be the inhibition of vascular endothelial growth factor (VEGF). Short-term results indicate that intravitreal application of the VEGF inhibitor bevacizumab is associated with a reduction in ectatic capillaries in early-phase fluorescein angiography as well as in late-phase leakage in type 2 IMT (Fig. 12.7) [8a, 8b]. These findings imply that VEGF plays a pathophysiological role in type 2 IMT. Furthermore, intravitreal bevacizumab was found to improve visual acuity in a subset of patients.

As atrophy indicated by "retinal black holes" on OCT imaging implies cell death in the neurosensory retina, administration of neuroprotective agents may be a rational therapeutic approach in the future (Mark Gillies, personal communication).

In the *vasoproliferative stage* the development of secondary neovascularization is a major cause of severe vision loss in type 2 IMT [14, 18, 50] and various therapeutic approaches have been undertaken to tackle this stage of the disease. Park and co-workers found little change in the

Early phase fluorescein angiography

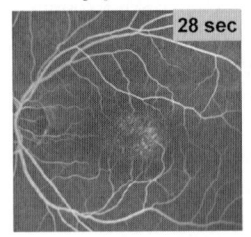

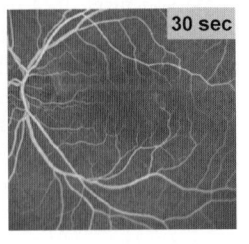

28 sec | 30 sec

Late phase fluorescein angiography

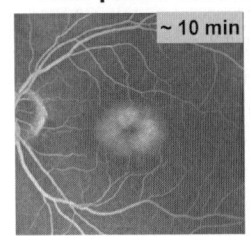

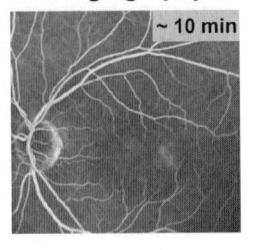

~ 10 min | ~ 10 min

Fig. 12.7 Effects of intravitreal applications of the vascular endothelial growth factor (VEGF) antagonist bevacizumab on the appearance in early and late phase fluorescein angiography in OS of a 52-year-old woman. Fluorescein angiography at baseline is shown on the *left*. Two intravitreal injections of 1.5 mg (0.06 ml) bevacizumab were performed with an interval of 4 weeks. The *right* images show the angiographic results at 4 weeks after the first injection and at 4 weeks after the second injection. Early phase angiography shows a decrease in ectatic parafoveal capillaries and late phase angiography shows a marked decrease in fluorescein leakage. Visual acuity improved from 20/80 to 20/63

size of the fibrovascular tissue and therefore questioned the usefulness of treatment in stage 5 eyes [39]. Therefore, interventions appear to be most beneficial in early and active disease stages before the development of fibrotic membranes. There are two reports on the surgical removal of subfoveal vascular membranes in two eyes with type 2 IMT [4, 11]. Due to the adherence of the membranes to the neurosensory retina, removal proved to be difficult and visual outcome was poor. Visual stabilization and deterioration have been reported after argon laser photocoagulation in stage 5 type 2 IMT [18, 27, 49].

Photodynamic therapy (PDT) was shown to result in functional and angiographic stabilization within a follow-up period of 7–23 months [23, 44, 48]. However, one patient's vision deteriorated from 20/50 to 20/200 after four sessions of PDT [48]. Interestingly, fluorescein angiography showed no leakage specific to the subretinal neovascular membrane after treatment, while leakage from the juxtafoveal telangiectasia continued.

In a retrospective report studying the effect of *transpupillary thermotherapy* (TTT), 92% of 14 eyes showed stabilization or improvement in visual acuity, as well as regression of the vascular membrane [46].

Posterior juxtascleral administration of *anecortave acetate* resulted in the stabilization or improvement of lesion size, resolution of leakage, and stabilization of vision [13].

Intravitreal application of *bevacizumab* in patients with vascular membranes [26] resulted in an absence of signs of activity and improvement of visual acuity in one of the patients presenting with an extrafoveal membrane [26].

In summary, there is yet insufficient information on potential treatment benefits to make any general recommendations. There are obviously promising approaches that need assessment in extensive clinical trials.

Summary for the Clinician

- Focal laser photocoagulation appears to be ineffective in the nonproliferative disease stages of type 2 IMT.
- Preliminary short term observations demonstrate positive effects of intravitreally administered anti-VEGF agents.
- In proliferative stage 5, photodynamic therapy, transpupillary thermotherapy, juxtascleral anecortave, and intravitreal anti-VEGF therapy have been applied in small case series.

12.4 Type 3: Idiopathic Macular Telangiectasia

Type 3 occlusive IMT occurs much less frequently than other types of IMT. It is characterized by, minimal exudation and relatively preserved visual acuity despite extensive occlusion in the juxtafoveolar capillary network [18]. There seems to be a familial tendency. However, none of the other larger case series of patients with IMT reported similar patients [1, 50].

12.5 Perspectives

Recently, based on new findings using OCT imaging and high-speed indocyanine green angiography, Yannuzzi and co-workers presented a simplified classification (Table 12.2) [50]. Gass and Blodi's groups 1A and B were combined as aneurysmatic telangiectasia (or type 1) since they believe that a small focal area in the juxtafoveal region simply represents a less severe variant in the spectrum of the disease and progresses to more extensive disease over time. Group 2 was named perifoveal telangiectasis (or type 2) and divided into only two categories: nonproliferative, representing Gass and Blodi's stages 1–4, and proliferative, representing stage 5. They argued that staging on this anatomical basis would have a functional significance since vision loss is due to progressive atrophy in the nonproliferative stage and due to development

Table 12.2 Idiopathic macular telangiectasia: comparison of the classification by Gass and Blodi [18] and the new simplified classification proposed by Yannuzzi and co-workers [50]

Gass and Blodi [18] Idiopathic juxtafoveolar retinal telangiectasis			Yannuzzi et al. [50] Idiopathic macular telangiectasia	
Group 1	A		Aneurysmatic telangiectasia	
	B			
Group 2	A	Stages 1–4	Nonproliferative	Perifoveal telangiectasia
		Stage 5	Proliferative	
	B		Ø	
Group 3	A			
	B		Ø	

of subretinal vascular membranes in the proliferative stages. Due to the rarity of occlusive telangiectasis (group 3), it was deleted from the classification.

Further insights into the pathophysiology and natural history of type 2 IMT (perifoveal telangiectasis) are expected to be gained from the international IMT Project (MacTel study, www.mactelresearch.com). It is the first longitudinal multicenter trial to investigate the natural history and risk factors of type 2 IMT in a large patient cohort. It will help to further characterize the disease, to determine genetic factors, and to identify novel therapeutic targets.

References

1. Abujamra S, Bonanomi MT, Cresta FB, Machado CG, Pimentel SL, Caramelli CB (2000) Idiopathic juxtafoveolar retinal telangiectasis: clinical pattern in 19 cases. Ophthalmologica 214:406–411
2. Alldredge CD, Garretson BR (2003) Intravitreal triamcinolone for the treatment of idiopathic juxtafoveal telangiectasis. Retina 23:113–116
3. Bakke EF, Drolsum L (2006) Iris microhaemangiomas and idiopathic juxtafoveolar retinal telangiectasis. Acta Ophthalmol Scand 84:818–822
4. Berger AS, McCuen BW, Brown GC, Brownlow RL Jr (1997) Surgical removal of subfoveal neovascularization in idiopathic juxtafoveolar retinal telangiectasis. Retina 17:94–98
5. Cahill M, O'Keefe M, Acheson R, Mulvihill A, Wallace D, Mooney D (2001) Classification of the spectrum of Coats' disease as subtypes of idiopathic retinal telangiectasis with exudation. Acta Ophthalmol Scand 79:596–602
6. Cakir M, Kapran Z, Basar D, Utine CA, Eroglu F, Perente I (2006) Optical coherence tomography evaluation of macular edema after intravitreal triamcinolone acetonide in patients with parafoveal telangiectasis. Eur J Ophthalmol 16:711–717
7. Casswell AG, Chaine G, Rush P, Bird AC (1986) Paramacular telangiectasis. Trans Ophthalmol Soc UK 105 (Pt 6):683–692
8. Charbel Issa P, Helb HM, Rohrschneider K, Holz FG, Scholl HPN (2007) Microperimetric assessment of patients with type II IMT. Invest Ophthalmol Vis Sci (in press)
8a. Charbel Issa P, Holz FG, Scholl HPN (2007) Findings in fluorescein angiography and optical coherence tomography after intravitreal bevacizumab in type 2 IMT, Ophthalmology (in press)
8b. Charbel Issa P, Scholl HPN, Holz FG (2007) Short-term effects of intravitreal bevacizumab in type 2 IMT, Retinal Cases and Brief Reports (in press)

9. Chew EY, Murphy RP, Newsome DA, Fine SL (1986) Parafoveal telangiectasis and diabetic retinopathy. Arch Ophthalmol 104:71–75
10. Chopdar A (1978) Retinal telangiectasis in adults: fluorescein angiographic findings and treatment by argon laser. Br J Ophthalmol 62:243–250
11. Davidorf FH, Pressman MD, Chambers RB (2004) Juxtafoveal telangiectasis—a name change? Retina 24:474–478
12. De Lahitte GD, Cohen SY, Gaudric A (2004) Lack of apparent short-term benefit of photodynamic therapy in bilateral, acquired, parafoveal telangiectasis without subretinal neovascularization. Am J Ophthalmol 138:892–894
13. Eandi CM, Ober MD, Freund KB, Klais CM, Slakter JS, Sorenson JA, Yannuzzi LA (2006) Anecortave acetate for the treatment of idiopathic perifoveal telangiectasia: a pilot study. Retina 26:780–785
14. Engelbrecht NE, Aaberg TM Jr, Sung J, Lewis ML (2002) Neovascular membranes associated with idiopathic juxtafoveolar telangiectasis. Arch Ophthalmol 120:320–324
15. Fitzsimons RB, Gurwin EB, Bird AC (1987) Retinal vascular abnormalities in facioscapulohumeral muscular dystrophy. A general association with genetic and therapeutic implications. Brain 110 (Pt 3):631–648
16. Friedman SM, Mames RN, Stewart MW (1993) Subretinal hemorrhage after grid laser photocoagulation for idiopathic juxtafoveolar retinal telangiectasis. Ophthalmic Surg 24:551–553
17. Gass JD (2003) Chorioretinal anastomosis probably occurs infrequently in type 2A idiopathic juxtafoveolar retinal telangiectasis. Arch Ophthalmol 121:1345–1346
18. Gass JD, Blodi BA (1993) Idiopathic juxtafoveolar retinal telangiectasis. Update of classification and follow-up study. Ophthalmology 100:1536–1546
19. Gass JD, Oyakawa RT (1982) Idiopathic juxtafoveolar retinal telangiectasis. Arch Ophthalmol 100:769–780
20. Gaudric A, Ducos de LG, Cohen SY, Massin P, Haouchine B (2006) Optical coherence tomography in group 2A idiopathic juxtafoveolar retinal telangiectasis. Arch Ophthalmol 124:1410–1419
21. Green WR, Quigley HA, de la CZ, Cohen B (1980) Parafoveal retinal telangiectasis. Light and electron microscopy studies. Trans Ophthalmol Soc UK 100:162–170
22. Gurwin EB, Fitzsimons RB, Sehmi KS, Bird AC (1985) Retinal telangiectasis in facioscapulohumeral muscular dystrophy with deafness. Arch Ophthalmol 103:1695–1700
23. Hershberger VS, Hutchins RK, Laber PW (2003) Photodynamic therapy with verteporfin for subretinal neovascularization secondary to bilateral idiopathic acquired juxtafoveolar telangiectasis. Ophthalmic Surg Lasers Imaging 34:318–320
24. Hutton WL, Snyder WB, Fuller D, Vaiser A (1978) Focal parafoveal retinal telangiectasis. Arch Ophthalmol 96:1362–1367
25. Isaacs TW, McAllister IL (1996) Familial idiopathic juxtafoveolar retinal telangiectasis. Eye 10 (Pt 5):639–642
26. Jorge R, Costa RA, Calucci D, Scott IU (2006) Intravitreal bevacizumab (Avastin) associated with the regression of subretinal neovascularization in idiopathic juxtafoveolar retinal telangiectasis. Graefes Arch Clin Exp Ophthalmol (published online doi: 10.1007/s00417-006-0468-2)
27. Lee BL (1996) Bilateral subretinal neovascular membrane in idiopathic juxtafoveolar telangiectasis. Retina 16:344–346
28. Lee HC, Liu M, Ho AC (2004) Idiopathic juxtafoveal telangiectasis in association with celiac sprue. Arch Ophthalmol 122:411–413
29. Leys A, Gilbert HD, Van De SW, Verougstraete C, Devriendt K, Lagae L, Gass JD (2000) Familial spastic paraplegia and maculopathy with juxtaveolar retinal telangiectasis and subretinal neovascularization. Retina 20:184–189
30. Li KK, Goh TY, Parsons H, Chan WM, Lam DS (2005) Use of intravitreal triamcinolone acetonide injection in unilateral idiopathic juxtafoveal telangiectasis. Clin Exp Ophthalmol 33:542–544
31. Maberley DA, Yannuzzi LA, Gitter K, Singerman L, Chew E, Freund KB, Noguiera F, Sallas D, Willson R, Tillocco K (1999) Radiation exposure: a new risk factor for idiopathic perifoveal telangiectasis. Ophthalmology 106:2248–2252
32. Martinez JA (2003) Intravitreal triamcinolone acetonide for bilateral acquired parafoveal telangiectasis. Arch Ophthalmol 121:1658–1659
33. Menchini U, Virgili G, Bandello F, Malara C, Rapizzi E, Lanzetta P (2000) Bilateral juxtafoveolar telangiectasis in monozygotic twins. Am J Ophthalmol 129:401–403

34. Millay RH, Klein ML, Handelman IL, Watzke RC (1986) Abnormal glucose metabolism and parafoveal telangiectasia. Am J Ophthalmol 102:363–370
35. Moisseiev J, Lewis H, Bartov E, Fine SL, Murphy RP (1990) Superficial retinal refractile deposits in juxtafoveal telangiectasis. Am J Ophthalmol 109:604–605
36. Nishimura M, Taniguchi Y (1982) Retinal vascular patterns in the macula and the perimacular area in premature and full-term infants. Ophthalmologica 185:147–157
37. Oh KT, Park DW (1999) Bilateral juxtafoveal telangiectasis in a family. Retina 19:246–247
38. Olson JL, Mandava N (2006) Macular hole formation associated with idiopathic parafoveal telangiectasia. Graefes Arch Clin Exp Ophthalmol 244:411–412
39. Park D, Schatz H, McDonald HR, Johnson RN (1996) Fibrovascular tissue in bilateral juxtafoveal telangiectasis. Arch Ophthalmol 114:1092–1096
40. Park DW, Schatz H, McDonald HR, Johnson RN (1997) Grid laser photocoagulation for macular edema in bilateral juxtafoveal telangiectasis. Ophthalmology 104:1838–1846
41. Parodi MB, Iacono P, Ravalico G (2006) Subretinal neovascular membrane associated with type 2a idiopathic juxtafoveolar telangiectasis in pseudoxanthoma elasticum. Graefes Arch Clin Exp Ophthalmol (published online doi: 10.1007/s00417-006-0402-7)
42. Patel B, Duvall J, Tullo AB (1988) Lamellar macular hole associated with idiopathic juxtafoveolar telangiectasia. Br J Ophthalmol 72:550–551
43. Paunescu LA, Ko TH, Duker JS, Chan A, Drexler W, Schuman JS, Fujimoto JG (2006) Idiopathic juxtafoveal retinal telangiectasis: new findings by ultrahigh-resolution optical coherence tomography. Ophthalmology 113:48–57
44. Potter MJ, Szabo SM, Chan EY, Morris AH (2002) Photodynamic therapy of a subretinal neovascular membrane in type 2A idiopathic juxtafoveolar retinal telangiectasis. Am J Ophthalmol 133:149–151
45. Reese AB (1956) Telangiectasis of the retina and Coats' disease. Am J Ophthalmol 42:1–8
46. Shukla D, Singh J, Kolluru CM, Kim R, Namperumalsamy P (2004) Transpupillary thermotherapy for subfoveal neovascularization secondary to group 2A idiopathic juxtafoveolar telangiectasis. Am J Ophthalmol 138:147–149
47. Siddiqui N, Fekrat S (2005) Group 2A idiopathic juxtafoveolar retinal telangiectasia in monozygotic twins. Am J Ophthalmol 139:568–570
48. Snyers B, Verougstraete C, Postelmans L, Leys A, Hykin P (2004) Photodynamic therapy of subfoveal neovascular membrane in type 2A idiopathic juxtafoveolar retinal telangiectasis. Am J Ophthalmol 137:812–819
49. Watzke RC, Klein ML, Folk JC, Farmer SG, Munsen RS, Champfer RJ, Sletten KR (2005) Long-term juxtafoveal retinal telangiectasia. Retina 25:727–735
50. Yannuzzi LA, Bardal AM, Freund KB, Chen KJ, Eandi CM, Blodi B (2006) IMT. Arch Ophthalmol 124:450–460

Chapter 13

Artificial Vision

Peter Walter

Core Messages

- Artificial vision is created by implants in the visual system operating by electrical stimulation via multielectrode arrays
- The retina, the optic nerve, and the visual cortex are targeted by chronic implants in pilot clinical trials
- Blind patients reported visual sensations, object localization, and simple geometries
- Animal experiments showed that the possible resolution using retinal implants will be about 1° of visual field and about 25 frames per second
- The quality of artificial vision in the future will be improved by increasing the number of implanted electrodes and by optimizing stimulation paradigms

13.1 Introduction

The term "artificial vision" comprises approaches for restoring vision in blind individuals using devices or implants. Although other approaches could be assumed under the term artificial vision using nonvisual senses such as tactile devices [44], nowadays artificial vision means restoring vision using implants interfacing with neurons of the visual system [10, 38]. Currently, some prototypes for such implants are under investigation in animal experiments, but also in pilot clinical trials. These systems are based on the electrical stimulation of groups of neurons at several levels of the visual system with multielectrode arrays placed onto or underneath the retina, onto the visual cortex, around the optic nerve, on the sclera or in the suprachoroidal space.

The history of artificial vision began when Brindley implanted several electrical stimulators close to the visual cortex in a woman who was blind due to retinitis pigmentosa (RP). After surgery, this patient was able to see spots of lights—electrically evoked phosphenes. Large efforts were undertaken to characterize the kind of phosphenes that were elicited with this system [3, 4, 54]. The Brindley approach was later continued by Dobelle, who implanted several patients with his cortical stimulator. The stimulator was connected to an external power source and to a visual processor with a cable. The information for the visual processor was taken from a camera chip mounted on one glass of spectacles and from an ultrasound sensor giving distance information. The Dobelle group reported that the patients were able to see phosphenes, to identify obstacles and to recognize high contrast objects [14, 15].

As technology advanced, especially in the field of microsystem technology and integration, but also with the advances in microsurgery new concepts were considered. Much smaller devices were designed and fabricated, devices that were remotely controlled, and devices that could be much more efficient in terms of spatial and temporal resolution compared with the historic approach of Brindley. The final goal of artificial vision is not to elicit phosphenes, but to restore vision with spatial and temporal properties similar to natural vision, vision that can be used by blind individuals to improve their daily life and performance, not only to restore spatial and temporal resolution in a picture, but also to restore the emotional content of vision, such as the recognition of a beautiful landscape, a colorful sunset or the face of a beloved friend, to make them also be able to participate in the emotional side of our visually dominated life.

13.2 Current Concepts for Restoring Vision Using Electrical Stimulation

Artificial vision uses electrical stimulation to drive neurons of the visual system, which are depleted from their natural input. Usually, electrical stimulation is provided in such concepts by implants consisting of an array of stimulating electrodes and electronic components, e.g., for pulse generation. Two main concepts evolved, one is that the optic path of the eye is still used to transmit visual information. In the second concept, visual information is obtained by a camera system. This information is then further processed depending on the level of the visual system where the stimulation is intended.

In the original idea of subretinal stimulation the implantation of thousands of very small microphotodiodes in the subretinal space was planned. These elements should transform light coming naturally through the optical path of the eye in electric current strong enough to drive postsynaptic cells. The microphotodiodes were intended to replace the photoreceptors. In this concept additional data processing or energy supply was not required. It was thought that the postreceptoral retinal data processing would be done by the postsynaptic neural network, which was thought to be more or less intact [6, 37, 55]. Chow et al. implanted several patients with such a system, an artificial silicon retina (ASR) in the subretinal space [8]. The surgery was carried out without complications and the patients reported visual sensations in the first year. Unfortunately, after a longer follow-up the patients reported that the percepts disappeared, and they were as blind as before the implantation. It turned out that the devices did not generate enough power to drive postsynaptic cells. Most likely, the primary percepts were the result of an unspecific effect of mediators and other cell signal molecules released after surgery [35, 36].

In approaches interfacing with ganglion cells or cells in the visual cortex, camera systems and data processing algorithms with application-specific hardware are used to obtain visual information and to calculate optimal stimulation pulses. Furthermore, in such approaches data processing algorithms will be modified by the percepts of the user in a training procedure.

13.3 Interfacing the Neurons

In RP the photoreceptors degenerate. However, postsynaptic neurons also show considerable changes in the degenerated retina with a loss of cell bodies and a chaotic de-organization. In advanced cases of RP a certain amount of ganglion cells remain alive [40, 47], but a huge amount of remodeling occurs in which new circuits are established and in which neurons migrate along glial structures forming microneuromas. The typical layered structure of the retina with known functional connections is destroyed [28, 31]. Electrical stimulation to restore neural function uses charge delivery from a stimulating electrode to adjacent cell membranes so that their membrane potential is considerably modulated. By changing this membrane potential a neuron may fire action potentials or release neurotransmitters at its synaptic terminal, thus making the neuronal chain functioning again as a response to stimulating pulses emitted from electrodes of a implanted stimulation device. However, making predictions which cells will be stimulated and which postsynaptic cells will be activated is nearly impossible because of the structural and functional remodeling of the degenerated retina and because in the clinical situation it cannot be exactly planned where stimulating electrodes will be placed with regard to the position of target cells (Fig. 13.1). If specific activation of cells is the goal, then it is desirable to have as many electrodes as possible to contact as many neurons as possible in a 1:1 ratio. Electrodes should be placed as near to the target cell as possible. Charge delivery may induce adverse events in the target tissue or in the material of the electrode; therefore, certain safety ranges of charge delivery should be taken into account. As a consequence electrodes could not be made as small as possible because the charge density would be enhanced, which is the main parameter in terms of electrode material stability and safety. Currently, in approaches using electrodes on the retinal surface electrodes are fabricated in diameters of

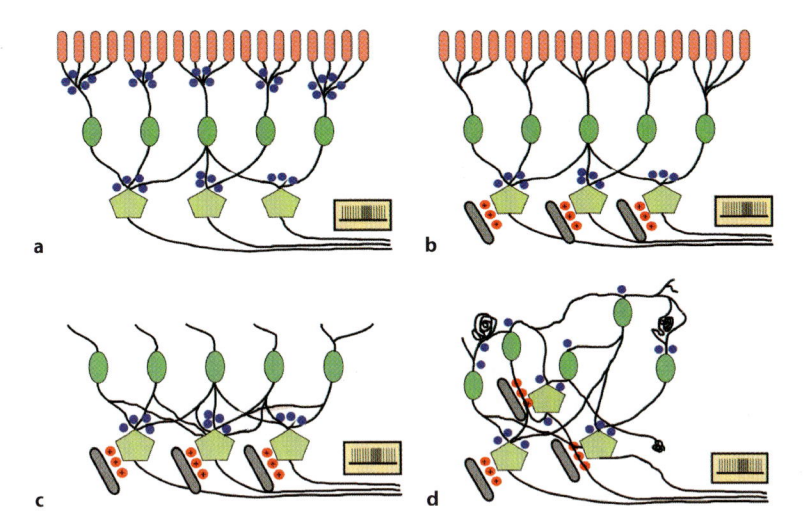

Fig. 13.1 a Simplified cone pathway in the healthy vertebrate retina. Action potentials measured in the axons of the retinal ganglion cells (RGC) are evoked by the release of neurotransmitters (*blue bubbles*) from the terminals of presynaptic cells. **b** Electrical stimulation in a normal cone pathway in the dark. Action potentials were elicited by changing the membrane potential of RGC with charge delivery from stimulating electrodes. Receptors are quiet in darkness; neurotransmitter action is still present from interneurons. **c** The original idea of ganglion cell stimulation in advanced retinitis pigmentosa: no receptors present. Action potentials should be elicited as in **b**. **d** More realistic model of electric stimulation in the retina with advanced receptor degeneration. Ganglion cell bodies are in unpredicted positions of the retina as well as interneurons being in different positions. The circuitry may be completely remodeled and chaotic. Electrode positioning maybe very variable with regard to ganglion cell position

40–200 µm. Electrode materials are platinum or gold with or without regular or sputtered iridium oxide. Surface modification of these electrodes is used to increase the surface area of the electrode without increasing the electrode diameter in order to reduce the charge density to protect both the material and also the tissue against side-effects of chronic electrical stimulation. These large electrodes could be placed close to the outer surface of the retina as well as underneath the retina. However, compared with the cell the electrodes are still very large and single-cell stimulation is not possible. Whole cell clusters will be activated with such large electrodes.

However, by intelligent selection of stimulus parameters the activation of certain cell types may be possible even when the electrode is adjacent to a cell cluster [23, 45, 46]. Technical difficulties are explained by the power needed to individually activate thousands of electrodes and by the electronics to transmit such very high density signals within a biologically safe range of power.

Summary for the Clinician

- Electrical stimulation acts by changing the membrane potential of neurons
- Electrodes should be as close to the neurons as possible
- Retinal remodeling may have a significant impact on stimulation protocols

13.3.1 Epiretinal Stimulation

Based on the early experiments of Dawson and Radtke [12], but also on the consideration that in RP more damage is in the outer retina than in the inner retina, strategies were developed based on multielectrode arrays fixed onto the inner retinal surface. The aim of this concept is to stimulate ganglion cells [18–20, 27, 39]. The electrodes are usually mounted on a flexible substrate, usually polyimide is used for this purpose. The electrodes are driven by power sources either outside the eye or inside the eye. If the power source is inside the eye, then it has to be controlled remotely via inductive or optoelectronic signal end energy transfer. If the power source is outside the eye, it is necessary to connect the multielectrode array with a cable to the power source. The cable has to cross the wall of the globe, usually through the choroid and sclera. Such an implant with a transscleral cable connection to an epiretinal multielectrode array was fabricated by Mahadevappa and colleagues and has been evaluated in a pilot clinical trial [30]. Theoretically, a transretinal cable may be at risk of intraocular infection or the risk of shearing forces transmitted to the implant and its anatomical interface with the inner retinal surface when the eye is moved. However, no reports exist on such potentially adverse events. The approach being used by Hornig et al. also consists of an epiretinal multielectrode array, a transscleral cable connection, and a data and energy system in which a receiver coil is mounted onto the scleral surface [25]. The group of Walter and Mokwa fabricated an epiretinal device in which the transponder coil is implanted in the capsular bag, meaning that no cable passes the wall of the globe (Fig. 13.2) [1, 49].

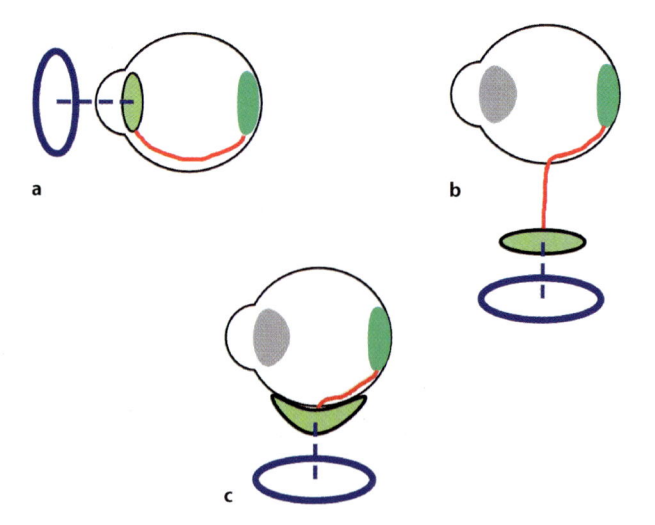

Fig. 13.2 Possible approaches to data and energy transfer in epiretinal stimulation. **a** Receiver for data and signal is implanted in the capsular bag. The sending coil is outside in front of the eye. **b** Receiver coil is implanted far from the eye, e.g. subcutaneously behind the ear. A cable connects the receiver to the multielectrode array and passes through the globe wall. This system is comparable to the data transmission system of cochlea implants. **c** Receiver is implanted onto the ocular surface, e.g. onto the sclera with a transscleral cable connecting the receiver to the multielectrode array. the sending coil is outside lateral to the eye.

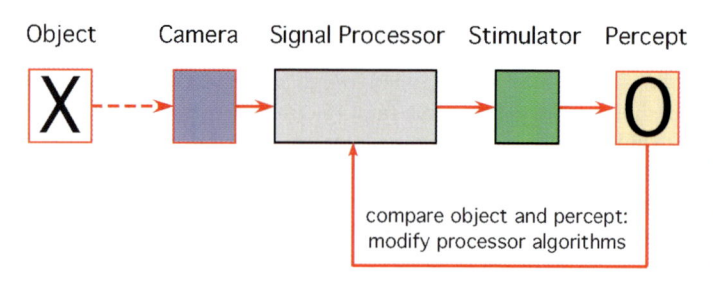

Fig. 13.3 Simplified concept of a visual preprocessing loop. The patient compares the percept and the object that he should see and modifies the characteristics of the filters implemented in the data processing unit. In several feedback loops the percept should be improved and as close to the object as possible

A crucial problem in epiretinal stimulation is the stimulus paradigm. Usually, ganglion cells receive preprocessed data from retinal interneurons and not only information on which receptor is activated by light. Therefore, camera data resembling receptor activation have to be processed in an encoder simulating retinal data processing. Adaptive spatiotemporal filters are used to process the camera data and the output of this processing is then used to stimulate the ganglion cells [21]. Because it is previously not known which ganglion cells are stimulated, the encoder properties have to be modified in a learning procedure based on the percepts of the patient, which should be as near to the input signal as possible (Fig. 13.3).

Summary for the Clinician

- In epiretinal stimulation electrodes are placed onto the inner retinal surface.
- The target cells are ganglion cells.
- Fixation is achieved with retinal tacks.
- Camera signals must be preprocessed using visual encoder technology.
- Signal and energy transmission concepts include both wire and wireless solutions.
- The first clinical trials are underway.

13.3.2 Subretinal Approach

In the subretinal approach microphotodiodes are implanted underneath the retina. The original idea of Chow et al. and Zrenner et al. was that thousands of such photodiodes would act as artificial receptors and change the light into a current large enough to drive postsynaptic cells in the retina [7, 8, 43, 55, 56]. However, it was found that the current generated by the currently available microphotodiodes was not strong enough to drive these cells. Therefore, implants are now fabricated with an additional power supply [24]. Zrenner and his group was able to demonstrate in patients that direct subretinal electrical stimulation can elicit phosphenes in patients over a certain time period and that patients were able to detect some basic geometries [53].

At present, it is not exactly clear what cells are activated in subretinal stimulation in advanced cases of RP because the retina shows a significant amount of destruction of the original layer structure making ganglion cells reach even as far as the outer retinal surface. It may be disclosed in the future that with both approaches ganglion cells and postsynaptic cells were activated from the epiretinal or from the subretinal side. That may also mean that the preprocessing of the input is maybe necessary for both approaches.

Summary for the Clinician

- In subretinal stimulation electrodes are placed underneath the retina.
- Target cells are postsynaptic neurons.
- No specific fixation procedures are necessary.
- First clinical trials are underway.

13.3.3 Transchoroidal, Transscleral, and Suprachoroidal Stimulation

In both the epiretinal and subretinal approaches major surgical steps have to be taken, meaning that both approaches have a certain risk profile. Therefore, approaches are considered to minimize the surgical risk. Electrode arrays may be placed with their basic structure onto the outer scleral surface or in an intrascleral pocket [9, 33]. Needle-type electrodes should penetrate into the suprachoroidal or into the subretinal space to get close to the target cells. Such approaches are not free of surgical risk because placement of such structures at the posterior pole may cause trouble with the ciliary arteries and sharp electrodes may penetrate deep within the retina. In concepts in which the electrodes remain on the scleral surface or in the suprachoroidal space the main problem remains in the distance between the electrodes and the target tissue. However, in a pilot trial Kanda was able to demonstrate in normal volunteers that they have phosphenes with stimulus intensities similar to those reported in epiretinal stimulation and that they were also able to differentiate different sizes of phosphenes, depending on stimulus parameters [29].

> **Summary for the Clinician**
>
> - Stimulation concepts are developed to reduce the surgical risk.
> - Electrodes are not very close to the target cells.
> - Clinical trials are planned.

13.3.4 Optic Nerve Approach

There is some experience in connecting peripheral nerves with cuff electrodes. Therefore, such cuff electrodes were used to contact the optic nerve in two experiments by Delbeke et al. [13]. They found that they could elicit phosphenes in their patients. Patients were able to recognize objects after a long learning period and the object identification took several minutes of scanning.

The optic nerve was contacted first in a neurosurgical approach at the level behind the orbit and in a second experiment within the orbit. Thresholds for electrical stimulation differed significantly and were much lower in the cranial approach than in the orbital approach [2, 13, 16, 48].

From a theoretical point of view, a prosthesis using stimulating electrodes around the optic nerve fibers may have the problem of good spatial resolution because the optic nerve fibers are very densely packed and therefore a large amount of fibers could have been stimulated. Whether perforating electrodes are a solution to that theoretical problem remains unanswered at present.

> **Summary for the Clinician**
>
> - Two patients were operated upon.
> - Both had visual percepts with different thresholds.
> - The intracranial approach yielded better results than the intraorbital approach.
> - Spatial resolution may be limited by dense packing of optic nerve fibers.

13.3.5 Cortical Prosthesis

A large portion of the central nervous system is involved in the processing of visual information and the primary target of fibers from the lateral geniculate nucleus is layer 4 of area V1 at the occipital pole of the brain.

In V1 good retinal topography is found with the large representation of the fovea at the most posterior parts and the peripheral representation in the more inwardly located, smaller areas of V1. Researchers intended to contact neurons in V1 to bypass other parts of the visual systems [22]. Such approaches may also be helpful in restoring vision in patients suffering from glaucoma or trauma to the optic nerve in contrast to retinal prostheses.

Multielectrode arrays have been developed by Normann and his group based on silicon needle arrays [34]. Such multielectrode arrays can be used for stimulation as well as for recording [52]. Animal experiments showed relatively little fibrotic response around the electrode tips [32]. The electrodes could be placed very near to the somata of the neurons in V1. Silicon-based multielectrode arrays were also already implanted in an acute trial in 6 patients who underwent brain surgery. It was shown that the stimulators could be inserted with a pneumatic shooter. Excised brain tissue showed only minor alteration such as small bleeds and deformations [26].

> **Summary for the Clinician**
>
> - Electrodes are placed near neurons in the V1 area
> - Placement is feasible.
> - In normal-sighted patients phosphenes were elicited.
> - Clinical trials in blind individuals are planned.

13.4 Pixel Vision and Filters

The possible resolution of artificial vision using retinal implants was evaluated in animal experiments in which cortical responses were obtained from the cat's visual cortex or by optical imaging. These data show a possible spatial resolution of about 1° in space and 25 images per second [17, 41, 42, 50]. However, relatively little data are known on the percepts of patients wearing the first available prototypes with regard to picture quality. In the pilot trials that are currently running threshold measurements are taken and standardized tests are used where single electrodes or groups of electrodes are activated. Patients are asked if they can see something, or if they can see separate spots of light or a line. Patients are also asked if they can identify the orientation of a line, whether it is a horizontal or vertical line. A systematic analysis of the presentation of real pictures has not yet been carried out. Patients who are implanted with the 16-electrode array used by Humayun's group and who are already connected to a camera system reported that they can identify high contrast obstacles or that they can now find the door in the wall of a house. To learn more about this kind of artificial vision with only a few implanted electrodes, simulations were performed based on certain assumptions. The simplest simulation is pixel vision where each electrode is considered as a pixel in a rectangular montage. Such a simulation can be seen in Fig. 13.4. It becomes obvious that the percept depends on the complexity of the real picture. For very simple pictures, e.g., a dark door in a bright room, only a few electrodes are necessary to identify the door, for complex pictures such as the face of a person, many electrodes are necessary for face recognition.

To point to a person 48 electrodes are necessary, but for face recognition in the example shown in Fig. 13.4, 864 electrodes are necessary. In contrast, to identify the door in Fig. 4b, i.e., to move to the door, only 12 electrodes are necessary. To identify the obstacle right in front of the door to the right and to enable free movement to the door 48 electrodes are needed, but to find the door opener again 864 electrodes are necessary.

For paragraph reading Dagnelie and coworkers found that 256 electrodes placed on a 3×3 mm retinal implant are necessary [11].

Performance with such a low number of electrodes in similar tests can be further improved by the design of the multielectrode array. It may be useful to place electrodes with a high density in the center of the device if it is implanted onto the macula and with a low density in the peripheral area of the multielectrode array. Performance will also depend on the size of the electrode array and the efficacy with which the electrodes make contact with retinal neurons.

Also, the application of filters to simulate the characteristics of receptive fields of ganglion cells is a useful tool to enhance the perceptual performance. The concepts for data preprocessing have been described [5, 21]. However, experimental data on its application in humans are still not available.

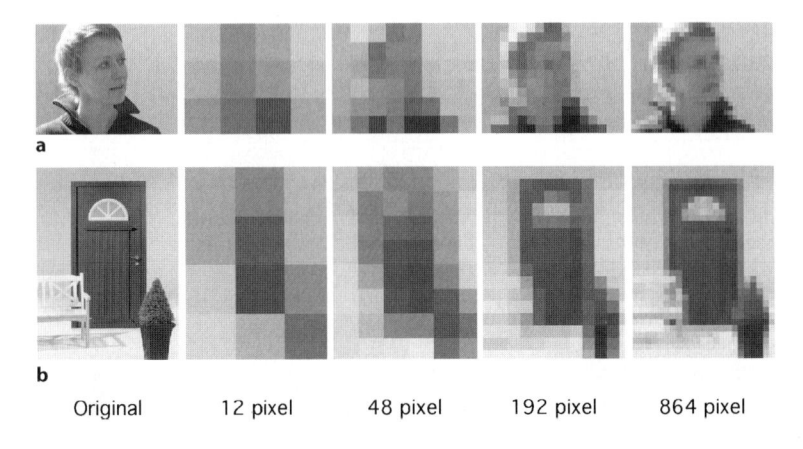

Fig. 13.4 Simulation of pixel vision assuming that each electrode will provide for a pixel. **a** Face recognition. **b** Identification of a dark door on a bright background. The number of electrodes needed to succeed with a task depends on the complexity of the picture

> **Summary for the Clinician**
>
> - Visual tasks can be performed with a limited number of electrodes.
> - Performance can be improved by the application of filters.
> - The requirement for a high number of electrodes depends on the complexity of the visual task; reading and face recognition requires many more electrodes than moving around.

Stimulation can take place at the level of the retina with either subretinal or epiretinal electrodes, but also with electrodes placed onto the scleral surface or electrodes in the suprachoroidal space. Stimulation has also been effected at the level of the optic nerve and in the visual cortex. These concepts are currently being evaluated in pilot clinical trials providing safety data. Future developments will concentrate on increasing the number of implanted electrodes, on reducing the surgical risk, on optimizing stimulus paradigm strategies, and on modulating the degenerative process by electrical stimulation.

13.5 Outlook

Several clinical trials have been started and will start in the near future of devices with a comparable low number of electrodes. With such devices only phosphene vision can be stimulated, but not artificial vision with useful spatial and temporal resolution. However, these trials will generate human data on the safety of the general concepts. They will also provide some data on efficacy, but the currently developed systems should not be considered as real visual prostheses because patients' expectations cannot be fully met.

However, these implants will serve as the technological basis for the development of further, more advanced devices that are much more likely to do what we are all aiming at, i.e., restoring vision in blind patients who cannot be treated with other modalities.

It might also be expected that electrical stimulation will be combined with treatment modalities currently subsumed under the term "regenerative therapies," meaning the use of stem cells and the genetic modification of transplanted cells. Both strategies, together with the finding that in the mature cortex reorganization may also occur due to chronic electrical stimulation, may lead to a brighter light at the end of the tunnel [51].

13.6 Conclusion

Artificial vision comprises approaches to electrically stimulating the neurons of the visual system to bypass degenerated receptors or other neurons to restore vision in otherwise blind individuals.

References

1. Alteheld N, Rossler G, Vobig M, Walter P (2004) The retina implant—a new approach to a visual prosthesis. Biomed Tech 49(4):99–103
2. Brelen ME, DePotter P, Gersdorff M, Cosnard G, Veraart C, Delbeke J (2006) Intraorbital implantation of a stimulating electrode for an optic nerve visual prosthesis. Case report. J Neurosurg 104(4):593–597
3. Brindley GS (1970) Sensations produced by electrical stimulation of the occipital poles of the cerebral hemispheres, and their use in constructing visual prostheses. Ann R Coll Surg Engl 47(2):106–108
4. Brindley GS, Lewin WS (1968) The sensations produced by electrical stimulation of the visual cortex. J Physiol 196:479–493
5. Buffoni LX, Coulombe J, Sawan M (2005) Image processing strategies dedicated to visual cortical stimulators: a survey. Artif Organs 29(8):658–664
6. Chow AY, Chow VY (1997) Subretinal electrical stimulation of the rabbit retina. Neurosci Lett 225(1):13–16
7. Chow AY, Pardue MT, Chow VY, Peyman GA, Liang C, Perlman JI, Peachey NS (2001) Implantation of silicon chip microphotodiode arrays into the cat subretinal space. IEEE Trans Neural Syst Rehabil Eng 9(1):86–95
8. Chow AY, Chow VY, Packo KH, Pollack JS, Peyman GA, Schuchard R (2004) The artificial silicon retina microchip for the treatment of vision loss from retinitis pigmentosa. Arch Ophthalmol 122(4):460–469

9. Chowdhury V, Morley JW, Coroneo MT (2005) Evaluation of extraocular electrodes for a retinal prosthesis using evoked potentials in cat visual cortex. J Clin Neurosci 12(5):574–579
10. Dagnelie G (2006) Visual prosthetics 2006: assessment and expectations. Expert Rev Med Devices 3(3):315–325
11. Dagnelie G, Barnett D, Humayun MS, Thompson RW Jr (2006) Paragraph text reading using a pixelized prosthetic vision simulator: parameter dependence and task learning in free viewing conditions. Invest Ophthalmol Vis Sci 47(3):1241–1250
12. Dawson WW, Radtke ND (1977) The electrical stimulation of the retina by indwelling electrodes. Invest Ophthalmol Vis Sci 16(3):249–252
13. Delbeke J, Oozeer M, Veraart C (2003) Position, size and luminosity of phosphenes generated by direct optic nerve stimulation. Vision Res 43(9):1091–1102
14. Dobelle WH (1994) Artificial vision for the blind. The summit may be closer than you think. ASAIO J 40(4):919–922
15. Dobelle WH (2000) Artificial vision for the blind by connecting a television camera to the visual cortex. ASAIO J 46(1):3–9
16. Duret F, Brelen ME, Lambert V, Gerard B, Delbeke J, Veraart C (2006) Object localization, discrimination, and grasping with the optic nerve visual prosthesis. Restor Neurol Neurosci 24(1):31–40
17. Eckhorn R, Wilms M, Schanze T, Eger M, Hesse L, Eysel UT, Kisvarday ZF, Zrenner E, Gekeler F, Schwahn H, Shinoda K, Sachs H, Walter P (2006) Visual resolution with retinal implants estimated from recordings in cat visual cortex. Vision Res 46(17):2675–2690
18. Eckmiller R (1995) Towards retina implants for improvement of vision in human with RP—challenges and first results. Proc WCNN, vol 1. INNS Press/Erlbaum, Hillsdale, pp 228–233
19. Eckmiller R (1996) Retina implants with adaptive retina encoders. RESNA Research Symposium, pp 21–24
20. Eckmiller R (1997) Learning retina implants with epiretinal contacts. Ophthalmic Res 29(5):281–289
21. Eckmiller R, Neumann D, Baruth O (2005) Tunable retina encoders for retina implants: why and how. J Neural Eng 2(1):S91–S104
22. Fernandez E, Pelayo F, Romero S, Bongard M, Marin C, Alfaro A, Merabet L (2005) Development of a cortical visual neuroprothesis for the blind: the relevance of neuroplasticity. J Neural Eng 2(2):R1–R12
23. Fried SI, Hsueh HA, Werblin FS (2006) A method for generating precise temporal patterns of retinal spiking using prosthetic stimulation. J Neurophysiol 95(2):970–978
24. Gekeler F, Szurman P, Grisanti S, Weiler U, Claus R, Greiner TO, Volker M, Kohler K, Zrenner E, Bartz-Schmidt KU (2006) Compound subretinal prostheses with extraocular parts designed for human trials: successful long term implantation in pigs. Graefes Arch Clin Exp Ophthalmol (published online doi: 10.1007/s00417-006-0339-x)
25. Hornig R, Velikay-Parel M, Feucht M, Zehnder T, Richard G (2006) Early clinical experience with a chronic retinal implant system for artificial vision. Invest Ophthalmol Vis Sci 47:E-Abstract 3216
26. House PA, MacDonald JD, Tresco PA, Normann RA (2006) Acute microelectrode array implantation into human neocortex: preliminary technique and histological considerations. Neurosurg Focus 20(5):E4
27. Humayun MS, de Juan E, Dagnelie G, Greenberg RJ, Probst RH, Phillips DH (1996) Visual perception elicited by electrical stimulation of retina in blind subjects. Arch Ophthalmol 114:40–46
28. Jones BW, Marc RE (2005) Retinal remodelling during retinal degeneration. Exp Eye Res 81(2):123–137
29. Kanda H, Morimoto T, Fujikado T, Tano Y (2006) Localized phosphene elicited by transscleral electrical stimulation in normal subjects. Invest Ophthalmol Vis Sci 47: E-Abstract 3201
30. Mahadevappa M, Weiland JD, Yanai D, Fine I, Greenberg RJ, Humayun MS (2005) Perceptual thresholds and electrode impedance in three retinal prosthesis subjects. IEEE Trans Neural Syst Rehabil Eng 13(2):201–206
31. Marc RE, Jones BW (2003) Retinal remodelling in inherited photoreceptor degeneration. Mol Neurobiol 28(2):139–147
32. Maynard EM, Fernandez E, Normann RA (2000) A technique to prevent dural adhesions to chronically implanted microelectrode arrays. J Neurosci Methods 97(2):93–101

33. Nakauchi K, Fujikado T, Kanda H, Morimoto T, Choi JS, Ikuno Y, Sakaguchi H, Kamei M, Ohji M, Yagi T, Nishimura S, Sawai H, Fukuda Y, Tano Y (2005) Transretinal electrical stimulation by an intrascleral multichannel electrode array in rabbit eyes. Graefes Arch Clin Exp Ophthalmol 243(2):169–174
34. Normann RA, Maynard EM, Rousche PJ, Warren DJ (1999) A neural interface for a cortical vision prosthesis. Vision Res 39(15):2577–2587
35. Pardue MT, Phillips MJ, Yin H, Fernandes A, Cheng Y, Chow AY, Ball SL (2005) Possible sources of neuroprotection following subretinal silicon chip implantation in RCS rats. J Neural Eng 2(1):S39–S47
36. Pardue MT, Phillips MJ, Yin H, Sippy BD, Webb-Wood S, Chow AY, Ball SL (2005) Neuroprotective effects of subretinal implants in the RCS rat. Invest Ophthalmol Vis Sci 46(2):674–682
37. Peyman G, Chow AY, Liang C, Chow VY, Perlman JI, Peachey NS (1998) Subretinal semiconductor microphotodiode array. Ophthalmic Surg Lasers 29:234–241
38. Rizzo JF III, Wyatt J, Humayun M, de Juan E, Liu W, Chow A, Eckmiller R, Zrenner E, Yagi T, Abrams G (2001) Retinal prosthesis: an encouraging first decade with major challenges ahead. Ophthalmology 108(1):13–14
39. Rizzo JF III, Wyatt J, Loewenstein J, Kelly S, Shire D (2003) Methods and perceptual thresholds for short term electrical stimulation of human retina with microelectrode arrays. Invest Ophthalmol Vis Sci 44(12):5355–5361
40. Santos A, Humayun MS, deJuan E Jr, Greenburg RJ, Marsh MJ, Klock IB, Milam AH (1997) Preservation of the inner retina in retinitis pigmentosa: a morphometric analysis. Arch Ophthalmol 115(4):511–515
41. Schanze T, Wilms M, Eger M, Hesse L, Eckhorn R (2002) Activation zones in cat visual cortex evoked by electrical retina stimulation. Graefes Arch Clin Exp Ophthalmol 240(11):947–954
42. Schanze T, Greve N, Hesse L (2003) Towards the cortical representation of form and motion stimuli generated by a retina implant. Graefes Arch Clin Exp Ophthalmol 241(8):685–693
43. Schwahn HN, Gekeler F, Kohler K, Kobuch K, Sachs HG, Schulmeyer F, Jakob W, Gabel VP, Zrenner E (2001) Studies on the feasibility of a subretinal visual prosthesis: data from Yucatan micropig and rabbit. Graefes Arch Clin Exp Ophthalmol 239(12):961–967
44. Segond H, Weiss D, Sampaio E (2005) Human spatial navigation via a visuo-tactile sensory substitution system. Perception 34(10):1231–1249
45. Sekirnjak C, Hottowy P, Sher A, Dabrowski W, Litke AM, Chichilnisky EJ (2006) Electrical stimulation of mammalian retinal ganglion cells with multielectrode arrays. J Neurophysiol 95(6):3311–3327
46. Shah HA, Montezuma SR, Rizzo JF III (2006) In vivo electrical stimulation of rabbit retina: effect of stimulus duration and electrical field orientation. Exp Eye Res 83(2):247–254
47. Stone JL, Barlow WE, Humayun MS, deJuan E Jr, Milam AH (1992) Morphometric analysis of macular photoreceptors and ganglion cells in retinas with Retinitis pigmentosa. Arch Ophthalmol 110(11):1634–1639
48. Veraart C, Raftopoulos C, Mortimer JT, Delbeke J, Pins D, Michaux G, Vanlierde A, Parrini S, Wanet-Defalque MC (1998) Visual sensations produced by optic nerve stimulation using an implanted self-sizing spiral cuff electrode. Brain Res 813(1):181–186
49. Walter P, Mokwa W (2005) Epiretinal visual prostheses. Ophthalmologe 102(10):933–940
50. Walter P, Kisvarday ZF, Gortz M, Altheld N, Rossler G, Stieglitz T, Eysel UT (2005) Cortical activation via an implanted wireless retinal prosthesis. Invest Ophthalmol Vis Sci 46(5):1780–1785
51. Warren DJ, Normann RA (2005) Functional reorganization of primary visual cortex induced by electrical stimulation in the cat. Vision Res 45(5):551–565
52. Warren DJ, Fernandez E, Normann RA (2001) High-resolution two-dimensional spatial mapping of cat striate cortex using a 100-microelectrode array. Neuroscience 105(1):19–31
53. Wilke R, Kuttenkeuler C, Wilhelm B, Sailer H, Sachs H, Gabel VP, Besch D, Bartz-Schmidt KU, Zrenner E (2006) Subretinal chronic multielectrode arrays in blind patients: perception of dots and patterns. Invest Ophthalmol Vis Sci 47: E-Abstract 3202

54. Wolff JG, Delacour J, Carpenter RH, Brindley GS (1968) The patterns seen when alternating electric current is passed through the eye. Q J Exp Psychol 20(1):1–10
55. Zrenner E, Miliczek KD, Gabel VP, Graf HG, Guenther E, Haemmerle H, Hoefflinger B, Kohler K, Nisch W, Schubert M, Stett A, Weiss S (1997) The development of subretinal microphotodiodes for replacement of degenerated photoreceptors. Ophthalmic Res 29(5):269–280
56. Zrenner E, Stett A, Weiss S, Aramant RB, Guenther E, Kohler K, Miliczek KD, Seiler MJ, Haemmerle H (1999) Can subretinal microphotodiodes successfully replace degenerated photoreceptors? Vision Res 39(15):2555–2567

Subject Index

11-cis-retinol
  dehydrogenase 178
16-electrode array 205

A

A2E oxiranes 178
ABCA4 gene 15, 27, 37, 165,
  174, 175, 177
abcr-/- mice 178
absolute scotoma 191
active flecks 167
advanced glycosylation end
  products (AGE) 136
ADVANCE study 63
AG-013958 63
Age-Related Eye Disease Study
  (AREDS) 105
– categories 106
– formulation 108
age-related macular
  degeneration (AMD) 4, 35,
  90, 105
– atrophic form 113
– candidate gene studies 36
– gene–environment
  interaction 46
– gene–gene interaction 45
– treatment 67
Ala69Ser 43
aldose reductase 132, 136
all-trans-retinal 175, 176
all-trans-retinol 176
all-trans-retinol
  dehydrogenase 177
Alport's disease 192
AMD–see age-related macular
  degeneration (AMD)
– linkage studies 38

amikacin 74, 78
aminoglycosides 78
Amsler grid examination 189
ANCHOR study 61
ANCHOR trial 57, 73, 75, 79
anecortave acetate 97, 98, 194
anemia 136
aneurysmatic
  telangiectasia 183, 194
angiogenesis 61, 90, 92
– cancer studies 91
angiographic leakage 191
angioscopy 29
angioscotoma 12
anterior segment
  neovascularization 150
anti-VEGF agents 151
anti-VEGF therapies 60
anti-VEGF treatment 93
antioxidant vitamin 119
Appropriate Blood Pressure
  Control in Diabetes
  (ABCD) study 135
aptamer 55
argon laser photocoagulation
  (ALP) 192, 193
arteriovenous
  sheathotomy 156
artificial silicon retina
  (ASR) 200
artificial vision 199, 205, 206
asthma 139
atherosclerotic disease 158
ATP Binding Cassette 174
atrophy 28, 116, 165
– baseline 117
– family history 118
– junctional zone 117, 119,
  124
– progression 117, 120

autofluorescence 24
autofluorescence imaging 8

B

bacterial infections 81
baseline atrophy 117, 122
Best's disease (see also
  vitelliform macular
  dystrophy) 16, 24, 116
betacarotene 106, 108
bevaciranib 62
bevacizumab 53, 56, 58, 61,
  74, 79, 84, 91, 93, 94, 97,
  140, 155, 194
– pharmacokinetics 59
biconvex aspheric lenses 29
binocular stereoscopic
  ophthalmoscopy 131, 133
blepharitis 76, 85
blind patients 199, 206
blind spot 10
blood glucose levels 137
blood pressure control 135
blood vessel density 93
body mass index (BMI) 46
bovine hyaluronidase 75
branch retinal vein occlusion
  (BRVO) 147
– intravitreal
  triamcinolone 153
Branch Vein Occlusion Study
  (BVOS) 148, 149
breast cancer 92, 192
Brindley approach 199
Bruch's membrane 22, 40, 44,
  115, 156
BRVO–see branch retinal vein
  occlusion (BRVO)

bull's eye 166, 167
BVOS–*see* Branch Vein Occlusion Study (BVOS)

C

C-reactive protein (CRP) 38
C3/C5 convertase 40
calcium dobesilate 136
cancer therapy 95, 98
cardiovascular disease 192
CARE study 63
cataract 22, 67, 121
– extraction 119
– progression 73
– steroid-induced 142
– surgery 75, 140, 141
CATT study 59
ceftazidime 78
celiac sprue 192
central retinal vein occlusion (CRVO) 147
central serous chorioretinopathy (CSC) 14, 21, 27
Central Vein Occlusion Study (CVOS) 148, 149
central visual acuity 1
central vitreal vein occlusion
– intravitreal triamcinolone 153
cephalosporins 78
CFH–*see* complement factor H
– gene cluster 41
– haplotype block structure 42
CFH (Y402H) 43
CFHR1 41
CFHR3 41
cholesterol 107
choriocapillaris 94, 115, 170
choriocapillaris atrophy 174
chorioretinal anastomosis (CRA) 156
chorioretinal atrophy 172
chorioretinopathy 1
choroidal neovascularization (CNV) 1, 5, 10, 39, 53, 89, 90, 168, 189

choroidal neovascular lesions 57
choroidal silence 169, 170, 171, 175
choroidal stroma 45
choroidal vessels 23
chromosome 1 (1p) 165, 174
chromosome 10q26 38
circinata rings 12
circinate exudates 134
CLEAR-AMD 1 Study 62
CLEAR-IT 1 Study 62
clinically significant macular edema (CSME) 134, 138
CNV–*see* choroidal neovascularization (CNV)
– development 91
– two-component system 94
coagulopathies 158
Coats' syndrome 186
color vision deficits 174
compartment syndrome 157
complement cascade 40
complement component 2 44
complement factor H (CFH) 38
complement system 39
cone rod dystrophy 15
confocal fluorometry 24
confocal imaging 21
confocal scanning laser ophthalmoscope (cSLO) 170
confocal scanning laser ophthalmoscopy (cSLO) 117
conjunctival hemorrhage 69
conjunctival scarring 72
conjunctivitis 76, 85
conventional cupola perimetry 4, 5
convex-concave contact lens 29
copper 106
copper-deficient anemia 106
corneal edema 72
corticosteroids 89, 95, 98, 151, 155
CRP–*see* C-reactive protein
CRVO–*see* central retinal vein occlusion

crystalline deposit 188
CSC–*see* central serous chorioretinopathy (CSC)
cSLO recordings 21
CSME–*see* "clinically significant macular edema"
cuff electrodes 204
cupola perimetry 6, 17
CVOS–*see* Central Vein Occlusion Study (CVOS)
cytokine 91, 95
cytotoxic edema 151

D

dark adaptation 124
dark choroid 27, 169, 170
deutan axis 174
diabetes 158
Diabetes Control and Complications Trial (DCCT) 135
diabetes mellitus 131, 191
diabetic macular edema 10, 14, 131
– laser treatment 138
– treatment 135
– treatment recommendations 141
diabetic microvascular disease 133
diabetic retinal disease 132
diabetic retinopathy 10, 131
Dicer 62
Dietary omega-3 fatty intake 107
docosahexaenoic acid (DHA) 178
Doyne honeycomb retinal dystrophy 36
drusen 23, 25, 40, 44, 108, 119

E

"egg yolk" lesion 16
Early Treatment of Diabetic Retinopathy Study (ETDRS) 134, 138
EFEMP1 36

eicosapentaenoic acid (EPA) 107
electrical stimulation 200, 206
electro-oculogram (EOG) 172
electrode arrays 203
electrodes 200
electroretinogram (ERG) 74, 172
ELOVL4 178
endolaser 158
endophthalmitis 57, 58, 60, 67, 69, 75, 77
- infectious 76
- postoperative 76
enucleation 77
epiretinal stimulation 202, 203
epistasis 45
Equator-plus camera 30
ETDRS (Early Treatment Diabetic Retinopathy Study) 55
exon 42 175
extracellular matrix proteins 36

F

"flippase" 177
face recognition 205
facioscapulohumeral muscular dystrophy 192
factor B (BF) 44, 118
factor X 53
FAF–see fundus autofluorescence (FAF)
FFA–see fundus fluorescein angiography
fibroblasts 95
fibrocytes 94
fibronectin 96
fibulin5 36, 37
fixation pattern 124
flecks 27, 28, 165, 166
- active 167, 170, 171
- resorbed 167, 171
florid diabetic retinopathy 137
fluocinolone acetonide implant 154
fluorescein angiogram 149

fluorescein angiography (FFA) 28, 62, 96, 114, 131, 133, 165, 185
fluorescence
- retinal pigment epithelium 24
fluorophores 24, 28
focal deposits (drusen) 22
focal edema 134, 142
focal hyperpigmentation 25
focal laser treatment 138
focal leaks 138
FOCUS study 58, 96
forceps injury 69
fovea 28, 115, 123
foveal atrophy 183, 188
free radicals 95
fundus
- contrast 23
- features 23
fundus-related perimetry 4, 6
fundus autofluorescence (FAF) 21, 37, 113, 114, 116
- abnormalities 25
- central serous chorioretinopathy 27
- choroidal neovascularization 26
- classification system 25
- geographic atrophy 26
- patterns 25
- Stargardt's disease 170
fundus cameras 30
funduscopy 81, 85
fundus examination 168
fundus flavimaculatus 15, 24, 166
fundus flecks 166, 168
fundus fluorescein angiography (FFA) 26
fundus perimetry (FP) 1, 2, 17, 124
- kinetic 3, 6
- static 3, 4

G

galactose 133
ganglion cells 203
genetic studies 46

genome-scan meta-analysis (GSMA) 38, 39
geographic atrophy 26, 39, 44, 113
- bilateral 123
- pathogenesis 119
- unilateral 123
geographic atrophy (GA) 8, 10, 11
glaucoma 2, 77, 79, 80
- medication 140
- surgery 67
glial cells 94
glucocorticoids 139
Gly1961Glu 175
glycosylated hemoglobin 135
glycosylated hemoglobin levels 137
Goldmann kinetic perimetry 2
gonioscopic gel 29
gonioscopy 159
gram-positive bacteria 78
grid laser photocoagulation 149
grid photocoagulation 138

H

haplotype block structure in CFH 42
heart disease 192
Heidelberg perimetry software 3
Heidelberg retina angiograph (HRA) 21
Heidelberg retina angiograph, HRA 2 37
helium neon laser beam 2
hematopoiesis 55
hemorrhage 22
herceptin antibody 56
histidine alteration in different populations 43
Humphrey static perimetry 2
hyaluronidase 74, 79
hydrostatic pressure 92
hyperfluorescence 123, 188
hyperglycemia 136
hyperlipidemia 118, 158
hyperopia 192

hypertension 118, 158
hypopyon 75
hypoxia 54
hypoxic stress 132

I

ICGA–see indocyanine green angiography (ICGA)
idiopathic juxtafoveolar telangiectasis 183, 184
idiopathic macular telangiectasia 183
- type 2 186
- type 3 194
indirect ophthalmoscopy 84
indocyanine green angiography (ICGA) 21, 165, 194
- Stargardt's disease 170
infliximab 96
infrared (IR) imaging 22
infrared diode laser 2
insulin 132
insulin-like growth factor 1 (IGF-1) 137
intraocular inflammation 74, 96
intraocular pressure (IOP) 69, 79
intraretinal lipid exudates 185
intraretinal neovascularization 189
intravitreal injection 67, 151
- complications 68
- guidelines 81, 82
- methodology 69
- pain 72
- perioperative complications 69
- postoperative endophthalmitis 77
- surgical technique 80
- technique 152
intravitreal steroids 139
intravitreal triamcinolone 139, 153, 159

intravitreal triamcinolone acetonide (IVTA) 131
iritis 75
ischemia 94
isopters 10
isotonic sodium chloride solution 29
isotretinoin 178

J

Jablonnski diagram 24

K

kinetic fundus perimetry 3, 7, 11

L

lamina cribrosa 23, 148
laser photocoagulation 105
laser scanning ophthalmoscopy (SLO) 28
laser scanning tomography 8
laser therapy 131
Leber's miliary aneurysms 186
lens
- biconvex aspheric 29
- convex-concave 29
lens damage 57
lens opacities 125
lens trauma 60
lidocaine 60
lid speculum 76
light sensitivity threshold values 12
linkage disequilibrium (LD) 38
linoleic acid 107
lipid peroxidation 119
lipofuscin 24, 26, 113, 116, 165, 167, 170, 171, 174
LOC387715 44, 118, 121
LOC387715 gene 43
lutein 105, 106, 188

M

macrophages 96
MacTel study 194
macular disease 1, 4, 8
macular edema 12, 13, 132
- cystoid 134
- diffuse 134
- ischemic 134
macular hole 8, 9, 28
macular ischemia 149
macular pigment 22
macular pseudoholes 28
macular telangiectasia 183
- focal laser photocoagulation 186
- intravitreal triamcinolone 187
- nonproliferative stage 193
- vasoproliferative stage 193
major histocompatibility complex class III 44
Malattia leventinese 36
MAP kinase pathways 55
MARINA study 61
MARINA trial 56, 73, 74, 75, 79
matrix metalloproteinases 90
mean defect (MD) 6
melanin 22, 23, 24
melano-lipofuscin fluorescence 24
melanolipofuscin 174
metamorphopsia 185, 188
metastatic colon cancer 61
metastatic colorectal cancer 58
methotrexate 74
microaneurysms 138, 185
microneuromas 200
microperimetry 2
microphotodiodes 200, 203
Millipore filter 53
mitochondria 177
monocyte chemotactic protein (MCP) 94
multielectrode array 201, 202, 204
- silicon-based 204
mutated alleles 38
myofibroblasts 94

N

N-retinylidene-N-retinyl-
  ethanolamine (A2E) 177
N-retinylidene-PE 176
N-retinylidene-phosphatidylethanolamine 165, 175
negative scotoma 185
neovascular glaucoma 159
neovascular membranes 192
nephropathy 136
neuro-ophthalmological
  disorders 2
neurosensory retina 27, 115
nictalopia 166
nitrous oxide synthase
  (NOS) 55
noninfectious
  endophthalmitis–
  see pseudo-endophthalmitis
nonproliferative diabetic
  retinopathy 13
NOS–see nitrous oxide
  synthase

O

OCT–see optical coherence
  tomography (OCT)
Octopus static perimetry 2
ocular adnexa 74, 81
ocular hypertension 67, 80
ocular neovascularization 91
omega-3 long-chain
  polyunsaturated fatty
  acids 105, 107
opacity 29
ophthalmoscopy 29
opsin 177
optical coherence tomography
  (OCT) 8, 12, 13, 58, 131,
  133, 134, 149, 185
- Stargardt's disease 172
optic nerve fibers 204
optic nerve head 7
optic nerve sheath
- external
  decompression 157
oral hypoglycemic agents 132
oxidative stress 105, 106, 132
oxygenated hemoglobin
  (choroidal blood) 22

P

paclitaxel 92
panretinal photocoagulation
  (PRP) 138, 150
paracentesis 78, 85
paracentral scotomata 10
paragraph reading 205
pars plana vitrectomy 74, 77,
  139, 156, 158
pattern electroretinogram
  (PERG) 166
pattern electroretinography
  (PERG) 27
PDT–see photodynamic
  therapy (PDT)
pegaptanib 53, 55, 59, 61, 69,
  74, 78, 79, 94, 96, 140, 155
- ocular adverse events 70
pentoxifylline 150
PERG–see pattern
  electroretinography
pericytes 92
perifoveal telangiectasia 183
periocular steroid 140
periorbital swelling 76
phacoemulsification 141
phosphatidylethanolamine
  (PE) 175, 176
phosphenes 199, 203
photodynamic therapy
  (PDT) 10, 57, 89, 97, 98,
  105, 193
photomontages of static
  images 30
photophobia 76, 85, 166
photoreceptor 106
photoreceptor cells 27
phototransduction
  cascade 177
phthisis 77
physiologic hypoxia 94
PIER study 57
pigment epithelial-derived
  factor (PEDF) 91
pigment epithelium-
  neuroretina complex 191
pixel vision 205
platelet-derived growth
  factor 89
platelet-derived growth factor
  receptor (PDGFR) 95
pneumatic shooter 204
poly(lactic-co-glycolic) acid
  (PLGA) 56
polycythemia vera 192
polyimide 201
posterior vitreous detachment
  (PVD) 142
povidine-iodine solution 60
povidine-iodine sticks 60
povidone-iodine
- anti-VEGF therapy 81
preferred retinal locus
  (PRL) 4, 5, 8
PRL–see preferred retinal
  locus
pro-apoptotic proteins 177
PRONTO study 58
prostate cancer 192
protan axis 174
PROTECT 96
protein C 55
protein kinase C
- isoform 136
proteinuria 62
proteoglycans 96
pseudo-endophthalmitis 75
- pain 76
pseudohypopyon 16
pseudophakia 121
pseudoxanthoma
  elasticum 192
PTK787 63
punctate keratitis 72

R

radial optic neurotomy
  (RON) 157, 158
ranibizumab 53, 56, 57, 58, 61,
  69, 74, 78, 79, 94, 96, 97, 140
- ocular adverse events 70
- pharmacokinetics 59

reactive oxygen species 136
reading speed 124, 126
recombinant tissue plasminogen activator (rt-PA) 157, 158
regenerative therapies 206
renal disease 137
resorbed flecks 167
retinal-retinal anastomosis 186
retinal artery occlusions 78
retinal detachment 60, 78
retinal diseases 2
retinal dystrophy 165
retinal ganglion cells (RGC) 201
retinal hypoxia
– triggers 151
– venous occlusion-induced 148
retinal injuries 73
retinal interneurons 203
retinal neovascularization 159
retinal oxygenation 159
retinal pigment epithelial (RPE) 74
retinal pigment epithelial (RPE) cells 94
retinal pigment epithelium (RPE) 8, 36, 165, 169
– fluorescence 24
retinal sensitivity 125, 126
retinal telangiectasis 183
retinal toxicity 74
retinal vasculature 192
retinal vein occlusion (RVO) 78, 147, 147–160
– management strategies 148
– risk factors 158
– systemic factors 158
retinitis pigmentosa (RP) 199
rhodopsin 172, 175
RISC 62
RNA
– gene-specific double-stranded 62
– interference 62
RNAs (siRNAs)
– small interfering 62

RON–*see* radial optic neurotomy
RPE 44
ruboxistaurin mesylate 136
RVO–*see* retinal vein occlusion (RVO)

S

scanning laser ophthalmoscope (SLO) 2, 9, 21, 24
scleral ring sectioning 157
SCORE study 147, 148, 155
– inclusion and exclusion criteria 155
scotoma 6, 13, 15, 120, 123, 191
– size 7
scotomata
– paracentral 10
scrambled egg formation 16
septic shock 96
sheathotomy 156
single-cell stimulation 201
single nucleotide polymorphisms (SNPs) 40, 41
singlet oxygen 95
slit-lamp biomicroscopy 169, 171
slit-lamp examination 85
SLO–*see* scanning laser ophthalmoscope
smoking 46, 105, 119, 121, 136
Snellen visual acuity 58
sorbitol 136
spastic paraplegia 192
Staphylococcus aureus 77
staphyloma 23
Stargardt-like macular dystrophy 178
Stargardt's disease (STGD) 1, 4, 15, 116, 118, 165–178
Stargardt's macular dystrophy 37, 38
Stargardt's macular dystrophy-fundus flavimaculatus (STGD-FFM) 27, 165

static fundus perimetry 3, 12
sterile endophthalmitis–*see* pseudo-endophthalmitis
sterile lid speculum 60
steroid glaucoma 186
steroid injection 153
STGD–*see* Stargardt's disease (STGD)
STGD-FFM–*see* Stargardt's disease-fundus flavimaculatus
stimulus diameters 3
strabismus 4
streptotocin 133
stroke 192
sub-threshold laser coagulation 139
subconjunctival injection
– pain 72
subretinal approach 203
subretinal fibrosis 168
subretinal hemorrhage 23
sunlight exposure 119
synchysis scintillans 192
systematic evolution of ligands by exponential enrichment (SELEX) 55
systemic arterial hypertension 191

T

TDMO study 140
tetracaine 60
tight blood glucose control 135
tissue hydrostatic pressure 92
tissue oxygen tension 53
toxic endophthalmitis–*see* pseudo-endophthalmitis
trabeculectomy 140
transpupillary thermotherapy (TTT) 194
traumatic cataract 72
triamcinolone 56, 67, 68, 73, 74, 75, 77, 79, 84, 89, 95, 97, 98
triamcinolone acetonide 151

tritan axis 174
tuberculin syringe 60
tumor necrosis factor alpha (TNFα) 89, 96, 98
tumor vascular permeability factor (VPF) 53

U

UK Prospective Diabetes Study (UKPDS) 135
untreatable blindness 35
uveitis 57, 63, 75

V

vancomycin 78
vascular disease 137
vascular endothelial growth factor (VEGF) 53, 89, 151, 193
vascular endothelial growth factor (VEGF-A) 54
vascular endothelial growth factor (VGEF)
– receptor tyrosine kinase activity 63
– VEGF trap 62

vascular endothelial growth factor-A (VEGF-A) 90
Vascular leakage 55
vascular normalization 93
vasculogenesis 61
vasoplegia 96
VEGF–*see* vascular endothelial growth factor
VEGF Inhibition Study in Ocular Neovascularization (VISION) 55
venous thrombosis 156
VERITAS study 56
verteporfin 55, 57
verteporfin PDT 58
viral retinitis 67
VISION study 61
VISION trial 69, 72, 74, 78, 79
visual acuity 57, 62, 113, 124, 135, 157, 165, 168
visual acuity loss 166
visual acuity measurement 123
visual function questionnaire (VFQ) 133
visual loss 77
visual prostheses 206
vitamin E 107
vitelliform macular dystrophy 16
vitrectomy 9, 75, 142, 156

vitreous floaters 74
vitreous hemorrhage 74, 79, 149
vitreous reflux 72, 78
VMD2 gene 16
VPF–*see* tumor vascular permeability factor

W

warfarin sodium 150
wide-field camera systems 30
wide-field contact lens system 29
wide-field fluorescein angiogram 30, 31

X

xanthophylls 107

Z

zeaxanthin 105, 106, 188
zinc 106, 108

Printing: Krips bv, Meppel
Binding: Stürtz, Würzburg